Consumers Guide to Cancer Drugs

SECOND EDITION

Jones and Bartlett Series in Oncology

Consumers Guide to Cancer Drugs

SECOND EDITION

Authors

Gail M. Wilkes, RNC, MS, AOCN
Boston Medical Center
Boston, Massachusetts

Terri B. Ades, MS, APRN-BC, AOCN
American Cancer Society
Atlanta, Georgia

JONES AND BARTLETT PUBLISHERS
Sudbury, Massachusetts
BOSTON   TORONTO   LONDON   SINGAPORE

World Headquarters
Jones and Bartlett Publishers
40 Tall Pine Drive
Sudbury, MA 01776
978-443-5000
info@jbpub.com
www.jbpub.com

Jones and Bartlett Publishers Canada
2406 Nikanna Road
Mississauga, ON L5C 2W6
CANADA

Jones and Bartlett Publishers International
Barb House, Barb Mews
London W6 7PA
UK

Production Credits
Chief Executive Officer: Clayton Jones
Chief Operating Officer: Don W. Jones, Jr.
Executive V.P. & Publisher: Robert W. Holland, Jr.
V.P., Sales and Marketing: William Kane
Acquistions Editor: Penny M. Glynn
Manufacturing Buyer: Amy Bacus
Production Editor: Anne Spencer
Cover Design: Anne Spencer
Associate Editor: Karen Zuck

Library of Congress Cataloging-in-Publication Data
Wilkes, Gail M.
    Consumers guide to cancer drugs / Gail M. Wilkes, Terri B. Ades.
        p.   cm.
    At head of title: American Cancer Society
    Includes bibliographical references and index.
    ISBN 0-7637-2254-5
        1. Antineoplastic agents—Popular works. I. Ades, Terri B. II. American Cancer Society.
    III. Title.
    RC271.C5W544 2003
    616.99'4061—dc21

                                                                                    2003040079

Cover Photo Credits: Copyright © AbleStock

Printed in the United States of America
07 06 05 04 03   10 9 8 7 6 5 4 3 2 1

Contents

Disclaimer

The drug information presented in the *Consumers Guide to Cancer Drugs, Second Edition* has been derived from standard reference sources, recently published data, and respected pharmaceutical texts. The writers and publishers of this book have made every effort to ensure that information presented is accurate and in accord with current labeling at the time of publication. However, in view of the constant and rapid flow of information resulting from ongoing research and clinical experience, as well as changes in government regulations, readers are urged to talk with their doctor, check the package insert, and consult with a pharmacist, if necessary, for each drug to be certain that changes have not been made in its indications, contraindications, or precautions for each use. While the drugs included in this publication were chosen on the basis of frequency of use and appropriate indications, the publisher and authors do not necessarily advocate, and take no responsiblility for, the use of products herein.

How to Use This Book

The *Consumers Guide to Cancer Drugs, Second Edition* was developed with the cancer patient in mind and provides answers to patients' most common drug-related questions. The guide lists the most common drugs on the market today, and provides basic information on drug action, how the drug is given, precautions, side effects, and other important facts.

The *Consumers Guide to Cancer Drugs, Second Edition* is intended as a reference for cancer patients and the people who care about them. It is not intended as a self-diagnostic tool, and should be used only as a supplement to the information you receive from your doctor.

Book Organization

The drug information within the *Consumers Guide to Cancer Drugs, Second Edition* can be found in two distinct sections: Section 1—Cancer Treatment Drugs, Section 2—Symptom Management Drugs. Within each section drugs are listed alphabetically by generic name. All generic and trade names are listed in the index for easy cross-referencing.

Drug Listings

For every drug listed in the *Consumers Guide to Cancer Drugs, Second Edition* an initial profile is given that includes drug name, drug type, and action of the drug. Following the initial profile is a more in-depth description of the drug, including common side effects, precautions, and circumstances in which taking this particular drug may not be in the patient's best interest.

The following is a brief overview of the organization of the listing for each drug in the *Consumers Guide to Cancer Drugs, Second Edition*. The organization and/or information provided may differ slightly depending on the particular drug.

Drug Name

The drug name is the generic name of the drug. The generic name is the common name approved by the Food and Drug Administration (FDA).

Trade Name

This is the brand name of the drug, as it is referred to by the manufacturer. This name will be more familiar to you.

Type of Drug

This identifies the type of drug and the group to which the drug belongs.

How Drug Works

This section provides important information on how the drug actually works.

How Drug Is Given

Some drugs are given in the vein, some are taken by mouth once a day, while others are taken by mouth several times a day. This section will let you know how to take this drug.

How Should I Take This Drug?

Some drugs have special instructions on how they should be taken. This section describes these special instructions.

Before taking this drug, tell your doctor

Many factors can affect a drug's effectiveness and physical results, including but not limited to other drugs being taken, physical condition (pregnancy, for example), and other medical problems. This cautionary section describes conditions that you must be aware of before taking this drug and that you must bring to the attention of your doctor.

Should I avoid any other medicines, foods, alcohol, and/or activities?

This section provides you with specific information on possible interactions and measures you should take to ensure that your medicine will be the most effective.

Precautions

Certain special precautions need to be followed with specific drugs, and these special precautions are described in this section.

More Common Side Effects

Almost every drug available can cause some sort of negative reaction; some, however, occur more frequently with one kind of drug than with another. This section details the most commonly reported side effects experienced with this particular drug. Keep in mind, however, that even the most common side effects appear in only a small percentage of patients.

Less Common Side Effects

These are side effects that occur less frequently, in fewer people, but these side effects can sometimes be serious. If you are concerned about any side effects, you should talk with your doctor before starting the medicine.

Rare Side Effects

These side effects rarely occur; still, it is necessary to consider them when starting a new drug.

Side Effects/Symptoms of This Drug

When certain side effects do occur, please report them to your doctor. This section will alert you to what to be concerned about.

FDA Approval

This section tells you whether the drug is FDA approved or if it has an investigational status (still being studied).

Chemotherapy Principles:
An In-Depth Discussion of the Techniques and Their Role in Cancer Treatment

INTRODUCTION

The thought of having chemotherapy frightens many people. Almost everyone has heard stories about someone who was "on chemo." But we believe that knowing what chemotherapy is, how it works, and what to expect can often help calm your fears and give you more of a sense of control.

WHAT IS CHEMOTHERAPY?

To doctors, nurses, pharmacists, and health professionals, the word *chemotherapy* means any drug (such as aspirin or penicillin) used for treating people with any disease. Most of us, however, think of anticancer medicines to treat cancer when we hear the term chemotherapy. Two other medical terms often used to describe cancer chemotherapy are *antineoplastic* (meaning anticancer) and *cytotoxic* (cell-killing).

History of Chemotherapy

The first drug used for cancer chemotherapy was not originally intended for that purpose. Mustard gas was used as a chemical warfare agent during World War I and was studied further during World War II. During a military operation in World War II, a large number of military personnel was accidentally exposed to mustard gas and were later found to have abnormally low white blood cell counts. It was reasoned that an agent that damaged the rapidly growing white blood cells might have a similar effect on cancer. Therefore, in the 1940s, several patients with advanced lymphomas (cancers of certain white blood cells) were given the drug by vein, rather than by breathing the irritating gas. Their improvement, although temporary, was remarkable. That experience started researchers studying other substances that might have similar effects against cancer. As a result, many drugs have been developed to treat many other types of cancer.

Why Chemotherapy Is Different from Other Treatments

Chemotherapy is sometimes the first choice for treating many cancers. It differs from surgery or radiation in that it is almost always used as a systemic treatment. This means the medicines travel throughout the whole body or system rather than being confined or localized to one area such as the breast, lung, or colon. This is important because chemotherapy can reach cancer cells that may have spread to other parts of the body.

More than 100 drugs are currently used for chemotherapy—either alone or in combination. Many more are expected to become available. These chemotherapy medicines vary widely in their chemical composition, how they are taken, their usefulness in treating specific forms of cancer, and their side effects. New medications are first developed through laboratory research in test tubes and animals. Then, their safety and effectiveness are tested in three phases of clinical trials in humans.

Chemotherapy in Clinical Trials

Clinical trials are studies of new or experimental medicines (or other new treatments). The studies are done when there is a reason to believe a new drug or a new combination of drugs may be of value in curing or controlling cancer.

If you wish to take part in a clinical trial, the researchers will fully explain to you and your family what is required. You always have the chance to refuse to take part in the study. Being in a clinical trial does not keep you from getting other medical or nursing care that you need.

People who take part in clinical trials make an important contribution to medical care because the study results will also help future patients. At the same time, these participants may also be among the first to benefit from these new treatments.

To learn more about clinical trials, you may contact the American Cancer Society at 1-800-ACS-2345 or visit the Web site (www.cancer.org). The American Cancer Society can match you to clinical trials appropriate for your specific cancer. You may also contact the National Cancer Institute at 1-800-4-CANCER or visit the Web site (www.cancer.gov). The National Cancer Institute provides a listing of clinical trials for people with cancer.

HOW DOES CHEMOTHERAPY WORK?

To understand how chemotherapy works as a treatment, it is helpful to understand the normal life cycle of a cell in the body. All living tissue is composed of cells. Cells grow and reproduce to replace cells lost during injury or normal "wear and tear." The cell cycle is a series of steps that both normal cells and abnormal cancer cells go through in order to grow and reproduce to form new cells.

This discussion is somewhat technical, but it can help you understand how doctors predict which drugs are likely to work well together and how doctors decide how often doses of each drug should be given.

There are five phases in the cell cycle, designated by letters and numbers in the following figure:

G_0 = Resting stage
G_1 = RNA and protein synthesis
S = DNA synthesis
G_2 = Construction of mitotic apparatus
M = Mitosis

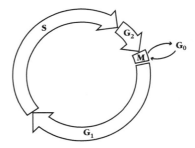

G_0 Phase (resting stage):	Cells have not yet started to divide. Depending on the type of cell, this step can last for a few hours to a few years. When the cell is signaled to reproduce, it moves into the G_1 phase.
G_1 Phase:	During this phase, the cell starts making more proteins to prepare to divide. This phase lasts about 18 to 30 hours.
S Phase:	In the S phase, the material containing the genetic code (DNA, or deoxyribonucleic acid) is copied so that both of the new cells formed will have the right amount of DNA. This phase lasts about 18 to 20 hours.
G_2 Phase:	The G_2 phase occurs just before the cell starts splitting into two cells. It lasts from 2 to 10 hours.
M Phase:	In this phase, which lasts only 30 to 60 minutes, the cell actually splits into two new cells.

This cell cycle is important to oncologists (cancer doctors) because many chemotherapy drugs work only on actively reproducing cells (not on cells in the resting phase, G_0). These drugs specifically attack cells in a particular phase of the cell cycle (the M or S phases, for example). Understanding how these drugs work helps oncologists predict which drugs are likely to work well together. Doctors can effectively plan how often doses of each drug should be given.

Although chemotherapy drugs attack reproducing cells, they cannot tell the difference between reproducing cells of normal tissues (that are replacing worn-out normal cells) and cancer cells. The damage to normal cells can result in side effects.

Each time chemotherapy is given, it involves an attempt to balance between destroying the cancer cells (in order to cure or control the disease) and sparing the normal cells (to lessen undesirable side effects).

WHAT ARE THE GOALS OF TREATMENT WITH CHEMOTHERAPY?

There are three goals for chemotherapy treatment:

- *Cure*: If possible, chemotherapy is used to cure the cancer, meaning that the tumor or cancer disappears and does not return.
- *Control*: If cure is not possible, the goal is to control the disease (stop the cancer from growing and spreading) in order to extend your life and provide you the best quality of life while you live with cancer.
- *Palliation*: Sometimes control is unlikely if the cancer is in an advanced stage. At this point the goal is called palliation. This means that chemotherapy drugs will be used to relieve symptoms caused by the cancer, thereby improving your quality of life, even though the drugs may not lengthen your life.

For some people, chemotherapy is the only treatment used in an attempt to cure, control, or palliate their cancer. In other cases, chemotherapy may be given as neoadjuvant therapy (before surgery or radiation) or as adjuvant therapy (after surgery or radiation).

- *Neoadjuvant chemotherapy* may be used to shrink a large tumor so that it can then be removed by surgery or a less extensive operation, or so it can be treated more effectively with radiation.
- *Adjuvant chemotherapy* is given to prevent the growth of stray cancer cells remaining in the body after surgery or radiation. In most cases, these stray cancer cells cannot be seen in routine tests such as computed tomography (CT) scans but may still be present.

WHAT ARE THE DIFFERENT TYPES OF CHEMOTHERAPY DRUGS?

Chemotherapy drugs are divided into several categories based on how they affect specific chemical substances within cancer cells, which cellular activities or processes the drugs interfere with, and which specific phases of the cell cycle they affect. Knowing this helps oncologists decide which drugs are likely to work well together and, if more than one drug will be used, to plan exactly when each of the drugs should be given (in which order and how often).

Alkylating Agents

Alkylating agents work directly on DNA to prevent the cancer cell from reproducing. As a class of drugs, these agents are not phase specific (in other words, they work in all phases of the cell cycle). These drugs are active against chronic leukemias, non-Hodgkin's lymphoma, Hodgkin's disease, multiple myeloma, and certain cancers of the lung, breast, and ovary.

Examples of alkylating agents include busulfan, cisplatin, carboplatin, chlorambucil, cyclophosphamide, ifosfamide, dacarbazine (DTIC), mechlorethamine (nitrogen mustard), and melphalan.

Nitrosoureas

Nitrosoureas act in a similar way to alkylating agents. They interfere with enzymes that help repair DNA. These agents are able to travel to the brain so they are used to treat brain tumors as well as non-Hodgkin's lymphomas, multiple myeloma, and malignant melanoma.

Examples of nitrosoureas include carmustine (BCNU) and lomustine (CCNU).

Antimetabolites

Antimetabolites are a class of drugs that interfere with DNA and RNA growth. These agents work during the S phase and are used to treat chronic leukemias as well as tumors of the breast, ovary, and the gastrointestinal tract.

Examples of antimetabolites include 5-fluorouracil, capecitabine, methotrexate, gemcitabine, cytarabine (ara-C), and fludarabine.

Antitumor Antibiotics

Antitumor antibiotics interfere with DNA by stopping enzymes and mitosis or by altering the membranes that surround cells. (They are not the same as antibiotics used to treat infections.) These agents work in all phases of the cell cycle. Thus, they are widely used for a variety of cancers.

Examples of antitumor antibiotics include dactinomycin, daunorubicin, doxorubicin (Adriamycin), idarubicin, and mitoxantrone.

Mitotic Inhibitors

Mitotic inhibitors are plant alkaloids and other compounds derived from natural products. They can inhibit, or stop, mitosis or inhibit enzymes for making proteins needed for reproduction of the cell. These inhibitors work during the M phase of the cell cycle.

Examples of mitotic inhibitors include paclitaxel, docetaxel, etoposide (VP-16), vinblastine, vincristine, and vinorelbine.

Corticosteroid Hormones

Steroids are natural hormones and hormone-like drugs that are useful in treating some types of cancer (lymphoma, leukemias, and multiple myeloma) as well as other illnesses. When these drugs are used to kill cancer cells or slow their growth, they are considered chemotherapy drugs. They are often combined with other types of chemotherapy drugs to increase their effectiveness.

Examples include prednisone and dexamethasone.

Sex Hormones

Sex hormones, or hormone-like drugs, alter the action or production of female or male hormones. They are used to slow the growth of breast, prostate, and endometrial (lining of the uterus) cancers, which normally grow in response to hormone levels in the body. These hormones do not work in the same ways as standard chemotherapy drugs.

Examples include antiestrogens (tamoxifen, fulvestrant), aromatase inhibitors (anastrozole, letrozole), progestins (megestrol acetate), antiandrogens (bicalutamide, flutamide), and LHRH agonists (leuprolide, goserelin).

Immunotherapy

Some drugs are given to people with cancer to stimulate their immune systems to more effectively recognize and attack cancer cells. These drugs offer a unique method of treatment and are often considered to be separate from chemotherapy.

Others

Some chemotherapy drugs act in slightly different ways and do not fit into any of the other categories.

Examples include such drugs as L-asparaginase and tretinoin.

SELECTING WHICH DRUGS TO USE FOR CHEMOTHERAPY TREATMENTS

In some cases, the best choice of doses and schedules for giving each drug are relatively clear, and most oncologists would recommend the same treatment. In other cases, less may be known about the best way to treat people with certain types and stages of cancer. Different cancer doctors might choose different drug combinations with different schedules.

Factors to consider choosing drugs for a chemotherapy regimen include the following:

- Type of cancer
- Stage of the cancer (how far it has spread)
- Age
- General state of health
- Other serious health problems (such as liver or kidney diseases)
- Other types of anticancer treatments given in the past

Doctors consider these factors in the context of information published in medical journals and textbooks describing the outcomes of similar patients treated with various chemotherapy drugs.

Chemotherapy regimens or treatment plans may use a single drug or a combination of drugs. Oncologists usually recommend a combination of drugs for most people with cancer. This is often more effective than a single drug, as the cancer cells can be attacked in several ways. Doctors must also consider side effects of each drug and any potential interactions among the drugs.

Side Effects

Different drugs may have different side effects, so it is often better to use moderate doses that cause bearable side effects rather than very high doses of a single drug that might cause severe side effects and possible permanent damage to organs. However, there are important exceptions to this rule, and a single chemotherapy drug may be the best option for some people with certain types of cancer.

Doctors try to give chemotherapy at levels high enough to cure or control the cancer while keeping side effects to a minimum. They also try to avoid drugs with similar and additive side effects.

Drug Interactions

In addition to considering how best to combine two or more chemotherapy drugs, doctors must also consider potential interactions between chemotherapy drugs and other medications, including vitamins and nonprescription medicines. In some cases these interactions may make side effects worse. In others they may interfere with the effectiveness of the chemotherapy. Therefore, it is important that you tell your doctor about all vitamins and nonprescription medicines you are taking.

For example, many chemotherapy drugs temporarily slow down the bone marrow's production of blood platelets (clotting cells). Aspirin or related drugs can weaken blood platelets. This is not a problem for healthy people with normal platelet counts. But for people with low platelet counts due to chemotherapy, this interaction may increase the risk of a serious bleeding problem. Avoid taking these medications while receiving chemotherapy unless your oncologist says it is safe to do so.

Vitamins. Many people want to take an active role in improving their general health in order to help their body's natural defenses fight the cancer and to speed up their recovery from the side effects of chemotherapy.

Because most people think of vitamins as a safe way to improve health, it is not surprising that many people with cancer take high doses of one or more vitamins. But few realize that some vitamins might make their chemotherapy less effective.

Certain vitamins, such as A, E, and C, act as antioxidants, meaning that they can prevent formation of ions that damage DNA. This damage is thought to have an important role in causing cancer. There is some evidence that getting enough of these vitamins (through a balanced diet and, perhaps, by taking vitamin supplements) may help reduce the risk of developing some types of cancer.

On the other hand, some chemotherapy drugs (and radiation) work by producing these same types of ions to severely damage the DNA of cancer cells so the cells are unable to grow and reproduce. Some scientists believe that taking high doses of antioxidant vitamins during treatment may make these drugs less effective. Few studies have been done to thoroughly test this theory. Until more is known about the effects of vitamins on chemotherapy drugs, many oncologists recommend the following during chemotherapy:

- If your doctor has not prescribed vitamins for a specific reason, it is best not to take any.
- A simple multivitamin is probably acceptable if you want to take a vitamin supplement, but check with your doctor first.
- It is safest to avoid taking high doses of antioxidant vitamins during chemotherapy treatment. Ask your doctors when it might be safe to start such vitamins after treatment is finished.
- If you are concerned about nutrition, you can usually get plenty of vitamins by eating a well-balanced diet.

PLANNING DRUG DOSES AND SCHEDULES

Some drugs, especially those available to people without a prescription, have a fairly wide *therapeutic index*. This means that wide ranges of doses can be used effectively and safely. For example, the label on a bottle of aspirin may suggest taking 2 tablets for a mild headache. But 1 tablet (half the dose) will probably help many people with a mild headache.

Most chemotherapy drugs, on the other hand, have a narrow range of safe and effective doses. Taking too little of the drug will not effectively treat the cancer and taking too much may cause life-threatening side effects. For this reason, doctors must calculate chemotherapy doses very precisely.

Doses

Chemotherapy doses, usually measured in milligrams (mg), are sometimes based on a person's body weight in kilograms (1 kilogram is 2.2 pounds). For instance, if the standard dose of a drug is 10 milligrams per kilogram (usually abbreviated as 10 mg/kg), a person weighing 50 kilograms (110 pounds) would receive 500 milligrams (5 x 10).

Chemotherapy doses are most commonly determined based on body surface area (BSA), which doctors calculate using your height and weight. Dosages for children and adults differ, even after BSA is taken into account. This is because children's bodies process drugs differently. They may have different levels of sensitivity to the drugs as well.

For similar reasons, dosages of some drugs may also be adjusted for people who are elderly, have poor nutritional status, have already taken or are currently taking other medications, have already received or are currently receiving radiation therapy, have low blood cell counts, or have liver or kidney diseases.

Schedule (Cycles)

Chemotherapy is generally given at regular intervals called cycles. A cycle may involve one dose followed by several days or weeks without treatment. This allows normal tissues time to recover from the side effects. Alternatively, doses may be given several days in a row, or every other day for several days, followed by a period of rest. Some drugs work best when given continuously over several days.

If more than one drug is used, the treatment plan will specify how often and exactly when each drug should be given. The number of cycles you receive may be determined before treatment starts (based on the type and stage of cancer) or may be flexible, to take into account how quickly the tumor is shrinking.

Certain serious side effects may also require doctors to adjust chemotherapy plans (dosage or schedule) to allow time to recover.

WHERE ARE CHEMOTHERAPY TREATMENTS GIVEN?

Chemotherapy treatments may be given in the following locations:

- Hospital
- Doctor's office
- Outpatient clinic
- Home
- Workplace

Both convenience and how the drugs are to be given must be considered in deciding the best place to administer chemotherapy. For example, a chemotherapy regimen that requires placement of a special intravenous catheter and infusion over 24 hours or longer may need to be done in a hospital. The specific drugs and their doses, as well as your general state of health, will determine the expected side effects and whether you need to be monitored more closely during treatment.

WHAT ARE THE DIFFERENT WAYS TO TAKE CHEMOTHERAPY?

Drugs used in chemotherapy regimens can be given in many ways.

- Oral (by mouth, or PO)
- Topical (on top of the skin as a cream or lotion)

- Intravenous (into a vein or IV)
- Intramuscular (into a muscle, or IM)
- Subcutaneous (under the skin, or SQ)
- Intra-arterial (into an artery)
- Intrathecal (into the central nervous system via the cerebrospinal fluid)
- Intrapleural (into the chest cavity)
- Intraperitoneal (into the abdominal cavity)
- Intravesical (into the bladder)
- Intralesional/intratumoral (into the tumor)

Some chemotherapy drugs are never taken by mouth because the digestive system cannot absorb them or because they are very irritating to the digestive system. Even when a drug is available in an oral form (such as a pill), this method may not be the best choice. For example, some people with certain digestive system symptoms (vomiting, diarrhea, or severe nausea) cannot swallow liquids or pills. Some people may have trouble remembering when or how many pills to take.

The term *parenteral* is used to describe drugs given intravenously, intramuscularly, or subcutaneously. The IV route is most common. Intramuscular and subcutaneous injections are less frequently used because many drugs can be very irritating or even damaging to the skin or muscle tissue.

The IV route gets the drug quickly throughout the body. IV therapy may be given through a vein in the arm or hand or through a vascular access device (VAD), which includes a catheter implanted into a larger vein in the chest, neck, or arm.

There are different types of VADs with different types of catheters and implantable ports. VADs are used for these reasons:

- To give several drugs at one time
- For long-term therapy (to reduce the number of needle sticks)
- For continuous infusion chemotherapy
- To give drugs that can cause serious damage to skin and muscle tissue if they leak outside of a vein (drugs that are vesicants). Delivering them through a VAD provides more stable access in a vein than a regular IV, thus reducing the risk of the drug leaking outside of the vein.

The type of VAD used is based on the length of chemotherapy planned, your preference and what your doctor may suggest, the care required to maintain the VAD, and its cost.

Types of Vascular Access Devices

Type of Device	Comments
PICC (peripherally inserted central catheter) (Per-Q-Cath, Groshong PICC)	Placed in the arm and threaded up through the vein to near the heart. Allows for continuous access to peripheral vein for several weeks. No surgery needed. Care of catheter needed.
Midline catheter (Per-Q-Cath Midline, Groshong Midline)	Also placed in the arm, but the catheter is not inserted as far as a PICC. Used for intermediate-length therapy when a regular peripheral IV is not advisable or available. No surgery needed. Care of catheter needed.
TCVC (tunneled central venous catheter) (Hickman, Broviac, Groshong)	Catheter with multiple lumens surgically placed in large central vein in the chest and with catheter tunneled under the skin. Care of catheter needed.

Types of Vascular Access Devices cont.

Type of Device

Implantable venous access port
    (Port-A-Cath, BardPort, PassPort, Medi-port)

Comments

A port of plastic, stainless steel, or titanium with a silicone septum with catheter surgically placed under the skin of the chest or arm in a large or central vein. The port is accessed by a needle to give chemotherapy.

Implantable pump

A titanium pump with an internal power source surgically implanted to give continuous infusion chemotherapy, usually at home. There is a refillable reservoir for continuous infusions.

Chemotherapy for Specific Areas of the Body (Regional Chemotherapy)

When there is a need to give high doses of chemotherapy to a specific area of the body, it may be given by a regional method. Regional chemotherapy involves directing the anticancer drugs into the tumor-bearing part of the body. The purpose is to achieve greater exposure to the cancer than could be achieved by chemotherapy drugs that go to all parts of the body while minimizing side effects elsewhere. Examples of regional chemotherapy include drugs given into the body through these routes:

- Intra-arterial (into an artery)
- Intracavitary (into a body cavity)
- Intravesical (into the bladder)
- Intrapleural (into the chest)
- Intraperitoneal (into the abdomen)
- Intrathecal (into the central nervous system via spinal fluid)

Intra-arterial infusions gained some popularity during the 1980s. An intra-arterial infusion allows a chemotherapy drug to be given directly through a catheter in an artery to an organ such as the liver (isolated hepatic perfusion) or to an extremity such as the leg (isolated limb perfusion). The catheter is attached to an implanted or portable pump. Although this approach sounds like a good idea for increasing effectiveness and reducing side effects, most studies have not found it to be as useful as was anticipated. Although clinical trials continue to improve this approach to chemotherapy, it is not widely used except in these studies.

Intracavitary is a broad term used to describe chemotherapy given directly into a body cavity, such as intravesical (into the bladder), intraperitoneal (abdominal cavity), or intrapleural (chest cavity) chemotherapy. The drug is given through a catheter placed directly into one of these areas.

Intravesical chemotherapy is especially effective for early-stage bladder cancer. The chemotherapy is usually given weekly for 4 to 12 weeks. For each treatment, a urinary catheter is placed into the bladder to give the drug. The drug is kept in the bladder for 2 hours and then drained. The urinary catheter is removed after each treatment.

Intrapleural and **intraperitoneal** chemotherapy are not used very often but are useful for some people with mesothelioma (cancer that develops in the lining of the lung), ovarian cancer that has spread to the peritoneum, and lung or breast cancers that have spread to the pleura.

Intrapleural chemotherapy is given through large or small chest catheters that may be connected to an implantable port. These catheters can be used to administer drugs as well as to drain fluid that often accumulates in the pleural or peritoneal cavity when cancer has spread to these tissues.

Intraperitoneal chemotherapy is given through a *Tenckhoff catheter* (a catheter specially designed for removing or adding large amounts of fluid from or into the peritoneum) or through an implanted port. Cancers of the appendix that spread extensively within the abdomen are sometimes treated with intraperitoneal chemotherapy.

Intrathecal chemotherapy is given directly into the cerebrospinal fluid (fluid that surrounds the brain and spinal cord) and can reach cancer cells in the central nervous system. Most chemotherapy drugs that are given into veins are unable to cross the barrier between the bloodstream and the central nervous system (brain and spinal cord) called the blood–brain barrier. Intrathecal chemotherapy may be necessary for some people with leukemia or other cancers that have spread to the brain or spinal cord.

Intrathecal chemotherapy may use one of 2 methods:

- In one method, chemotherapy is given by a *lumbar puncture* (spinal tap) daily or weekly into the space around the spinal cord.
- The second method uses a special device called an *Ommaya reservoir*, which is placed into the skull and has a catheter inserted into a ventricle (a space inside the brain filled with cerebrospinal fluid).

SAFETY PRECAUTIONS FOR HEALTH CARE PROFESSIONALS

Many chemotherapy drugs are considered hazardous, so the nurses and doctors who give chemotherapy will take precautions to avoid direct contact with the drugs while giving them to you.

Some chemotherapy drugs are dangerous to others in these ways:

- They can cause abnormal changes in DNA (mutagenic).
- They may be able to alter development of a fetus or embryo, leading to birth defects (teratogenic).
- They may be able to cause another type of cancer (carcinogenic).
- Some may cause localized skin irritation or damage.

Nurses may wear special gloves and gowns when preparing and giving you the chemotherapy drugs. Additionally, pharmacists or nurses prepare the drugs in areas with special ventilation systems.

If you are hospitalized, nurses and health care professionals may take special precautions in handling your urine and stool for a few days after treatment, as they may contain the drugs. If you are receiving chemotherapy drugs at home, you will be given special instructions and precautions to ensure the safety of caregivers in the home.

Special procedures are used for disposing of materials after mixing and administering the drugs. There are separate plastic containers to dispose of sharp items, syringes, IV tubing, and medication bags. Gowns and gloves are disposed of in special bags. If any drug leaks or spills, special precautions are used to clean it up.

WHAT ARE THE SIDE EFFECTS OF CHEMOTHERAPY?

If after reading this section you want more information about managing the side effects of chemotherapy, please call the American Cancer Society at 1-800-ACS-2345 and ask for the booklet *Understanding Chemotherapy: A Guide for Patients and Their Families* or visit the Web site at www.cancer.org.

Although chemotherapy is given to kill cancer cells, it can also damage normal cells. Most likely to be damaged are normal cells that divide rapidly, such as:

- Bone marrow/blood cells
- Cells of hair follicles

- Cells in the reproductive and digestive tracts

Damage to these cells accounts for many of the side effects of chemotherapy drugs. Side effects are different for each chemotherapy drug, and they also differ based on the dosage, the route through which the drug is given, and how the drug affects you individually.

Bone Marrow Suppression

The bone marrow is the tissue inside some bones that produces white blood cells (WBCs), red blood cells (RBCs), and blood platelets. Damage to the blood cell–producing tissues of the bone marrow is called bone marrow suppression, or *myelosuppression*, and is one of the most common side effects of chemotherapy.

Cells produced in the bone marrow tissue are growing rapidly and are sensitive to the effects of chemotherapy. Until your bone marrow cells recover from this damage, you may have abnormally low numbers of WBCs, RBCs, and/or blood platelets.

While you are getting chemotherapy, your blood will be regularly sampled, sometimes daily when necessary, so the numbers of these cells can be counted by a complete blood count (CBC). Bone marrow samples may also be taken periodically to check on the blood-forming marrow cells that develop into WBCs, RBCs, and blood platelets.

The decrease in blood cell counts does not occur immediately after chemotherapy because the drugs do not destroy the cells already in the bloodstream (which are not dividing rapidly). Instead, the drugs temporarily prevent formation of new blood cells by the bone marrow.

Each type of blood cell has a different life span.

- White blood cells average a 6-hour life span.
- Platelets average 10 days.
- Red blood cells average 120 days.

As blood cells normally wear out, they are constantly replaced by the bone marrow. Following chemotherapy, as these cells wear out, they are not replaced as they would be normally, and the blood cell levels begin to drop. The type and dosage of the chemotherapy influences how low the blood cell counts drop and how long it takes for the drop to occur.

The lowest count to which blood cell levels fall is called the *nadir*. The nadir for each blood cell type occurs at different times, but usually WBCs and platelets reach their nadirs within 7 to 14 days. RBCs live longer and do not reach a nadir for several weeks.

Knowing what the 3 types of blood cells normally do can help you understand the effects of low blood cell counts.

- White blood cells help the body fight off infections.
- Platelets help prevent bleeding by forming plugs to seal up damaged blood vessels.
- Red blood cells bring oxygen to tissues so cells throughout the body can use that oxygen to turn certain nutrients into energy.

The side effects caused by low blood cell counts will likely be at their worst when the WBC, blood platelet, and RBC are at their nadirs, or lowest values.

Low white blood cell counts. The medical term for a low WBC count is *leukopenia*. Blood normally has between 4,000 and 10,000 WBCs per cubic millimeter. WBCs are divided into 2 main categories based on how they appear under the microscope:

- *Granulocytes*, which contain granules (visible specks) in the cytoplasm of the cell, include 3 subtypes: neutrophils, eosinophils, and basophils.
- *Agranulocytes*, which do not contain granules in the cytoplasm of the cell, include 3 subtypes: lymphocytes, monocytes, and macrophages.

Granulocytes, especially neutrophils, provide an important defense against infections and are the most numerous type of WBC. *Neutropenia*, an abnormally low number of neutrophils, is the most common factor that puts people with cancer at risk for infection. The normal range of neutrophils is between 2,500 and 6,000 cells per cubic millimeter. Your doctor will likely watch your neutrophil count closely.

To determine how likely someone is to develop an infection, health care providers calculate a number called the *absolute neutrophil count* (ANC). Someone with an ANC of 1,000 or less is considered to be *neutropenic* and at risk of developing an infection. An ANC lower than 500 is considered severe neutropenia.

Even though your WBC count or the neutrophil count may be low, it does not mean you will get an infection. But you need to watch for these signs and symptoms:

- Fever
- Sore throat
- New cough or shortness of breath
- Nasal congestion
- Burning during urination
- Shaking chills
- Redness, swelling, and warmth at the site of an injury

Fever is a very important sign and may be the first sign of an infection. Usually, you will be instructed to call your doctor or nurse if you have a fever greater than or equal to 100.5°F, any signs or symptoms of infection, or shaking chills.

Your health care team may take preventive care measures to reduce your risk of infection and exposure to others with infections. When WBC counts are very low, doctors often prescribe antibiotics as a preventive measure. These anti-infection drugs may be given intravenously or by mouth.

Because of the risk of infections, additional chemotherapy doses may be delayed when you have a very low white blood cell count. In some situations, so that chemotherapy can be given on schedule, doctors may prescribe growth factors to keep the WBC from falling too low.

Your body normally produces several growth factors (also called colony-stimulating factors) to stimulate the production of various types of blood cells. But the levels of these factors in the body are often not enough to keep up with demands during chemotherapy. Scientists have recently learned how to produce these growth factors in the laboratory, so they are now available as drugs.

The two growth factors that stimulate production of white blood cells are granulocyte–macrophage colony-stimulating factor (GM-CSF, sargramostim, Leukine) and granulocyte colony-stimulating factor (G-CSF, filgrastim, Neupogen). These drugs are often given daily, starting the day after you receive chemotherapy, for up to 2 weeks. A newer, longer-lasting form of G-CSF (pegfilgrastim, Neulasta) is now available and may need to be given only once each chemotherapy cycle.

These drugs help bone marrow recover more quickly and reduce your risk of getting a serious infection. They are given intravenously (IV) or as injections under the skin (SQ). Nurses give the injections if you are in the hospital or at the doctor's office, but you or your family members can learn how to give these injections at home.

Low red blood cell counts. Not having enough red blood cells is called *anemia*. Doctors use 2 measurements to determine whether you have enough RBCs.

- The red pigment in RBCs that carries oxygen is *hemoglobin*. If there are not enough RBCs, the blood hemoglobin concentration will be less than its usual range of 12 to 16 grams per deciliter (g/dL) in women or 14 to 18 g/dL in men.
- Hematocrit is the percentage of total blood volume occupied by red blood cells. Its normal range is between 37% and 52%. Levels are normally higher for men than for women.

With anemia, you may experience the following symptoms:

- Fatigue
- Dizziness
- Headaches
- Irritability
- Shortness of breath
- An increase in heart rate or rate of breathing, or both

Anemia caused by chemotherapy is usually temporary. But bleeding caused by surgery or the cancer (a common occurrence with colorectal cancers, for example) can make anemia even worse.

Blood transfusions may be needed until the bone marrow is healthy enough to replace worn-out RBCs. Because blood transfusions have some risks, doctors use this procedure only if they see significant signs and symptoms, such as shortness of breath and/or very low RBC counts. Other factors also affect this decision. For example, people with heart or lung diseases are more sensitive to anemia.

A newer option for treating anemia caused by chemotherapy is erythropoietin (EPO, Procrit, Epogen). This naturally occurring growth factor stimulates RBC production by bone marrow cells. It can relieve symptoms of anemia and reduce the need for blood transfusions. Erythropoietin is generally given 3 times per week by injection under the skin (SQ) until the hemoglobin level increases to 12 g/dL. A newer, longer-lasting form, known as darbepoietin (Aranesp), may reduce the number of injections to every 1 to 2 weeks.

Low platelet counts. The normal range for platelet counts is between 150,000 and 450,000 per cubic millimeter. The medical term for a low platelet count is *thrombocytopenia*.

If your platelet count is low, you may show these signs:

- Bruise easily
- Bleed longer than usual after minor cuts or scrapes
- Bleeding gums or nose bleeds
- Develop ecchymoses (large bruises) and petechiae (multiple small bruises)
- Serious internal bleeding if the platelet count is very low

Although low platelet counts resulting from chemotherapy are temporary, they can cause serious blood loss from injury or bleeding that can damage internal organs. Sometimes a low platelet count will delay necessary surgery because doctors are concerned about blood loss during surgery. If platelet counts are very low (below 10,000) or if a person with moderately low counts has greater than normal bleeding or bruising, platelet transfusions may be given.

Transfused platelets last only a few days, and some people who have received many platelet transfusions can develop an immune reaction that destroys donor platelets. A platelet growth factor called oprelvekin (Neumega) can be given as a drug for people with severe thrombocytopenia. This decreases their need for platelet transfusions and can stop increased bleeding. It is given under the skin every day.

Hematopoietic stem cell transplantation. *Hematopoietic stem cell transplantation (HSCT)* is the term now used to include *bone marrow transplantation (BMT)* and *peripheral blood stem cell transplantation (PBSCT)*. These transplants permit the use of especially high doses of chemotherapy and/or *total body irradiation (TBI)* to kill the cancer cells. In the process of using these treatments to wipe out the cancer, your normal hematopoietic (blood-forming) stem cells in the bone marrow are also killed. Therefore, stem cells are removed from your blood or bone marrow before treatment and are given back to you once it is completed. Another option is to receive stem cells from another person (a donor).

Hair Loss

Chemotherapy affects the rapidly growing cells of hair follicles. Your hair may become brittle and break off at the surface of the scalp or it may simply fall out from the hair follicle.

Here are some basic facts about hair loss:

- Hair loss can be very individual. Some people may have complete loss of hair while others may see just a thinning of their hair. Loss of eyebrows, eyelashes, pubic hair, and body hair is usually less severe because the growth is less active in these hair follicles than in the scalp.
- Hair loss depends on which drugs are given, their doses, and the length of treatment.
- If hair is going to be affected, you may see it happen 2 to 3 weeks after treatment begins.
- Hair loss from chemotherapy is almost always temporary rather than permanent. When your hair grows back, its color or texture may be different. Hair may start to regrow near the end of your treatment or after the treatment is completed.
- Unlike some other side effects of chemotherapy, hair loss is never life-threatening. But it may have a substantial impact on your quality of life. Hair loss may cause depression, loss of self-confidence, and grief reactions.

Appetite Loss and Weight Loss

Anorexia is a decrease in or complete loss of appetite. Most chemotherapy medications cause some degree of anorexia. Anorexia may be mild, or it may lead to *cachexia*, a form of malnutrition. Loss of appetite, as well as weight loss, may result directly from effects of the cancer on the body's metabolism.

Proper nutrition helps strengthen the body to fight the disease and cope with cancer treatments. Decreased appetite is generally temporary and returns when chemotherapy is completed. It may take several weeks after chemotherapy is finished for your appetite to recover. Some chemotherapy may cause more severe loss of appetite.

Talk with your doctor or nurse if you experience anorexia or cachexia. Medications can be prescribed to help improve these conditions.

Taste Changes

Cancer treatments and the cancer itself can change the way some foods taste. Taste changes can contribute to anorexia and malnutrition. With taste changes caused by chemotherapy, you may notice the following:

- Either a dislike for or an increased desire for sweet foods
- Dislike of foods with bitter tastes
- Dislike of tomatoes and tomato products
- Dislike of beef or pork
- Constant metallic or medicinal taste in your mouth

These changes occur because chemotherapy drugs can change the taste-receptor cells in your mouth that tell you what flavor you are tasting. Changes in taste and smell may continue as long as chemotherapy treatments continue, or longer. Several weeks after chemotherapy has ended, taste and smell sensations usually (but not always) return to normal.

Stomatitis and Esophagitis

Stomatitis refers to the inflammation and sores within your mouth that may result from chemotherapy. Similar changes in the throat or the esophagus (the tube that leads from the throat to the stomach) are called *pharyngitis* and *esophagitis.* The term *mucositis* is used to refer to inflammation of the lining layer of the mouth, throat, and esophagus.

The first signs of mouth sores occur when the lining of the mouth appears pale and dry. Later, the mouth, gums, and throat may feel sore and become red and inflamed. The tongue may be coated and swollen, leading to difficulty swallowing, eating, or talking. Stomatitis, pharyngitis, and esophagitis can lead to bleeding, painful ulceration, and infection.

Mouth, throat, and esophagus sores are temporary and usually develop 5 to 14 days after receiving chemotherapy. They will heal completely once chemotherapy is finished.

Nausea and Vomiting

Although there are new medications to both prevent and treat nausea and vomiting, these symptoms are possible side effects of chemotherapy. Chemotherapy agents cause nausea and vomiting for a variety of reasons. One is that they irritate the lining of the stomach and duodenum (the first section of the small intestine). This irritation stimulates certain nerves that lead to the vomiting center in the brain.

Nausea is an unpleasant wavelike sensation in the stomach and back of the throat. It can be accompanied by symptoms such as sweating, light-headedness, dizziness, and weakness. It can lead to retching, vomiting, or both. *Retching* is a rhythmic movement of the diaphragm and stomach muscles that are controlled by the vomiting center. *Vomiting* is a process controlled by the vomiting center that causes the contents of the stomach to be forced out through the mouth. Vomiting can occur at various times. It can be *acute*, occurring within minutes to hours after chemotherapy, or *delayed*, developing or continuing for 24 hours after chemotherapy and sometimes lasting for days. *Anticipatory vomiting* occurs when you have had a bad experience with nausea and vomiting in the past that was not treated. As a result, you develop nausea and vomiting when placed in the same situation (for example, before receiving the next chemotherapy treatments).

Although it is not possible to predict the onset, severity, or duration of nausea and vomiting for any one person, certain chemotherapy medications are more likely to cause nausea and vomiting. Some examples of these are as follows:

- Cisplatin
- Dacarbazine
- Mechlorethamine
- Daunorubicin
- Streptozocin
- Cytarabine (high doses)
- Doxorubicin
- Carmustine
- Cyclophosphamide
- Ifosfamide
- Procarbazine
- Lomustine
- Dactinomycin
- Plicamycin
- Methotrexate (high doses)

- Carboplatin

Some factors that may affect the amount and severity of nausea and vomiting include:

- Prior experiences with motion sickness
- Previous bad experiences with nausea and vomiting
- Being young
- Heavy alcohol intake
- Being a woman of menstrual age (at greatest risk for severe and long-lasting nausea and vomiting)

Many drugs are used alone or in combination to prevent or decrease nausea and vomiting. They include the following:

- Lorazepam
- Prochlorperazine
- Promethazine
- Metoclopramide
- Dexamethasone
- Ondansetron
- Granisetron

The key to effective control is to prevent nausea and vomiting before it occurs. Consideration may also be given to nondrug methods to help with nausea and vomiting, such as the following:

- Ginger in tablets or in ginger ale
- Relaxation exercises
- Guided imagery
- Soothing music

Constipation

Constipation is the passage (usually with discomfort) of infrequent, hard, dry stool. If you experience constipation, you may also experience excessive straining, bloating, increased gas, cramping, or pain. Constipation affects about half of people with cancer and about 3 out of 4 of those with advanced disease.

Risk factors for developing constipation include:

- Taking opioid pain medications
- Decreased physical activity
- Poor diet
- Decreased fluid intake and dehydration
- Bed rest
- Depression
- Certain chemotherapy agents (such as vincristine and vinblastine)

If constipation develops, your doctor will try to determine the cause, then take appropriate measures to treat the problem.

Diarrhea

Diarrhea is the passage of loose or watery stools 3 or more times a day with or without discomfort. Along with diarrhea, you may have gas, cramping, and bloating. Diarrhea occurs in about 3 of 4 people who receive chemotherapy because of the damage to the rapidly dividing cells in the digestive (gastrointestinal) tract.

Factors affecting diarrhea during chemotherapy include:

- Drugs that cause diarrhea (examples include irinotecan, 5-fluorouracil, methotrexate, docetaxel, and actinomycin-D)
- Dosage
- Length of treatment
- Having a stomach tumor
- Receiving both radiation and chemotherapy
- Being lactose intolerant (can't drink milk, for example)

Diarrhea can be serious and become life-threatening if dehydration, malnutrition, and electrolyte imbalances occur. It is important to report any diarrhea to your doctor or nurse. Keep a record of the number of times you have diarrhea, the amount, and the appearance, and give this information to your doctor.

Fatigue

Fatigue is a common side effect of cancer and chemotherapy. With fatigue caused by chemotherapy, you may experience these feelings:

- Weariness
- Weakness
- Lack of energy
- Decreased ability for physical and mental work
- Difficulty thinking
- Forgetfulness
- Inability to concentrate

The fatigue a person with cancer feels is different from the fatigue of everyday life. It is unrelated to activity and may not be resolved with rest or sleep. Fatigue can be prolonged and can affect your quality of life.

Heart Damage

Certain chemotherapy drugs can damage the heart. The most common ones are daunorubicin and doxorubicin (Adriamycin). This occurs in about 1 in 10 people who receive these drugs and usually involves changes to the heart muscles.

With heart damage caused by chemotherapy, you may feel these symptoms:

- Puffiness or swelling in the hands and feet
- Shortness of breath
- Dizziness
- Erratic heartbeats
- Dry cough

If you have had radiation to the midchest area before, have existing heart problems, have uncontrolled high blood pressure, or are a smoker, you will be at higher risk for heart damage.

Before chemotherapy is started, your doctor will check your heart function to make sure that there are no major problems. During the treatments, your heart function will be checked to ensure that no changes have occurred. Tests such as an electrocardiogram (ECG), an echocardiogram, or a MUGA scan are done to check for any changes in heart function. With a MUGA scan, you receive a radioactive substance that is then traced through your heart with a special scanner.

If problems develop, the chemotherapy drug will be stopped to prevent further permanent damage. Notify your doctor or nurse if you notice changes in your heart rhythm or experience weight gain or fluid retention.

Nervous System Changes

Some chemotherapy drugs can cause direct or indirect changes in the central nervous system (brain and spinal cord), the cranial nerves, or peripheral nerves. The cranial nerves are connected directly to the brain and are important for movement and touch sensation of the head, face, and neck. Cranial nerves are also important for vision, hearing, taste, and smell. Peripheral nerves lead to and from the rest of the body and are important in movement, touch sensation, and regulating activities of some internal organs.

Side effects that are the result of nerve damage caused by chemotherapy can occur soon after chemotherapy or years later. Changes in the central nervous system could produce these symptoms:

- Stiff neck
- Headache
- Nausea and vomiting
- Lethargy or sleepiness
- Fever
- Confusion
- Depression
- Seizures

Peripheral nervous system changes usually affect the hands and feet and can include the following:

- Numbness
- Tingling
- Decreased sensation

This may make you feel clumsy and cause difficulty in daily activities, such as opening jars or squeezing toothpaste tubes.

One of the most commonly used drugs that causes peripheral nerve damage is vincristine. If the chemotherapy is decreased or stopped, the symptoms will usually decrease or disappear. However, there are times when the damage may be permanent.

Damage to the cranial nerves may cause these symptoms:

- Visual difficulties (such as blurred vision or double vision)
- Increased sensitivity to odors
- Hearing loss or ringing in the ears
- Dry mouth

Cognitive Changes

Recent research has shown that chemotherapy can also affect the way your brain functions many years after treatment. This occurs in a small number of patients and is often worse with larger doses of chemotherapy agents. Some of the brain's activities that are affected are concentration, memory, comprehension (understanding), and reasoning.

The changes that were discovered in patients are subtle, but the people who have problems notice the differences in their thinking. Patients who have had chemotherapy and have cognitive impairment call this experience "chemo-brain" or "chemo-fog." Researchers are not sure exactly why chemotherapy affects the brain in this way or exactly how much chemotherapy (or in what combinations) it takes to cause a problem.

Researchers are currently studying the problem to get more information to help prevent and treat cognitive impairment for chemotherapy patients. If you have problems with thinking that interfere with daily life, there are programs that can help you improve your memory and problem-solving abilities. Simply being aware that problems with thinking can occur may help patients and their family members feel less isolated and alone.

Lung Damage

It is possible for some chemotherapy drugs, such as bleomycin, to cause irreversible damage to the lungs. The likelihood of this occurring is increased if you receive radiation to the chest in addition to chemotherapy. Age seems to be an important factor in the development of lung damage. For example, people over 70 years old have 3 times the risk of developing lung problems from the drug bleomycin.

Lung damage may cause symptoms such as shortness of breath, a nonproductive (dry) cough, and possibly fever. If the chemotherapy drug is stopped early enough, the lung tissue can regenerate. Because early lung changes may not show up on a chest X-ray, your doctor may assess your lungs through pulmonary function tests and arterial blood gas tests.

Reproduction and Sexuality

Reproductive and sexual problems can occur after you receive chemotherapy. Which, if any, reproductive problems develop depends on your age when you are treated, the dose and duration of the chemotherapy, and the chemotherapy drug(s) administered.

The following are sexual changes men may experience:

- Most men on chemotherapy still have normal erections. A few, however, may develop problems.
- Erections and sexual desire often decrease just after a course of chemotherapy but usually recover in a week or two. A few chemotherapy drugs, for example, cisplatin or vincristine, can permanently damage parts of the nervous system. Although it is not yet proven, these drugs may interfere with the nerves that control erection.
- Chemotherapy can sometimes affect sexual desire and erections by slowing down the amount of testosterone produced. Some of the medications used to prevent nausea during chemotherapy can also upset a man's hormonal balance, but hormone levels should return to normal after treatments have ended.
- Many chemotherapy drugs can affect sperm and the parts of the body that produce them. Some of these effects may be permanent. Freezing sperm prior to chemotherapy is one option for men who wish to father children later in life. Although it is possible to conceive during chemotherapy, the toxicity of some drugs may cause birth defects. Therefore, it is suggested that all men and women take precautions and use a reliable type of birth control if they are sexually active during treatment.
- Chemotherapy may suppress your immune system. If you have had genital herpes or genital wart infections in the past, you may have flare-ups during chemotherapy.

The following are sexual changes women may experience:

- Many chemotherapy drugs can either temporarily or permanently damage a woman's ovaries, reducing their output of hormones. This affects a woman's fertility and libido. Ovarian function is less likely to return in women over age 30, and these women are therefore more likely to go into menopause.
- Although it is possible to conceive during chemotherapy, the toxicity of some drugs may cause birth defects. Therefore, it is suggested that all men and women take precautions and use a reliable type of birth control if they are sexually active during treatment.
- Symptoms of early menopause include hot flashes, vaginal dryness and tightness during intercourse, and irregular or no menstrual periods. As the lining of the vagina thins, light spotting

of blood after intercourse becomes common.

- Some chemotherapy drugs irritate all mucous membranes in the body. This includes the lining of the vagina, which often becomes dry and inflamed.
- Vaginal infections are common during chemotherapy, particularly in women taking steroids or the powerful antibiotics used to prevent bacterial infections. Yeast cells are a natural part of the vagina's cleansing system. If too many grow, however, you will notice itching inside your vagina. You may also have a whitish discharge that often looks like cottage cheese. Yeast infections inflame the lining of the vagina so that intercourse burns. Yeast infections can often be prevented by not wearing pantyhose, nylon panties, or tight pants. Loose clothing and cotton panties let the vagina breathe. The doctor may also prescribe a vaginal cream or suppository to reduce yeast cells or other organisms that grow in the vagina.
- If you have had genital herpes or genital wart infections in the past, you may have flare-ups during chemotherapy. It is especially important to have a vaginal infection treated if you are taking chemotherapy. Your body's immune system is not as strong because of the treatment, and any infection is a greater problem.
- Chemotherapy is often given through an IV tube into the bloodstream. However, new ways have been developed to bring drugs directly to a tumor. For cancer of the bladder, for example, a liquid is placed directly into the bladder through a catheter in the urethra. Such a treatment has only a minor effect on a woman's sex life. You may notice some pain if you have intercourse too soon after the treatment. This is because the bladder and urethra are still irritated.
- For tumors in the pelvis, you may be given chemotherapy by pelvic infusion. The drugs are put into the arteries that feed the tumor and give an extra strong dose to the genital area. Because this method is fairly new, doctors do not yet know the long-term effects on a woman's sex life. The immediate side effects are most likely similar to those of IV chemotherapy.
- For cancer of the ovaries or colon, the cavity around the intestines is filled with drugs in liquid form. This method of giving chemotherapy is called intraperitoneal "belly bath." Because the chemotherapy causes the area to swell temporarily, a woman looks as if she is pregnant, which may cause her more emotional distress.

Liver Damage

The liver is the organ that metabolizes, or breaks down, most of the chemotherapy drugs that enter the body. Unfortunately, some drugs can cause liver damage, including methotrexate, cytarabine (ara-C), high-dose cisplatin, high-dose cyclophosphamide, vincristine, vinblastine, and doxorubicin (Adriamycin). Most often the damage is temporary, and the liver recovers a few weeks after the drug is stopped.

Signs of liver damage include the following:

- A yellowing of the skin and the whites of the eyes (jaundice)
- Fatigue
- Pain under the lower part of the right ribs or right upper abdomen

Blood tests will be necessary to watch for possible liver damage. People who are older or who have hepatitis may be more likely to develop liver damage.

Kidney and Urinary System Damage

Many of the breakdown products of chemotherapy drugs are excreted through the kidneys. These drug by-products can damage the kidneys, ureters, and bladder. If you have a history of kidney problems, you may be at a higher risk for kidney damage.

Certain chemotherapy drugs such as cisplatin, high-dose methotrexate, ifosfamide, and streptozocin are more likely to cause kidney and urinary damage than other medications.

Signs of possible kidney problems include:

- Headache
- Pain in the lower back
- Fatigue
- Weakness
- Nausea
- Vomiting
- Increased blood pressure
- Increased rate of breathing
- Change in pattern of urination
- Change in color of urine
- Urgent need to urinate
- Swelling or puffiness of the body

Blood tests to measure kidney function are done regularly to watch for any changes.

Long-Term Side Effects of Chemotherapy

For many people with cancer, chemotherapy is the best option for controlling their disease. You may be faced, however, with long-term side effects related to your chemotherapy treatments.

Side effects related to specific chemotherapy drugs can continue after the treatment is completed. These effects can progress and become chronic, or new side effects may occur. Long-term side effects depend on the specific drugs received and whether you received other treatments such as radiation therapy.

- *Permanent organ damage*: Certain chemotherapy drugs may permanently damage the body's organs. If the damage is detected during treatment, the drug is stopped. However, some of the side effects may remain. Damage to some organs and systems, such as the reproductive system, may not show up until after chemotherapy is finished.
- *Delayed development in children*: When young children receive chemotherapy for cancer treatment, it may affect their growth and their ability to learn. Several factors affect long-term side effects, including the age of the child, the specific drugs that are given, the dosage and length of treatment, and whether chemotherapy is used along with other types of treatment, such as radiation.
- *Nerve damage*: Nervous system changes can develop months or years after treatment. Signs of nerve damage may include hearing loss or tinnitus (ringing in the ears), sensations in the hands and feet, personality changes, sleepiness, impaired memory, shortened attention span, and seizures.
- *Blood in the urine*: Hemorrhagic cystitis (blood in the urine), a side effect of cyclophosphamide and ifosfamide, can continue for some time after the drug is stopped, and symptoms may become worse.
- *Another cancer*: Development of a second cancer is a great concern for cancer survivors. Secondary cancers can include Hodgkin's disease and non-Hodgkin's lymphoma, leukemias, and some solid tumors. Follow-up care after all treatment is finished is an essential component of cancer care for all cancer survivors.

WHAT QUESTIONS SHOULD I ASK ABOUT CHEMOTHERAPY?

The doctor will decide on the appropriate chemotherapy plan based on your medical history, type of cancer, extent of cancer, current state of health, and current research.

You may want to ask your doctor or nurses the following questions about your treatment plan for chemotherapy:

- What chemotherapy medications will I be given?

- How will I take these drugs (by mouth or through a vein)?
- How frequently will I need to take chemotherapy?
- How long will I be receiving chemotherapy treatments?
- What side effects might I experience?
- What activities should I do or not do to take care of myself?
- What long-term effects might I expect?
- How can I contact you after office hours if I have signs or symptoms that you need to know about?

WHAT'S NEW IN CHEMOTHERAPY RESEARCH?

Over the years, many people have been successfully treated with chemotherapy drugs, thanks to ongoing development and research. Yet, despite the best treatments, some cancers still come back.

Several exciting uses of chemotherapy and other agents hold even more promise for curing or controlling cancer. New drugs, new combinations of chemotherapy drugs, and new delivery techniques hold significant promise for curing or controlling cancer and improving the quality of life for people with cancer. Expected advances in coming years include the following:

- New classes of chemotherapy medications and combinations of medications.
- New ways to give the drugs, such as using smaller amounts over longer periods of time.
- Chemotherapy medications that are specifically developed to attack a particular target on cancer cells. One such drug, imatinib mesylate (Gleevec), is already approved for use against a form of leukemia and gastrointestinal stromal tumors, and other drugs like it are now under study.
- Other approaches to targeting drugs more specifically at the cancer cells, such as attaching drugs to monoclonal antibodies to make them more effective and produce fewer side effects. *Monoclonal antibodies*, a special type of antibody produced in laboratories, can be designed to guide chemotherapy medications directly to the tumor. Such antibodies (without attached chemotherapy) can also be used as immunotherapy drugs, to strengthen the body's immune response against cancer cells.
- Liposomal therapy, using chemotherapy drugs that have been packaged inside *liposomes* (synthetic fat globules). The liposome, or fatty coating, helps the drugs penetrate the cancer cells more selectively and decreases possible side effects (such as hair loss and nausea and vomiting). Examples of liposomal medications already in use are Doxil (the encapsulated form of doxorubicin) and DaunoXome (the encapsulated form of daunorubicin).
- Newer drugs to reduce side effects, such as colony-stimulating factors to increase blood counts. Other *chemoprotective agents* are being developed to protect against specific side effects of certain chemotherapy drugs. For example, dexrazoxane helps prevent heart damage, amifostine helps protect the kidneys, and mesna protects the bladder.
- Agents that overcome multidrug resistance. Cancer cells often become resistant to chemotherapy by developing the ability to pump the drugs out of the cells. These new agents inactivate the pumps, allowing the chemotherapy to remain in the cancer cells longer and hopefully make it more effective.

REFERENCES

Burke MB, Wilkes GM, Ingwersen K, Bean CK, Berg D. *Cancer Chemotherapy: A Nursing Process Approach*. 2nd ed. Sudbury, MA: Jones and Bartlett; 1996.

Camp-Sorrell D. Chemotherapy: Toxicity management. In: Groenwald SL, Frogge MH, Goodman M, Yarbro CH, eds. *Cancer Nursing: Principles and Practice*. 4th ed. Boston, MA: Jones and Bartlett; 1997:385–425.

Goodman M, Riley MB. Chemotherapy: Principles of Administration. In: Groenwald SL, Frogge MH, Goodman M, Yarbro CH, eds. *Cancer Nursing: Principles and Practice*. 4th ed. Boston, MA: Jones and Bartlett; 1997:317–384.

Guy JL, Ingram BA. Medical oncology: The agents. In: McCorkle R, Grant M, Frank-Stromborg M, Baird SB, eds. *Cancer Nursing: A Comprehensive Textbook*. 2nd ed. Philadelphia, PA: W.B. Saunders; 1996:395–433.

Labriola D, Livingston R. Possible interactions between dietary antioxidants and chemotherapy. *Oncology* 1999; 13(6):1003–1008.

Martin VR, Walker FE, Goodman M. Delivery of cancer chemotherapy. In: McCorkle R, Grant M, Frank-Stromborg M, Baird SB, eds. *Cancer Nursing: A Comprehensive Textbook*. 2nd ed. Philadelphia, PA: W.B. Saunders; 1996:395–433.

Tenenbaum L. *Cancer Chemotherapy and Biotherapy: A Reference Guide*. 2nd ed. Philadelphia, PA: W.B. Saunders; 1994.

Trotice PV. Chemotherapy: Principles of therapy. In: Groenwald SL, Frogge MH, Goodman M, Yarbro CH, eds. *Cancer Nursing: Principles and Practice*. 4th ed. Boston, MA: Jones and Bartlett; 1997:283–316.

Varricchio C, Pierce M, Walter CL, Ades TB, eds. *A Cancer Source Book for Nurses*. 7th ed. Atlanta, GA: American Cancer Society; 1997.

Waibel-Rycek DA. *Cancer Chemotherapy: Basic Nursing Interventions*. Omaha, NE: American Cancer Society, Nebraska Division.

Yasko JM. *Nursing Management of Symptoms Associated with Chemotherapy*. Bala Cynwyd, PA: Meniscus Health Care Communications; 1998.

Molecularly Targeted Drugs

Scientific advances in molecular biology during the past few decades have begun to expose the inner workings of the cells in our bodies. Researchers can now look at the smallest parts of cancer cells to determine what makes them different from normal ones. More importantly, they are now learning how to exploit these differences to create therapies that are truly "targeted" only at these renegade cells.

In the middle of the 20th century, chemotherapy really was a breakthrough. For the first time, doctors could treat, and sometimes even cure, cancer that had spread to distant parts of the body.

But our understanding of cancer was much more limited at the time. Doctors knew that unlike normal cells, cancer cells grew and multiplied quickly. So, chemotherapy drugs were (and still largely are) based on the principle that chemotherapy kills quickly growing cells.

However, other cells in the body, such as those in the skin and the bone marrow, also grow quickly. Chemotherapy affects these cells as well, often leading to side effects such as hair loss and low blood cell counts, among others. Some of these effects are bothersome. But others can be life-threatening, limiting the amount of chemotherapy that can be given and, therefore, its effectiveness.

Beginning in the 1940s (and even today, to some extent), the development of chemotherapy drugs was largely based on the same types of experiments: put a new compound in a dish with cancer cells and see whether it stops them from growing or kills them. If it does either, the compound can go on to be tested in animal, and eventually human, studies.

This has proven to be a reliable way to find effective drugs, but unfortunately it tells us very little about exactly why the drug works. Without this knowledge, developing newer, safer drugs has been a tremendous challenge.

Until recent years, the approach was backwards—new drugs were developed and then their effectiveness was studied.

Advances in molecular biology have changed this. Knowing the differences among cancer cells allows us to design drugs specifically to attack these differences, leaving healthy cells largely untouched. These newer cancer therapies are not perfect, but because their targets are more specific, they are proving to be safer, and in many cases more effective, than conventional treatments.

WHAT ARE MOLECULAR TARGETS?

Researchers have discovered that there are many potential targets—where normal and cancer cells differ. Most of these are abnormal proteins that cancer cells make. These may be unique to the cancer cells or just made in much higher or lower amounts in cancer cells than in normal ones.

The cells in our bodies are made up of 3 main components: DNA (deoxyribonucleic acid), RNA (ribonucleic acid), and proteins. DNA makes up the material of our genes—the "blueprints" that tell our cells what to do. DNA sits (in the form of long strands called chromosomes) in the control center of each cell, which is called the nucleus. Here, something similar to carbon copies of certain genes are made out of material called RNA, which is very much like DNA.

Pieces of RNA then move into the main part of the cell (the cytoplasm). Here, the cell's machinery uses these instructions to make proteins. Proteins are the working parts of each cell, responsible for much of its structure and function.

Even though every cell has the same blueprints (DNA), obviously not every cell is the same. A heart muscle cell, for example, is very different from a skin cell. This is because not all of the genes in each cell are active—they're not all being used to make the same proteins. Some are shut off (either temporarily or permanently) in a process that is tightly controlled in normal cells.

But cancer cells are different. They often have one or more genes turned on that shouldn't be or have essential genes turned off. This leads to having the wrong kind or amount of proteins in the cell, which in turn can affect how the cell behaves.

These proteins are what make a cell cancerous. They may cause it to multiply uncontrollably, to ignore chemical signals from other cells telling it to slow down or to respect their space, and/or to travel to another part of the body to set up shop. Some proteins are inside the cell while others sit on its outer surface.

These types of proteins, and the genes that encode for them, are now the subjects of intense research. They are the targets doctors hope to hone in on when developing new ways to treat cancer.

Unfortunately, not all cells become cancerous by taking the same path. While some of the same abnormal genes and proteins appear in different types of cancer, many of the pathways appear to be unique to a certain type of cancer, or even to only a certain percentage of that type. Progress is being made, but it is becoming more and more evident that there will not be a single cure for all cancers.

TOOLS FOR A NEW AGE

The good news is that researchers are getting better not only at identifying the unique parts of cancer cells, but also at using new molecular tools to attack these targets. As new genes and proteins related to cancer are discovered and characterized, three-dimensional molecules are designed with computers that might interrupt their activities. With molecular techniques these molecules can now be built from scratch in large numbers and tested against cancer cells.

These techniques have already yielded huge dividends, enabling researchers to develop a highly effective, minimally toxic drug to treat certain forms of leukemia. The researchers were able to do this because they knew of the unique gene and its protein that set these particular cancer cells apart.

Several such targeted therapies against various cancers are now in the advanced stages of clinical trials and will likely be available in the next few years.

Another approach uses the principles of the body's own natural form of targeted therapy to attack specific objects. When a person is exposed to a foreign substance, the body's immune system responds by making a protein, called an antibody, that specifically attaches to and attacks that substance.

With a growing list of targets, researchers have learned how to expose laboratory animals to a particular target, such as a protein found on the surface of cancer cells. They can then isolate the antibody that attacks the target and produce it in the laboratory.

These substances, called *monoclonal antibodies,* have been found to be effective against many types of cancer. In fact, monoclonal antibodies are already in use in doctors' offices and hospitals to treat some leukemias, lymphomas, and breast cancers. Researchers have even been able to make some of these antibodies more effective by attaching them to toxins, radioactive particles, or even other chemotherapy drugs. The antibodies then deliver these substances directly to tumors, largely sparing other areas of the body from their effects.

Many other forms of targeted therapy are now being studied as well, including cancer vaccines, antiangiogenesis therapy (attacking a tumor's blood supply), and even forms of gene therapy. Some ideas are more promising in theory at this time, while others are already being studied in people. Most are likely still several years from being available outside of clinical trials.

Of course, many questions remain to be answered. Because molecularly targeted therapies are still relatively new, doctors are now trying to determine the best way to use them. They may prove to be most useful when given in combination with more traditional treatments such as chemotherapy. Only time will tell.

But while the field of molecular therapeutics is still in its infancy, the development of molecularly targeted drugs will undoubtedly play a much larger role in treating cancer in the future, allowing doctors to offer patients safer, more effective forms of therapy.

REFERENCES

Liotta LA, Liu ET. Essentials of molecular biology: Basic principles. In: DeVita VT, Hellman S, Rosenberg SA, eds. *Cancer: Principles and Practice of Oncology.* 6th ed. Philadelphia PA: Lippincott-Raven; 2001:3–15.

Marshall JL, Rizvi NA, Bhargava P, Wojtowicz-Praga S, Hawkins MJ. New developmental therapies. In: Abeloff MD, Armitage JO, Lichter AS, Niederhuber, JE, eds. *Clinical Oncology.* 2nd ed. New York, NY: Churchill Livingstone; 2000:242–278.

Shawver LK, Slamon D, Ullrich A. Smart drugs: Tyrosine kinase inhibitors in cancer therapy. *Cancer Cell* 2002; 2:117–123.

Cancer Treatment Drugs

5-azacytidine

Trade Names:
5AZ, Azacytidine

Type of Drug:
5-azacytidine belongs to the general group of chemotherapy drugs known as antimetabolites. It is being studied for the treatment of several types of cancer including acute myelocytic leukemia.

How Drug Works:
5-azacytidine prevents cells from making DNA and RNA (our body's genetic material). Antimetabolites look like needed chemicals in the body called metabolites. The antimetabolites fool the body into thinking they are metabolites. When the body tries to use them in place of the metabolite, the DNA and RNA cannot be made, thus stopping the growth of cancer cells.

How Drug Is Given:
5-azacytidine is given into a vein (intravenously) over a period of 20 to 60 minutes, or continuously for up to 5 days. It can also be given by an injection under the skin (subcutaneous or SQ), 1 or more times a day. The dose given will depend on your size, whether other medicines are given with it, and your blood counts. Since this drug is still being studied (investigational), the specific dose, how it is given, and schedule will be determined by the study (clinical trial).

 Read the following information. If you do not understand it or if any of it causes you special concern, check with your doctor.

Before taking this drug, tell your doctor:
- If you are trying to become pregnant, are pregnant, or breastfeeding. This drug may cause birth defects if either the male or female is taking it at the time of conception or during pregnancy. Men and women who are taking this drug need to use some kind of birth control. However, do not use oral contraceptives ("the pill") without checking with your doctor.
- If you think you may want to have children in the future. Many chemotherapy drugs can cause sterility.
- If you have any of the following medical problems: chickenpox or exposure to chickenpox, gout, heart disease, congestive heart failure, shingles, kidney stones, liver disease, or other forms of cancer.
- If you are taking any other prescription or over-the-counter drugs, including vitamins and herbals.

Should I avoid any other medicines, foods, alcohol, and/or activities?
Your prescription and nonprescription medicines may interact with other drugs, causing harm. Certain foods or alcohol can also interact with drug products. Never begin taking a new medicine—prescription or nonprescription—without asking your doctor or nurse if it will interact with alcohol, food, or other medicines. Some drug products can cause drowsiness and affect activities such as driving.

Precautions:
5-azacytidine can lower your blood counts (white blood cells, red blood cells, platelets). Your doctor will check your blood counts before and after each treatment to see how it affects your blood counts. Your doctor or nurse will give you specific instructions if your blood counts are low.

5-azacytidine can cause a decrease in your white blood cell count, especially 14 to 17 days after the drug is given. This can increase your risk of getting an infection. Report fever of 100.5°F or higher, or signs of infection such as pain in passing your urine, coughing and bringing up sputum.

5-azacytidine can cause a decrease in the platelet count. This can increase your risk of bleeding. DO NOT take any aspirin or aspirin-containing medicines. Report unusual bruising, or bleeding such as nosebleeds, bleeding gums when you brush your teeth, or black, tarry stools.

While you are being treated with 5-azacytidine, and after you stop treatment, do not have any immunizations (vaccinations) without your doctor's okay. Try to avoid contact with people who have recently taken the oral polio vaccine. Check with your doctor about this.

5-azacytidine can cause nausea and vomiting. Ask your doctor or nurse to give you medicines to prevent this or lessen it.

Tell all the doctors, dentists, and pharmacists you visit that you are taking this drug.
- -
• Most of the following side effects probably will not occur.
• Your doctor or nurse will want to discuss specific care instructions with you.
• They can help you understand these side effects and help you deal with them.

Side Effects:

More Common Side Effects
Decreased white blood cell count with increased risk of infection
Decreased platelet count with increased risk of bleeding
Nausea
Vomiting
Diarrhea

Less Common Side Effects
Decreased red blood cell count with increased risk of tiredness (fatigue)

Rare Side Effects
Increased liver function blood tests
Sores in mouth or on lips
Feeling sleepy or drowsy
Muscle aches
Coma (very rare)
Rash with itching
Fever
Decrease in blood pressure

Other side effects not listed above can also occur in some patients.
Tell your doctor or nurse if you develop any problems.

FDA Approval: This drug is being studied for cancer treatment.

5-fluorouracil

Trade Names:
5-FU, Adrucil, Efudex (topical), Fluorouracil

Type of Drug:
5-fluorouracil belongs to the general group of chemotherapy drugs known as antimetabolites. It is used to treat several types of cancer including colon and head and neck cancers.

How Drug Works:
5-fluorouracil prevents cells from making DNA and RNA by interfering with the synthesis of nucleic acids, thus disrupting the growth of cancer cells.

How Drug Is Given:
5-fluorouracil is given as a shot in the vein (intravenously) over 5 to 10 minutes, over 20 to 60 minutes, or as a continuous infusion over 22 to 24 hours for 1 to 4 days, or longer. The treatment can be repeated weekly, every other week, or every 3 weeks, depending on the treatment regimen. 5-fluorouracil is usually given after a special vitamin, called leucovorin, which increases the effect of the 5-fluorouracil on the cancer cells. The dose depends upon your size. The dose may need to be decreased if you have problems taking the drug (severe diarrhea, or low white blood cell or platelet count).

 Read the following information. If you do not understand it or if any of it causes you special concern, check with your doctor.

Before taking this drug, tell your doctor:
- If you are trying to become pregnant, are pregnant, or breastfeeding. This drug may cause birth defects if either the male or female is taking it at the time of conception or during pregnancy. Men and women who are taking this drug need to use some kind of birth control. However, do not use oral contraceptives ("the pill") without checking with your doctor.
- If you think you may want to have children in the future. Many chemotherapy drugs can cause sterility.
- If you have any of the following medical problems: chickenpox or exposure to chickenpox, gout, heart disease, congestive heart failure, shingles, kidney stones, liver disease, or other forms of cancer.
- If you are taking any other prescription or over-the-counter drugs, including vitamins and herbals.

Should I avoid any other medicines, foods, alcohol, and/or activities?
Your prescription and nonprescription medicines may interact with other drugs, causing harm. Certain foods or alcohol can also interact with drug products. Never begin taking a new medicine—prescription or nonprescription—without asking your doctor or nurse if it will interact with alcohol, food, or other medicines. Some drug products can cause drowsiness and affect activities such as driving.

Precautions:
While you are being treated with 5-fluorouracil, and after you stop treatment, do not have any immunizations (vaccinations) without your doctor's okay. Try to avoid contact with people who have recently taken the oral polio vaccine. Check with your doctor about this.

5-fluorouracil can lower your blood counts (white blood cells, red blood cells, platelets). Your doctor will check your blood counts before and after each treatment to see how it affects your blood counts. Your doctor or nurse will give you specific instructions if your blood counts are low.

5-fluorouracil can decrease your white blood cell count, especially 10 to 14 days after the drug is given. This can increase your chance of getting an infection. Report fever of 100.5°F or higher, or signs of infection such as pain in passing your urine, coughing and bringing up sputum.

5-fluorouracil can cause a decrease in the platelet count. This can increase your risk of bleeding. DO NOT take any aspirin or aspirin-containing medicines. Report unusual bruising, or bleeding such as nosebleeds, bleeding gums when you brush your teeth, or black, tarry stools.

Tell all the doctors, dentists, and pharmacists you visit that you are taking this drug.

- Most of the following side effects probably will not occur.
- Your doctor or nurse will want to discuss specific care instructions with you.
- They can help you understand these side effects and help you deal with them.

Side Effects:

More Common Side Effects
Decreased white blood cell count with increased risk of infection
Decreased platelet count with increased risk of bleeding
Darkening of skin and nail beds
Nausea
Vomiting
Sores in mouth or on lips
Thinning hair
Diarrhea
Brittle nails
Increased sensitivity to sun
Dry, flaky skin

Less Common Side Effects
Darkening and hardening of vein used for giving the drug
Decreased appetite
Headache
Weakness
Muscle aches

Rare Side Effects
Difficulty walking
Irritation of eyes
Increased tearing of eyes
Blurred vision

Other side effects not listed above can also occur in some patients.
Tell your doctor or nurse if you develop any problems.

FDA Approval: This drug is approved for cancer treatment.

90 yttrium (90 Y) ibritumomab tiuxetan

Trade Names:
Zevalin, IDEC-Y288

Type of Drug:
90 Y ibritumomab tiuxetan is a monoclonal antibody (antibodies made in the laboratory and designed to target substances called antigens, which are recognized by the immune system) with an attached radioactive substance (yttrium). It belongs to the class of chemotherapy drugs called radioimmunotherapeutic agents. It is used to treat certain non-Hodgkin's lymphomas.

How Drug Works:
90 Y ibritumomab tiuxetan is like a "smart bomb." The monoclonal antibody ibritumomab tiuxetan is directed against a certain receptor (CD20) located on B lymphocyte cells. This receptor is found on some normal lymphocytes and also on lymphocytes that are cancerous, as in non-Hodgkin's lymphoma. Once attached, the radiation in the antibody (90 yttrium) kills the cells by exposing them to radiation. This treatment seems to work better if another monoclonal medicine called rituximab is given first.

How Drug Is Given:
The drug is given in 4 steps. First, rituximab is given by an infusion into a vein over 4 or more hours. It attaches to the CD 20 receptor on B cell lymphocytes and helps clear some of the cancerous ones out of the blood. Second, a small dose of the 90 yttrium is given over 10 minutes into a vein. Then special x-rays are done to show where the yttrium has moved to in your body. This helps the doctors make sure that when the treatment dose of 90 Y ibritumomab tiuxetan is given it will go to all the right places. Third, about 7 to 9 days after the first dose of rituximab, another dose of rituximab is given over 4 or more hours, depending upon how well the dose is tolerated. Fourth, the 90 Y ibritumomab tiuxetan is given by a 10-minute injection into a vein. The doses given depend on your size, and the dose of rituximab is lower than if given alone.

 Read the following information. If you do not understand it or if any of it causes you special concern, check with your doctor.

Before taking this drug, tell your doctor:
- If you are trying to become pregnant, are pregnant, or breastfeeding. This drug may cause birth defects if either the male or female is taking it at the time of conception or during pregnancy. Men and women who are taking this drug need to use some kind of birth control. However, do not use oral contraceptives ("the pill") without checking with your doctor.
- If you think you may want to have children in the future. Many chemotherapy drugs can cause sterility.
- If you have any of the following medical problems: chickenpox or exposure to chickenpox, gout, heart disease, congestive heart failure, shingles, kidney stones, liver disease, or other forms of cancer.
- If you are taking any other prescription or over-the-counter drugs, including vitamins and herbals.

Should I avoid any other medicines, foods, alcohol, and/or activities?
Your prescription and nonprescription medicines may interact with other drugs, causing harm. Certain foods or alcohol can also interact with drug products. Never begin taking a new medicine—prescription or nonprescription—without asking your doctor or nurse if it will interact with alcohol, food, or other medicines. Some drug products can cause drowsiness and affect activities such as driving.

Precautions:
Many people get mild symptoms after receiving the treatment, including headache, feeling "blah" and without energy, nausea, abdominal pain, and feeling tired. Talk with your doctor or nurse about what to do for these symptoms.

While you are being treated with 90 Y ibritumomab tiuxetan, and after you stop treatment, do not have any immunizations (vaccinations) without your doctor's okay. Try to avoid contact with people who have recently taken the oral polio vaccine. Check with your doctor about this.

90 Y ibritumomab tiuxetan can lower your blood counts (white blood cells, red blood cells, platelets). Your doctor will check your blood counts before and after each treatment to see how it affects your blood counts. Your doctor or nurse will give you specific instructions if your blood counts are low.

90 Y ibritumomab tiuxetan can cause a decrease in your white blood cell count, reaching the lowest point about 6 to 7 weeks after treatment is given. This can increase your risk of getting an infection. Report fever of 100.5°F or higher, or signs of infection such as pain in passing your urine, coughing, or bringing up sputum.

90 Y ibritumomab tiuxetan can lower your platelet count. This can increase your risk of bleeding. DO NOT take any aspirin or aspirin-containing medicines. Report unusual bruising or bleeding, such as nosebleeds, bleeding gums when you brush your teeth, or black, tarry stools.

Rarely, you can have a severe allergic reaction to the monoclonal antibody. Your nurse or doctor will watch you very closely during the treatment.

 Tell all the doctors, dentists, and pharmacists you visit that you are taking this drug.

- Most of the following side effects probably will not occur.
- Your doctor or nurse will want to discuss specific care instructions with you.
- They can help you understand these side effects and help you deal with them.

Side Effects:

More Common Side Effects
Mild to moderate symptoms with nausea, feeling "blah," and feeling tired
Decreased white blood cell count with increased risk of infection
Decreased platelet count with increased risk of bleeding
Decreased red blood cell count with increased risk of tiredness

Rare Side Effects
Severe allergic reaction with rash, hives, fever and chills, swelling of face or lips, and difficulty breathing.

Side Effects / Symptoms of the Drug
You will be given the treatment as an outpatient. Your doctor or nurse will watch you closely for an allergic reaction.

Other side effects not listed above can also occur in some patients.
Tell your doctor or nurse if you develop any problems.

FDA Approval: This drug is approved for cancer treatment.

9-aminocamptothecin (9-AC)

Trade Name:
(Investigational)

Type of Drug:
9-aminocamptothecin (9-AC) belongs to the general group of chemotherapy drugs called topoisomerase inhibitors. It is being studied in several cancers, including colon and ovarian cancers.

How Drug Works:
9-aminocamptothecin (9-AC) stops the growth of cancer cells by blocking the development of DNA and RNA.

How Drug Is Given:
9-aminocamptothecin (9-AC) is given into a vein (intravenuously) for 3 days or as directed by the specific clinical study. The dose given will depend on your size, whether other medicines are given with it, and your blood counts. If you are also taking antiseizure medicines, the dose of 9-aminocamptothecin (9-AC) may be increased. Since this drug is still being studied (investigational), the specific dose, how it is given, and schedule will be determined by the study (clinical trial).

 Read the following information. If you do not understand it or if any of it causes you special concern, check with your doctor.

Before taking this drug, tell your doctor:
- If you are trying to become pregnant, are pregnant, or breastfeeding. This drug may cause birth defects if either the male or female is taking it at the time of conception or during pregnancy. Men and women who are taking this drug need to use some kind of birth control. However, do not use oral contraceptives ("the pill") without checking with your doctor.
- If you think you may want to have children in the future. Many chemotherapy drugs can cause sterility.
- If you have any of the following medical problems: chickenpox or exposure to chickenpox, gout, heart disease, congestive heart failure, shingles, kidney stones, liver disease, or other forms of cancer.
- If you are taking any other prescription or over-the-counter drugs, including vitamins and herbals.

Should I avoid any other medicines, foods, alcohol, and/or activities?
Your prescription and nonprescription medicines may interact with other drugs, causing harm. Certain foods or alcohol can also interact with drug products. Never begin taking a new medicine—prescription or non-prescription—without asking your doctor or nurse if it will interact with alcohol, food, or other medicines. Some drug products can cause drowsiness and affect activities such as driving.

Precautions:
9-aminocamptothecin (9-AC) can lower your blood counts (white blood cells, red blood cells, platelets). Your doctor will check your blood counts before and after each treatment to see how it affects your blood counts. Your doctor or nurse will give you specific instructions if your blood counts are low.

9-aminocamptothecin (9-AC) can cause a decrease in your white blood cell count. This can increase your chance of getting an infection. Report fever of 100.5°F or higher, or signs of infection such as pain in passing your urine, coughing and bringing up sputum.

9-aminocamptothecin (9-AC) can cause a decrease in the platelet count. This can increase your risk of bleeding. DO NOT take any aspirin or aspirin-containing medicines. Report unusual bruising, or bleeding such as nosebleeds, bleeding gums when you brush your teeth, or black, tarry stools.

9-aminocamptothecin (9-AC) can cause nausea and vomiting. Ask your doctor or nurse to give you medicines to prevent or lessen this side effect.

Tell all the doctors, dentists, and pharmacists you visit that you are taking this drug.
- Most of the following side effects probably will not occur.
- Your doctor or nurse will want to discuss specific care instructions with you.
- They can help you understand these side effects and help you deal with them.

Side Effects:

More Common Side Effects
Decreased white blood cell count with increased risk of infection
Decreased platelet count with increased risk of bleeding
Tiredness (fatigue)
Nausea
Vomiting
Diarrhea
Hair loss
Anemia

Side Effects / Symptoms of the Drug
Talk to your doctor or nurse about getting a wig before you start your chemotherapy.

Tell your doctor or nurse if you develop diarrhea and ask them how it should be treated.

Other side effects not listed above can also occur in some patients.
Tell your doctor or nurse if you develop any problems.

FDA Approval: This drug is being studied for cancer treatment.

acridinyl anisidide

Trade Names:
AMISA, AMSA, Amsacrine

Type of Drug:
Acridinyl anisidide belongs to a general group of chemotherapy drugs known as topoisomerase II inhibitors. It is used to treat several types of cancer including leukemia and lymphoma.

How Drug Works:
Acridinyl anisidide stops the growth of cancer cells by blocking the development of DNA and RNA.

How Drug Is Given:
Acridinyl anisidide is given into a vein (intravenously) as a 1-hour infusion. Tell the nurse immediately if you feel stinging or burning in the vein during or after the drug is given. The dose given will depend on your size, whether other medicines are given with it, and your liver blood tests. Since this drug is still being studied, the specific dose, how it is given, and schedule will be determined by the clinical trial.

 Read the following information. If you do not understand it or if any of it causes you special concern, check with your doctor.

Before taking this drug, tell your doctor:
- If you are trying to become pregnant, are pregnant, or breastfeeding. This drug may cause birth defects if either the male or female is taking it at the time of conception or during pregnancy. Men and women who are taking this drug need to use some kind of birth control. However, do not use oral contraceptives ("the pill") without checking with your doctor.
- If you think you may want to have children in the future. Many chemotherapy drugs can cause sterility.
- If you have any of the following medical problems: chickenpox or exposure to chickenpox, gout, heart disease, congestive heart failure, shingles, kidney stones, liver disease, or other forms of cancer.
- If you are taking any other prescription or over-the-counter drugs, including vitamins and herbals.

Should I avoid any other medicines, foods, alcohol, and/or activities?
Your prescription and nonprescription medicines may interact with other drugs, causing harm. Certain foods or alcohol can also interact with drug products. Never begin taking a new medicine—prescription or non-prescription—without asking your doctor or nurse if it will interact with alcohol, food, or other medicines. Some drug products can cause drowsiness and affect activities such as driving.

Precautions:
Acridinyl anisidide is given intravenously. If the drug accidentally leaks out of the vein where it is given, it can damage the tissue and cause scarring. Tell the nurse right away if you notice redness, pain, or swelling at the place of injection.

Acridinyl anisidide can lower your blood counts (white blood cells, red blood cells, platelets). Your doctor will check your blood counts before and after each treatment to see how it affects your blood counts. Your doctor or nurse will give you specific instructions if your blood counts are low.

Acridinyl anisidide can cause a decrease in your white blood cell count, especially 7 to 14 days after the drug is given. This can increase your chance of getting an infection. Report fever of 100.5°F or higher, or signs of infection such as pain in passing your urine, coughing, and bringing up sputum.

Acridinyl anisidide can cause a decrease in the platelet count. This can increase your risk of bleeding. DO NOT take any aspirin or aspirin-containing medicines. Report unusual bruising, or bleeding such as nosebleeds, bleeding gums when you brush your teeth, or black, tarry stools.

Acridinyl anisidide can cause nausea and vomiting. Ask your doctor or nurse to give you a medicine to prevent or lessen this side effect.

The dose of acridinyl anisidide will be decreased if your liver or kidneys are not working properly. Blood tests will be done before each treatment to check your blood counts, liver and kidney function, and potassium level. If the potassium level is low, you will receive some extra potassium.

While you are being treated with acridinyl anisidide, and after you stop treatment with it, do not have any immunizations (vaccinations) without your doctor's okay. Try to avoid contact with people who have recently taken the oral polio vaccine. Check with your doctor about this.

Tell all the doctors, dentists, and pharmacists you visit that you are taking this drug.

- Most of the following side effects probably will not occur.
- Your doctor or nurse will want to discuss specific care instructions with you.
- They can help you understand these side effects and help you deal with them.

Side Effects:

More Common Side Effects
Decreased white blood cell count with increased risk of infection
Decreased platelet count with increased risk of bleeding
Nausea
Vomiting
Irritation of vein used for giving the drug
Decrease in red blood cell counts with increased risk of tiredness

Less Common Side Effects
Sores in mouth or on lips
Damage to liver
Diarrhea
Skin rash

Rare Side Effects
Skin may turn yellow to orange
Seizures
Severe allergic reaction (anaphylaxis)
Hearing loss
Tingling sensations in hands and feet
Congestive heart failure in patients who have been treated with other anthracycline antibiotics
Cardiac arrest

Side Effects / Symptoms of the Drug
This drug may irritate your vein, so a special intravenous catheter may be placed for your treatment.

Other side effects not listed above can also occur in some patients.
Tell your doctor or nurse if you develop any problems.

FDA Approval: This drug is being studied for cancer treatment.

AG3340

Trade Name:
Prinometstat

Type of Drug:
AG3340 is a matrix metalloproteinase inhibitor used in molecular targeted therapy.

How Drug Works:
Matrix metalloproteinases (MMPs) are enzymes that provide structure between cells. In cancer, MMPs help the tumor grow, invade surrounding tissue, and develop blood vessels that help the cancer cells spread to distant tissues. Matrix metalloproteinase inhibitors (MMPIs) prevent the action of these enzymes, so that the tumor does not grow or spread to other tissues.

How Drug Is Given:
AG 3340 is given by mouth, twice a day, without regard to meals. The dose depends on your size. Since this drug is still being studied, the specific dose, how it is given, and schedule will be determined by the clinical trial. Keep the medicine in a tightly closed container, away from heat and moisture, and out of the reach of children and pets.

How Should I Take This Drug?
Take this drug exactly as directed by your doctor. If you do not understand the instructions, ask your doctor or nurse to explain them to you. This drug can be given at different strengths depending on the type of cancer being treated. Dosage may vary depending on your body weight and the type of cancer being treated.

 Read the following information. If you do not understand it or if any of it causes you special concern, check with your doctor.

Before taking this drug, tell your doctor:
- If you are trying to become pregnant, are pregnant, or breastfeeding. This drug may cause birth defects if either the male or female is taking it at the time of conception or during pregnancy. Men and women who are taking this drug need to use some kind of birth control. However, do not use oral contraceptives ("the pill") without checking with your doctor.
- If you think you may want to have children in the future. Many chemotherapy drugs can cause sterility.
- If you have any of the following medical problems: chickenpox or exposure to chickenpox, gout, heart disease, congestive heart failure, shingles, kidney stones, liver disease, or other forms of cancer.
- If you are taking any other prescription or over-the-counter drugs, including vitamins and herbals.

Should I avoid any other medicines, foods, alcohol, and/or activities?
Your prescription and nonprescription medicines may interact with other drugs, causing harm. Certain foods or alcohol can also interact with drug products. Never begin taking a new medicine—prescription or nonprescription—without asking your doctor or nurse if it will interact with alcohol, food, or other medicines. Some drug products can cause drowsiness and affect activities such as driving.

Precautions:
Taking this drug may increase the levels of some other drugs if they are given together. These drugs include codeine, rifampin, steroid medicines, and phenobarbitol. Be sure to tell your doctor about all medicines you are taking.

This can be given with chemotherapy to increase the effect on the cancer. This does not increase side effects of the chemotherapy.

AG3340 interferes with normal MMPs that help provide structure around joints and tendons. Most side effects are related to this action. Symptoms begin within the first 4 weeks of therapy, are mild, and affect the shoulders and hands first. By 8 weeks, the achiness may increase and affect other joints. The discomfort goes away within 3 to 5 weeks after the drug is stopped. Tell your doctor or nurse if the joint aches are uncomfortable.

Tell all the doctors, dentists, and pharmacists you visit that you are taking this drug.

- Most of the following side effects probably will not occur.
- Your doctor or nurse will want to discuss specific care instructions with you.
- They can help you understand these side effects and help you deal with them.

Side Effects:

More Common Side Effects
Arthralgias (joint pain) of shoulders, hands, knees, hips, ankles, elbows, neck, jaw, and back

Less Common Side Effects
Bone pain
Pain in other areas
Myalgia (muscle aches)
Dermatitis (skin inflammation)
Weakness

Rare Side Effects
Swelling of fingers
Thickening of finger joints, palms, fingertips
Nodules of the hand and wrist
Contractures of finger tendons
Changes in sense of smell and taste
Numbness and sensation of pins and needles in fingers and toes
Mild to moderate nausea and/or vomiting
Constipation
Decreased appetite
Swelling of the ankles
Calf tenderness and warmth of lower leg caused by blood clot in legs

---

Other side effects not listed above can also occur in some patients.
Tell your doctor or nurse if you develop any problems.

FDA Approval: This drug is being studied for cancer treatment.

alemtuzumab

Trade Name:
Campath-1H

Type of Drug:
Alemtuzumab is a monoclonal antibody that belongs to the general class of synthetic substances called biologic response modifiers. It is used to treat B cell chronic lymphocytic leukemia that no longer responds to fludarabine therapy. It is also being studied in some lymphomas and other diseases.

How Drug Works:
A monocloncal antibody is a protein that fits like a lock and key with a protein on the cancer cell. Alemtuzumab (antibody) attaches to the CD 52 protein (antigen) found on both normal and cancerous B and T cell lymphocytes as well as other immune cells. This attachment results in cell death. The drug cannot distinguish between normal and cancer cells, so some normal cells are affected (see Side Effects).

How Drug Is Given:
Alemtuzumab is given into a vein over 2 hours. People can have infusion reactions, so you may be given medicine to prevent a reaction. The drug is given in a lower dose on the first treatment, and gradually the dose is increased over 3 to 7 days. You will get treatments 3 times a week on alternating days. You will then receive "maintenance" treatments, again 3 times a week for up to 12 weeks. If you have a break in treatment of 7 days or more, you will need to be started with a smaller dose again, and gradually the dose will be increased. The dose depends upon your size, whether other medicines are given with it, and your blood counts.

 Read the following information. If you do not understand it or if any of it causes you special concern, check with your doctor.

Before taking this drug, tell your doctor:
- If you are trying to become pregnant, are pregnant, or breastfeeding. This drug may cause birth defects if either the male or female is taking it at the time of conception or during pregnancy. Men and women who are taking this drug need to use some kind of birth control. However, do not use oral contraceptives ("the pill") without checking with your doctor.
- If you think you may want to have children in the future. Many chemotherapy drugs can cause sterility.
- If you have any of the following medical problems: chickenpox or exposure to chickenpox, gout, heart disease, congestive heart failure, shingles, kidney stones, liver disease, or other forms of cancer.
- If you are taking any other prescription or over-the-counter drugs, including vitamins and herbals.

Should I avoid any other medicines, foods, alcohol, and/or activities?
Your prescription and nonprescription medicines may interact with other drugs, causing harm. Certain foods or alcohol can also interact with drug products. Never begin taking a new medicine—prescription or nonprescription—without asking your doctor or nurse if it will interact with alcohol, food, or other medicines. Some drug products can cause drowsiness and affect activities such as driving.

Precautions:
While you are being treated with alemtuzumab and after you stop treatment, do not have any immunizations (vaccinations) without your doctor's okay. Try to avoid contact with people who have recently taken the oral polio vaccine. Check with your doctor about this.

Allergic infusion reactions, such as fever and chills, may occur. Rarely, decreased blood pressure, swelling of the face, and coughing can occur. Tell your nurse right away if you get a fever or chills, hives, nausea, itching, headache, shortness of breath, or swollen tongue or throat during your treatment. Your nurse will stop your infusion and evaluate you.

Alemtuzumab can lower your blood counts (white blood cells, red blood cells, and platelets). Your doctor will check your blood counts before and after each treatment to see how it affects your blood counts. Your doctor or nurse will give you specific instructions if your blood counts are low.

Alemtuzumab can lower your white blood cell count, including lymphocytes, for an extended period of time. This will increase your chance of getting an infection. Your doctor will give you medicines to help protect you from bacterial and viral infections during treatment when your lymphocyte count is low. Report fever of 100.5°F or higher, or signs of infection such as pain in passing your urine, coughing, and bringing up sputum.

Alemtuzumab can cause a decrease in the platelet count, which can increase your risk of bleeding. DO NOT take any aspirin or aspirin-containing medicines. Report unusual bruising, or bleeding such as nosebleeds, bleeding of gums when brushing your teeth, or black, tarry stools.

 Tell all the doctors, dentists, and pharmacists you visit that you are taking this drug.
- • Most of the following side effects probably will not occur.
- • Your doctor or nurse will want to discuss specific care instructions with you.
- • They can help you understand these side effects and help you deal with them.

Side Effects:

More Common Side Effects
Nausea

Decreased white blood cell count with increased risk of infection	Decreased platelet count with increased risk of bleeding
Decreased red blood cell count with increased risk of fatigue (or tiredness)	Infusion reactions with fever, shaking chills, decreased blood pressure, nausea
	Rash

Less Common Side Effects

Tiredness (fatigue)	Headache
Pain	Dizziness
Loss of appetite	Vomiting
Feeling "blah"	Diarrhea
Swelling of the feet	Sores in the mouth
Chest pain	Abdominal pain
Decreased blood pressure	Heartburn
Increased blood pressure	Constipation
Rapid heartbeat	Nosebleeds
Difficulty sleeping	Muscle aches
Severe blood infection (sepsis)	Viral infections
Fungal infections	Shortness of breath
Cough	Pneumonia
Sore throat	Spasm in the breathing tube (bronchus)
Sweating	Itching
Back pain	

Rare Side Effects

Depression	Confusion
Sleepiness	Severe allergic reaction (anaphylaxis)
Damage to the bone marrow, which can be fatal, so no blood cells are made	Heart damage or arrest
	Coma
Itchy or runny nose	Hallucinations

Side Effects / Symptoms of the Drug
It is very important to take the medicine your doctor prescribes to prevent infection when your blood counts are down.

Your doctor may give you medicines to help prevent allergic reactions before you receive the treatment.

Other side effects not listed above can also occur in some patients.
Tell your doctor or nurse if you develop any problems.

FDA Approval: This drug is approved for cancer treatment.

alitretinoin gel 0.1%

Trade Name:
Panretin

Type of Drug:
Alitretinoin gel 0.1% is a retinoid used in molecular targeted therapy. A retinoid is a naturally occuring substance in the body that helps to regulate, or control, the work of genes. These retinoids work to help the cells to mature (differentiate) and divide.

How Drug Works:
Alitretinoin (in a gel form) "turns on" certain retinoid receptors on the cancer cell to control cancer cell growth and division. The gel has been found to stop the growth of Kaposi's sarcoma (KS) cells and is used to treat KS skin lesions.

How Drug Is Given:
Alitretinoin gel 0.1% is applied to skin lesions twice a day. When you tolerate it well, your doctor will tell you to apply the gel to the lesions 3 to 4 times a day. Let the gel dry for 3 to 5 minutes before covering the skin lesions with clothes. The dose depends upon the size of the lesions and how often you apply it depends upon how well you tolerate it.

How Should I Take This Drug?
Take this drug exactly as directed by your doctor. If you do not understand the instructions, ask your doctor or nurse to explain them to you.

 Read the following information. If you do not understand it or if any of it causes you special concern, check with your doctor.

Before taking this drug, tell your doctor:
• If you are trying to become pregnant, are pregnant, or breastfeeding. This drug may cause birth defects if either the male or female is taking it at the time of conception or during pregnancy. Men and women who are taking this drug need to use some kind of birth control. However, do not use oral contraceptives ("the pill") without checking with your doctor.
• If you think you may want to have children in the future. Many chemotherapy drugs can cause sterility.
• If you have any of the following medical problems: chickenpox or exposure to chickenpox, gout, heart disease, congestive heart failure, shingles, kidney stones, liver disease, or other forms of cancer.
• If you are taking any other prescription or over-the-counter drugs, including vitamins and herbals.

Should I avoid any other medicines, foods, alcohol, and/or activities?
Your prescription and nonprescription medicines may interact with other drugs, causing harm. Certain foods or alcohol can also interact with drug products. Never begin taking a new medicine—prescription or nonprescription—without asking your doctor or nurse if it will interact with alcohol, food, or other medicines. Some drug products can cause drowsiness and affect activities such as driving.

Precautions:
This drug causes increased sensitivity to the sun. Do not use sunlamps and reduce your exposure to the sun.

Store tube of gel at room temperature. Put on glove to apply gel to lesions. Be careful not to get the gel on skin around the lesion.

DO NOT apply gel to mucous membranes, such as on the inside of mouth. If skin irritation develops, your doctor or nurse may instruct you to stop using the gel for a few days until irritation goes away.

DO NOT use an occlusive dressing over gel.

DO NOT use insect repellent containing DEET with gel, as gel increases DEET toxicity.

Responses may be seen in 2 weeks but usually take longer, sometimes up to 14 weeks.

Side effects are related to skin reactions. These are usually mild to moderate and begin as redness of the skin. This may progress to swelling of the skin where the gel is applied. Rarely, some patients may have severe reactions, such as intense redness, severe swelling, or blister formation. Stop using the gel and call your doctor or nurse if this occurs.

DO NOT use when systemic therapy for Kaposi's sarcoma is needed—for example, if 10 or more KS lesions are present in prior month, or if you have lymphedema (swelling of arm or leg), or lung or organ KS involvement.

DO NOT use this gel if you are allergic to retinoids.

DO NOT use this gel if you are a nursing mother.

 Tell all the doctors, dentists, and pharmacists you visit that you are taking this drug.

- Most of the following side effects probably will not occur.
- Your doctor or nurse will want to discuss specific care instructions with you.
- They can help you understand these side effects and help you deal with them.

Side Effects:

More Common Side Effects
Redness (erythema) or swelling of the area where the gel is applied

Less Common Side Effects
Blister formation
Rash
Pain
Itching

Rare Side Effects
Peeling of the skin where the redness was
Cracking, crusting of the skin where the gel is applied
Oozing of the skin where the gel is applied
Stinging or tingling of the skin where the gel is applied

Side Effects / Symptoms of the Drug
If you develop severe skin reaction(s), stop using the gel and call your doctor or nurse right away.

Other side effects not listed above can also occur in some patients.
Tell your doctor or nurse if you develop any problems.

FDA Approval: This drug is approved for cancer treatment.

altretamine

Trade Names:
Hexalen, Hexamethylmelamine

Type of Drug:
Altretamine belongs to the general group of chemotherapy drugs known as alkylating agents. It is used to treat ovarian cancer that no longer responds to first-line drugs.

How Drug Works:
Altretamine disrupts the growth of cancer cells, which are then destroyed.

How Drug Is Given:
Altretamine is a capsule taken by mouth. The dose depends upon your size. The daily dose is split into 4 divided doses, taken after meals and at bedtime. Altretamine is taken for 14 or 21 days every 4 weeks (28 days). The dose may need to be decreased if you have problems taking the drug (stomach upset that doesn't respond to usual antinausea medicines, low white blood cell or platelet count, or neuropathy [sensations of pins and needles in hands and feet]) that seem to be worsening. Keep the medicine in a tightly closed container and out of the reach of children and pets.

 Read the following information. If you do not understand it or if any of it causes you special concern, check with your doctor.

Before taking this drug, tell your doctor:
• If you are trying to become pregnant, are pregnant, or breastfeeding. This drug may cause birth defects if either the male or female is taking it at the time of conception or during pregnancy. Men and women who are taking this drug need to use some kind of birth control. However, do not use oral contraceptives ("the pill") without checking with your doctor.
• If you think you may want to have children in the future. Many chemotherapy drugs can cause sterility.
• If you have any of the following medical problems: chickenpox or exposure to chickenpox, gout, heart disease, congestive heart failure, shingles, kidney stones, liver disease, or other forms of cancer.
• If you are taking any other prescription or over-the-counter drugs, including vitamins and herbals.

Should I avoid any other medicines, foods, alcohol, and/or activities?
Your prescription and nonprescription medicines may interact with other drugs, causing harm. Certain foods or alcohol can also interact with drug products. Never begin taking a new medicine—prescription or nonprescription—without asking your doctor or nurse if it will interact with alcohol, food, or other medicines. Some drug products can cause drowsiness and affect activities such as driving.

Precautions:
While you are being treated with altretamine and after you stop treatment with it, do not have any immunizations (vaccinations) without your doctor's okay. Try to avoid contact with people who have recently taken the oral polio vaccine. Check with your doctor about this.

Altretamine can lower your blood counts (white blood cells, red blood cells, and platelets). Your doctor will check your blood counts before and after each treatment to see how it affects your blood counts. Your doctor or nurse will give you specific instructions if your blood counts are low.

Altretamine can cause a decrease in your white blood cell count, especially 21 to 28 days after the drug is given. This can increase your chance of getting an infection. Report fever of 100.5°F or higher, or signs of infection such as pain in passing your urine, coughing, and bringing up sputum.

Altretamine can cause a decrease in your platelet count. This can increase your risk of bleeding. DO NOT take any aspirin or aspirin-containing medicines. Report unusual bruising, or bleeding such as nosebleeds, bleeding gums when you brush your teeth, or black, tarry stools.

Altretamine can cause nausea, diarrhea, and abdominal cramping. Your doctor or nurse will give you medicines to prevent these side effects. If you do get them, talk to your doctor or nurse right away about ways to prevent or lessen them.

Tell all the doctors, dentists, and pharmacists you visit that you are taking this drug.

- Most of the following side effects probably will not occur.
- Your doctor or nurse will want to discuss specific care instructions with you.
- They can help you understand these side effects and help you deal with them.

Side Effects:

More Common Side Effects
Decreased white blood cell count with increased risk of infection
Decreased platelet count with increased risk of bleeding
Nausea
Vomiting
Decreased production of sperm
Fetal abnormalities if pregnant

Less Common Side Effects
Sleepiness
Mood changes
Tiredness
Decreased appetite
Abdominal cramps
Diarrhea
Changes in kidney function

Rare Side Effects
Sensation of pins and needles in hands and/or feet due to affect of drug on the nerves
Difficulty walking
Skin rash, itching

Other side effects not listed above can also occur in some patients.
Tell your doctor or nurse if you develop any problems.

FDA Approval: This drug is approved for cancer treatment.

amifostine

Trade Name:
Ethyol

Type of Drug:
Amifostine belongs to the general group of drugs known as cytoprotective agents. It is used to prevent side effects, such as kidney damage, from platinum compounds. It is also used to protect the mouth, skin, bladder, and pelvic structures against radiation reactions.

How Drug Works:
Amifostine neutralizes the platinum in normal, noncancerous tissues so that DNA and RNA are not damaged. It protects the kidneys from damage by platinum chemotherapy. It also appears to protect the nervous system; it may protect the bone marrow; and it offers some protection from radiation therapy.

How Drug Is Given:
The day before treatment you will be asked to stop any blood pressure medicines you are taking. You will get an antinausea medicine, and amifostine will be given as a 15-minute injection into your vein about 30 minutes before your chemotherapy or radiation treatment. If you get low blood pressure during the treatment, you will be asked to lie flat on your back and get fluids through the vein to bring the pressure back up. This drug can be given at different strengths depending on the type of cancer being treated. Dosage may vary depending on your weight and your type of cancer.

 Read the following information. If you do not understand it or if any of it causes you special concern, check with your doctor.

Before taking this drug, tell your doctor:
• If you are trying to become pregnant, are pregnant, or breastfeeding. This drug may cause birth defects if either the male or female is taking it at the time of conception or during pregnancy. Men and women who are taking this drug need to use some kind of birth control. However, do not use oral contraceptives ("the pill") without checking with your doctor.
• If you think you may want to have children in the future. Many chemotherapy drugs can cause sterility.
• If you have any of the following medical problems: chickenpox or exposure to chickenpox, gout, heart disease, congestive heart failure, shingles, kidney stones, liver disease, or other forms of cancer.
• If you are taking any other prescription or over-the-counter drugs, including vitamins and herbals.

Should I avoid any other medicines, foods, alcohol, and/or activities?
Your prescription and nonprescription medicines may interact with other drugs, causing harm. Certain foods or alcohol can also interact with drug products. Never begin taking a new medicine—prescription or non-prescription—without asking your doctor or nurse if it will interact with alcohol, food, or other medicines. Some drug products can cause drowsiness and affect activities such as driving.

Precautions:
Amifostine can cause severe nausea and vomiting. Ask your doctor or nurse to give you medicines to prevent this or lessen it.

Amifostine can cause a decrease in blood pressure during treatment. Tell your doctor if you are taking any medicine for high blood pressure. Your blood pressure medicine will be stopped before you start amifostine. During the treatment, your blood pressure will be checked frequently. The drug will be stopped if your blood pressure falls.

Tell all the doctors, dentists, and pharmacists you visit that you are taking this drug.

- Most of the following side effects probably will not occur.
- Your doctor or nurse will want to discuss specific care instructions with you.
- They can help you understand these side effects and help you deal with them.

Side Effects:

More Common Side Effects

Nausea
Vomiting
Low blood pressure

Less Common Side Effects

Facial flushing
Chills
Sneezing
Hiccups
Sleepiness

Rare Side Effects

Decreased calcium in the blood

Other side effects not listed above can also occur in some patients.
Tell your doctor or nurse if you develop any problems.

FDA Approval: This drug is approved for cancer treatment.

aminoglutethimide

Trade Names:
Cytadren, Elipten

Type of Drug:
Aminoglutethimide belongs to a class of hormone and hormone-blocking drugs called adrenal steroid inhibitors. It is used to treat some cancers, including breast cancer.

How Drug Works:
Aminoglutethimide prevents the body's adrenal glands from making steroid hormones, including estrogen.

How Drug Is Given:
Aminoglutethamide is a pill taken by mouth. The starting dose is small and gradually increased. Take the daily dose in 2 to 3 divided doses, with meals. Your doctor will also give you a prescription for a steroid hormone like hydrocortisone that you must take with the aminoglutethimide. Keep the medicine in a tightly closed container and out of the reach of children and pets.

How Should I Take This Drug?
Take this drug exactly as directed by your doctor. If you do not understand the instructions, ask your doctor or nurse to explain them to you. This drug can be given at different strengths depending on the type of cancer being treated. Dosage may vary depending on your weight and your type of cancer.

 Read the following information. If you do not understand it or if any of it causes you special concern, check with your doctor.

Before taking this drug, tell your doctor:
- If you are trying to become pregnant, are pregnant, or breastfeeding. This drug may cause birth defects if either the male or female is taking it at the time of conception or during pregnancy. Men and women who are taking this drug need to use some kind of birth control. However, do not use oral contraceptives ("the pill") without checking with your doctor.
- If you think you may want to have children in the future. Many chemotherapy drugs can cause sterility.
- If you have any of the following medical problems: chickenpox or exposure to chickenpox, gout, heart disease, congestive heart failure, shingles, kidney stones, liver disease, or other forms of cancer.
- If you are taking any other prescription or over-the-counter drugs, including vitamins and herbals.

Should I avoid any other medicines, foods, alcohol, and/or activities?
Your prescription and nonprescription medicines may interact with other drugs, causing harm. Certain foods or alcohol can also interact with drug products. Never begin taking a new medicine—prescription or nonprescription—without asking your doctor or nurse if it will interact with alcohol, food, or other medicines. Some drug products can cause drowsiness and affect activities such as driving.

Precautions:
Aminoglutethimide must be taken together with hydrocortisone. Without this additional medicine, you might have nausea, loss of appetite, tiredness, dizziness, weakness, difficulty breathing, and pain in the joints (due to too little corticosteroids in the body).

A skin rash may develop, but it usually goes away within 1 to 2 weeks. Notify your doctor if the rash does not go away by the second week.

Do not take this drug if you are pregnant.

Tell all the doctors, dentists, and pharmacists you visit that you are taking this drug.

- Most of the following side effects probably will not occur.
- Your doctor or nurse will want to discuss specific care instructions with you.
- They can help you understand these side effects and help you deal with them.

Side Effects:

More Common Side Effects
Skin rash, together with malaise, low grade fever

Less Common Side Effects
Drowsiness
Lack of energy
Sleepiness
Blurred vision
Dizziness when standing or turning around
Mild nausea
Mild vomiting
Mild loss of appetite

Rare Side Effects
Rhythmic eye movements
Uncoordinated gait when walking
Lowered blood pressure

Other side effects not listed above can also occur in some patients.
Tell your doctor or nurse if you develop any problems.

FDA Approval: This drug is approved for cancer treatment.

anastrozole

Trade Name:
Arimidex

Type of Drug:
Anastrozole belongs to a general group of drugs called hormones or hormone antagonists. It is used as a treatment for postmenopausal women with locally advanced or metastatic breast cancer.

How Drug Works:
Anastrozole selectively prevents the body's adrenal glands from making estrogen. Other steroid hormones made by the adrenal glands are not affected.

How Drug Is Given:
Anastrozole is a pill taken once a day, about the same time each day. The dose is the same for all adults. Keep the medicine in a tightly closed container and out of the reach of children and pets.

How Should I Take This Drug?
Take this drug exactly as directed by your doctor. If you do not understand these instructions, ask your doctor or nurse to explain them to you. This drug can be given at different strengths depending on the type of cancer being treated. Dosage may vary depending on your weight and your type of cancer.

 Read the following information. If you do not understand it or if any of it causes you special concern, check with your doctor.

Before taking this drug, tell your doctor:
- If you are trying to become pregnant, are pregnant, or breastfeeding. This drug may cause birth defects if either the male or female is taking it at the time of conception or during pregnancy. Men and women who are taking this drug need to use some kind of birth control. However, do not use oral contraceptives ("the pill") without checking with your doctor.
- If you think you may want to have children in the future. Many chemotherapy drugs can cause sterility.
- If you have any of the following medical problems: chickenpox or exposure to chickenpox, gout, heart disease, congestive heart failure, shingles, kidney stones, liver disease, or other forms of cancer.
- If you are taking any other prescription or over-the-counter drugs, including vitamins and herbals.

Should I avoid any other medicines, foods, alcohol, and/or activities?
Your prescription and nonprescription medicines may interact with other drugs, causing harm. Certain foods or alcohol can also interact with drug products. Never begin taking a new medicine—prescription or nonprescription—without asking your doctor or nurse if it will interact with alcohol, food, or other medicines. Some drug products can cause drowsiness and affect activities such as driving.

Precautions:
Very rarely, this drug may cause blood clots to form. Call your doctor or nurse right away if you develop pain in your lower leg (calf), redness or swelling of your arm or leg, shortness of breath, or chest pain.

Tell all the doctors, dentists, and pharmacists you visit that you are taking this drug.

- Most of the following side effects probably will not occur.
- Your doctor or nurse will want to discuss specific care instructions with you.
- They can help you understand these side effects and help you deal with them.

Side Effects:

More Common Side Effects
Weakness
Decreased energy level

Less Common Side Effects
Headache
Nausea
Mild diarrhea
Increased or decreased appetite
Sweating
Hot flushes
Vaginal dryness

Rare Side Effects
Blood clots with redness or mild swelling of arms, legs and ankles, pain in leg calves, shortness of breath, difficulty breathing

Other side effects not listed above can also occur in some patients.
Tell your doctor or nurse if you develop any problems.

FDA Approval: This drug is approved for cancer treatment.

androgens

Trade Names:
Testex, Halotestin, Teslac

Type of Drug:
Androgens belong to the general group of drugs known as hormones or hormone antagonists. They are used to treat several types of cancer that are sensitive to hormones, including breast cancer.

How Drug Works:
Androgens appear to change the hormonal environment in the cancer cell. This takes away the stimulus to grow, and the cancer cell does not divide. The exact mechanism is unknown.

How Drug Is Given:
Androgens can be given as a pill every day by mouth or by an injection in the muscle weekly. Your doctor will decide the type of androgen, dose, and frequency. Keep the medicine in a tightly closed container and out of the reach of children and pets.

How Should I Take This Drug?
Take this drug exactly as directed by your doctor. If you do not understand the instructions, ask your doctor or nurse to explain them to you.

 Read the following information. If you do not understand it or if any of it causes you special concern, check with your doctor.

Before taking this drug, tell your doctor:
- If you are trying to become pregnant, are pregnant, or breastfeeding. This drug may cause birth defects if either the male or female is taking it at the time of conception or during pregnancy. Men and women who are taking this drug need to use some kind of birth control. However, do not use oral contraceptives ("the pill") without checking with your doctor.
- If you think you may want to have children in the future. Many chemotherapy drugs can cause sterility.
- If you have any of the following medical problems: chickenpox or exposure to chickenpox, gout, heart disease, congestive heart failure, shingles, kidney stones, liver disease, or other forms of cancer.
- If you are taking any other prescription or over-the-counter drugs, including vitamins and herbals.

Should I avoid any other medicines, foods, alcohol, and/or activities?
Your prescription and nonprescription medicines may interact with other drugs, causing harm. Certain foods or alcohol can also interact with drug products. Never begin taking a new medicine—prescription or nonprescription—without asking your doctor or nurse if it will interact with alcohol, food, or other medicines. Some drug products can cause drowsiness and affect activities such as driving.

Precautions:
Androgens may cause you to retain salt and water. Your doctor may prescribe a diuretic ("water pill"). Tell your doctor or nurse if you gain weight or your feet or ankles swell.

Increased blood calcium may occur when you start the drug if you have cancer in the bones. Your doctor will monitor your blood calcium levels.

Tell your doctor or nurse if you start becoming drowsy, are more thirsty, constipated, and have to urinate frequently.

Women receiving androgens will notice their voice deepening after a period of time. If you take the drug for more than 3 months, you may have less interest in sex, more body hair, and acne. Talk to your doctor or nurse about this.

Tell your doctor if you are taking blood-thinning medicines (anticoagulants such as Coumadin). Talk to your doctor about possible drug interactions.

Tell all the doctors, dentists, and pharmacists you visit that you are taking this drug.

- Most of the following side effects probably will not occur.
- Your doctor or nurse will want to discuss specific care instructions with you.
- They can help you understand these side effects and help you deal with them.

Side Effects:

More Common Side Effects
Fluid retention
Deepening of voice in women
Increased body hair and acne in women

Less Common Side Effects
Increased blood calcium level
Nausea

Rare Side Effects
Painful erections in men

Other side effects not listed above can also occur in some patients.
Tell your doctor or nurse if you develop any problems.

FDA Approval: This drug is approved for cancer treatment.

arsenic trioxide

Trade Name:
Trisenox

Type of Drug:
Arsenic trioxide is a chemotherapy drug.

How Drug Works:
The action of arsenic trioxide is not completely understood. Arsenic trioxide appears to cause changes in cancer cells that make them die. It also appears to correct the gene responsible for making a flawed protein (called the PML-RAR fusion protein) that causes acute promyelocytic leukemia. It is used to treat acute promyelocytic leukemia that no longer responds to first-line chemotherapy and ATRA (All-Trans-Retinoic Acid).

How Drug Is Given:
Arsenic trioxide is given by injection into a vein. The first set of treatments (induction) are given daily until the leukemic cells in the bone marrow disappear, up to 60 treatments. Then 3 to 6 weeks after induction, consolidation treatment is given 5 days a week for up to 5 weeks. The dose depends on your size.

 Read the following information. If you do not understand it or if any of it causes you special concern, check with your doctor.

Before taking this drug, tell your doctor:
- If you are trying to become pregnant, are pregnant, or breastfeeding. This drug may cause birth defects if either the male or female is taking it at the time of conception or during pregnancy. Men and women who are taking this drug need to use some kind of birth control. However, do not use oral contraceptives ("the pill") without checking with your doctor.
- If you think you may want to have children in the future. Many chemotherapy drugs can cause sterility.
- If you have any of the following medical problems: chickenpox or exposure to chickenpox, gout, heart disease, congestive heart failure, shingles, kidney stones, liver disease, or other forms of cancer.
- If you are taking any other prescription or over-the-counter drugs, including vitamins and herbals.

Should I avoid any other medicines, foods, alcohol, and/or activities?
Your prescription and nonprescription medicines may interact with other drugs, causing harm. Certain foods or alcohol can also interact with drug products. Never begin taking a new medicine—prescription or non-prescription—without asking your doctor or nurse if it will interact with alcohol, food, or other medicines. Some drug products can cause drowsiness and affect activities such as driving.

Precautions:
Arsenic trioxide can increase the time it takes for the heartbeat impulse to pass through the heart. You will have a baseline electrocardiogram (EKG), and this may be repeated during the treatment. In addition, you will have blood tests to make sure that the blood electrolyte values and the kidney function tests are normal. If they are abnormal, or if the EKG shows changes, your treatment will be stopped and the abnormalities corrected.

Tell your doctor if you are taking any medicines for an irregular heartbeat or fluid pills.

If you have acute promyelocytic leukemia (APL), the drug may cause APL differentiation syndrome, with fever, difficulty breathing, weight gain, fluid in or around the lung, and death. You will be watched very closely and need to report any of these symptoms right away so that treatment of the syndrome can begin.

Tell all the doctors, dentists, and pharmacists you visit that you are taking this drug.
- -
- Most of the following side effects probably will not occur.
- Your doctor or nurse will want to discuss specific care instructions with you.
- They can help you understand these side effects and help you deal with them.

Side Effects:

More Common Side Effects

Nausea

Vomiting

Diarrhea

Fever, shaking chills (rigors), hives, difficulty breathing

Constipation

Poor appetite

Tiredness (fatigue)

High sugar level in the blood

High white blood cell count

Skin redness

Weight gain

Itching

Headaches

Dizziness

Low blood levels of potassium

Low blood levels of magnesium

Difficulty sleeping

Cough

Skin inflammation

Less Common Side Effects

Heartburn

EKG changes, which can lead to slowing down of the heart

Dry mouth

Low red blood cell count with increased risk of anemia and tiredness (fatigue)

Low platelet count with increased risk of bleeding

Low white blood cell count with increased risk of infection

Chest pain

Pain, redness, and swelling at injection site

Aching of muscles and bones

High blood levels of potassium

Low blood level of calcium

Low blood sugar

Increased blood levels of liver function tests

Numbness or tingling of hands or feet

Tremor

Too little oxygen in the blood

Fluid around the lungs or heart

Wheezing

Breathing problems

Rare Side Effects

Fatal irregular heartbeats

Abdominal distention or tenderness

Seizures

Coma

Darkening of skin

Side Effects / Symptoms of the Drug

Call your doctor or nurse right away if you develop a rash, fever, chills, or difficulty breathing.

Report any bruising or bleeding, seizures, or chest pain immediately.

Other side effects not listed above can also occur in some patients.
Tell your doctor or nurse if you develop any problems.

FDA Approval: This drug is approved for cancer treatment.

asparaginase

Trade Name:
Elspar

Type of Drug:
Asparaginase is an enzyme chemotherapy drug. It is used to treat acute leukemia.

How Drug Works:
Asparaginase interferes with the growth of cancer cells, especially leukemia cells. Normal cells are unharmed.

How Drug Is Given:
Asparaginase is given by infusion into a vein over at least 30 minutes, or by injection into the muscle. The dose and frequency of asparaginase treatment depends on your size, liver function tests, and treatment plan.

 Read the following information. If you do not understand it or if any of it causes you special concern, check with your doctor.

Before taking this drug, tell your doctor:
- If you are trying to become pregnant, are pregnant, or breastfeeding. This drug may cause birth defects if either the male or female is taking it at the time of conception or during pregnancy. Men and women who are taking this drug need to use some kind of birth control. However, do not use oral contraceptives ("the pill") without checking with your doctor.
- If you think you may want to have children in the future. Many chemotherapy drugs can cause sterility.
- If you have any of the following medical problems: chickenpox or exposure to chickenpox, gout, heart disease, congestive heart failure, shingles, kidney stones, liver disease, or other forms of cancer.
- If you are taking any other prescription or over-the-counter drugs, including vitamins and herbals.

Should I avoid any other medicines, foods, alcohol, and/or activities?
Your prescription and nonprescription medicines may interact with other drugs, causing harm. Certain foods or alcohol can also interact with drug products. Never begin taking a new medicine—prescription or non-prescription—without asking your doctor or nurse if it will interact with alcohol, food, or other medicines. Some drug products can cause drowsiness and affect activities such as driving.

Precautions:
Do not take aspirin or any over-the-counter medicine without talking to your doctor first.

Asparaginase can cause a severe allergic reaction. Your doctor and nurse will be prepared to give you special medicine(s) if you have an allergic reaction when you receive the drug. You will probably receive a test dose before your first dose of the drug.

Tell your nurse or doctor if you feel short of breath, pain in your back, lightheaded or dizzy, or any sensation that is different.

Tell all the doctors, dentists, and pharmacists you visit that you are taking this drug.

- Most of the following side effects probably will not occur.
- Your doctor or nurse will want to discuss specific care instructions with you.
- They can help you understand these side effects and help you deal with them.

Side Effects:

More Common Side Effects
Mild nausea
Mild vomiting
Loss of appetite
Tiredness (fatigue)
Drowsiness
Depression
Increased liver function blood levels
Allergic reaction ranging from mild (most) to severe and life-threatening

Less Common Side Effects
Increased blood sugar level
Mild anemia

Rare Side Effects
Inflammation of the pancreas
Decreased white blood cell count with increased risk of infection
Decreased platelet count with increased risk of bleeding

Side Effects / Symptoms of the Drug
Tell your doctor or nurse right away if you have increased thirst, increased hunger, or increased urination (related to increased blood sugar).

Tell your doctor or nurse right away if you have any unusual bruising or bleeding.

Tell your doctor or nurse right away if you have a fever (higher than 100.5°F).

Other side effects not listed above can also occur in some patients.
Tell your doctor or nurse if you develop any problems.

FDA Approval: This drug is approved for cancer treatment.

bevacizumab

Trade Name:
Avastin

Type of Drug:
Bevacizumab is an antiangiogenesis drug, used in molecular targeted therapy to stop tumors from making new blood vessels.

How Drug Works:
Bevacizumab is a monoclonal antibody that fits like a lock and key into a receptor on the cell surface. It stops vascular endothelial growth factor (VEGF) from starting the growth of new blood vessels. Without new blood vessels, the tumor cannot grow. Bevacizumab is being studied for the treatment of many different cancers.

How Drug Is Given:
Bevacizumab is given by a shot in the vein. The dose, how long the infusion is, and how many treatments you get depends on the clinical trial treatment plan. Often the dose depends upon your size. Other drugs may be given first to help you tolerate the drug better.

 Read the following information. If you do not understand it or if any of it causes you special concern, check with your doctor.

Before taking this drug, tell your doctor:
- If you are trying to become pregnant, are pregnant, or breastfeeding. This drug may cause birth defects if either the male or female is taking it at the time of conception or during pregnancy. Men and women who are taking this drug need to use some kind of birth control. However, do not use oral contraceptives ("the pill") without checking with your doctor.
- If you think you may want to have children in the future. Many chemotherapy drugs can cause sterility.
- If you have any of the following medical problems: chickenpox or exposure to chickenpox, gout, heart disease, congestive heart failure, shingles, kidney stones, liver disease, or other forms of cancer.
- If you are taking any other prescription or over-the-counter drugs, including vitamins and herbals.

Should I avoid any other medicines, foods, alcohol, and/or activities?
Your prescription and nonprescription medicines may interact with other drugs, causing harm. Certain foods or alcohol can also interact with drug products. Never begin taking a new medicine—prescription or non-prescription—without asking your doctor or nurse if it will interact with alcohol, food, or other medicines. Some drug products can cause drowsiness and affect activities such as driving.

Precautions:
While you are being treated with bevacizumab and after you stop treatment, do not have any immunizations (vaccinations) without your doctor's okay. Try to avoid contact with people who have recently taken the oral polio vaccine. Check with your doctor about this.

Allergic reactions such as fever and chills may occur. Rarely, decreased blood pressure, swelling of the face, and coughing can occur. Tell your nurse right away if you get a fever or chills, hives, nausea, itching, headache, shortness of breath, or a swollen tongue or throat during treatment. Your nurse will stop your infusion and evaluate you.

Blood clots and bleeding have occured in clinical trials of this drug.

You should report shortness of breath, chest pain, severe headache, change in your mental status, loss of coordination, new weakness or numbness, or bleeding from any site.

Rarely, the drug can cause uncontrolled hypertension. If you are taking a drug for hypertension, talk to your doctor about this.

The drug may cause bleeding at tumor sites. If you have been told the cancer has spread to your brain, talk to your doctor about the risk of bleeding.

This drug is investigational, so new side effects may become known during the clinical studies.

Tell all the doctors, dentists, and pharmacists you visit that you are taking this drug.

- Most of the following side effects probably will not occur.
- Your doctor or nurse will want to discuss specific care instructions with you.
- They can help you understand these side effects and help you deal with them.

Side Effects:

More Common Side Effects
Allergic reactions
Infusion reaction with fever, shaking, or chills
Mouth sores
Constipation
Nausea
Vomiting
Headache
Feeling tired
Muscle aches

Less Common Side Effects
Nosebleed
Coughing up blood
Vomiting blood
Bleeding at tumor sites
Decreased platelet count
Sore throat
Intestinal blockage
Inflammation of intestines
Pain
Coughing
Shortness of breath
Decreased white blood cell count

Rare Side Effects
Rash with peeling of the skin
Uncontrolled high blood pressure
Blot clots in the lung
Bleeding in the brain or central nervous system
Decreased kidney function
Protein in the urine

Side Effects / Symptoms of the Drug
Call your doctor or nurse right away if you develop shortness of breath, chest pain, severe headache, change in your mental status, loss of coordination, new weakness or numbness, or bleeding from any site.

Other side effects not listed above can also occur in some patients.
Tell your doctor or nurse if you develop any problems.

FDA Approval: This drug is being studied for cancer treatment.

bexarotene

Trade Name:
Targretin

Type of Drug:
Bexarotene is a retinoid used in molecular targeted therapy. A retinoid is a naturally occuring substance in the body that helps to regulate, or control, the work of genes to help cells grow and divide.

How Drug Works:
Bexarotene "turns on" certain retinoid receptors on the cancer cell. The "turned on" receptor works with other substances to control cancer cell growth and division. Bexarotene capsules are used to treat skin lesions due to cutaneous T-cell lymphoma that has not responded to prior systemic treatment. The 1% topical gel is used for treatment of early stage skin lesions that no longer respond to other therapies in patients with cutaneous T-cell lymphoma.

How Drug Is Given:
Bexarotene is taken as a capsule by mouth with a meal. The dose depends on your size. To start, you will take a capsule daily until a response is seen, for up to 97 weeks. Sometimes the bexarotene dose needs to be lowered if you have a lot of side effects. If the side effects go away on a lowered dose, then your doctor may try to slowly increase the dose again. Keep the medicine in a tightly closed container and out of the reach of children and pets. Also, keep the container out of heat, light, and humidity. Bexarotene can also be given as a gel on skin lesions. The dose is just enough to cover the lesion.

How Should I Take This Drug?
Take this drug exactly as directed by your doctor. If you do not understand the instructions, ask your doctor or nurse to explain them to you.

 Read the following information. If you do not understand it or if any of it causes you special concern, check with your doctor.

Before taking this drug, tell your doctor:
- If you are trying to become pregnant, are pregnant, or breastfeeding. This drug may cause birth defects if either the male or female is taking it at the time of conception or during pregnancy. Men and women who are taking this drug need to use some kind of birth control. However, do not use oral contraceptives ("the pill") without checking with your doctor.
- If you think you may want to have children in the future. Many chemotherapy drugs can cause sterility.
- If you have any of the following medical problems: chickenpox or exposure to chickenpox, gout, heart disease, congestive heart failure, shingles, kidney stones, liver disease, or other forms of cancer.
- If you are taking any other prescription or over-the-counter drugs, including vitamins and herbals.

Should I avoid any other medicines, foods, alcohol, and/or activities?
Your prescription and nonprescription medicines may interact with other drugs, causing harm. Certain foods or alcohol can also interact with drug products. Never begin taking a new medicine—prescription or nonprescription—without asking your doctor or nurse if it will interact with alcohol, food, or other medicines. Some drug products can cause drowsiness and affect activities such as driving.

Precautions:
You must AVOID direct sunlight and artificial ultraviolet (UV) light while you are taking bexarotene. UV light exposure can cause a severe sunburn.

The drug may interact with other medicines. Make sure you tell your doctor about all other medicines you are taking.

DO NOT take gemfibrozil with bexarotene as it can increase blood levels of bexarotene. Also, avoid eating grapefruit when taking the capsules.

Bexarotene may change some of your blood test results: increased triglycerides and total cholesterol, decreased HDL, increased blood levels of liver function, decreased blood levels of thyroid function, increased LDH, and decreased white blood cells. All these levels will be checked before you start bexarotene capsules.

Women of childbearing age taking the capsules should use effective contraception. Bexarotene affects the unborn fetus, and pregnancy must be avoided. Pregnancy tests should be negative before starting therapy. Nursing mothers should not use bexarotene.

Bexarotene capsules should be used cautiously if at all in patients who have had allergic reactions to other retinoids and patients with liver problems. If you have pancreatitis (inflammation of the pancreas), or uncontrolled blood lipids or cholesterol in the blood, uncontrolled diabetes, or are taking drugs that may cause pancreatitis or increased blood lipids, you should not take this medicine. Talk with your doctor if you have any questions.

Bexarotene causes increased lipid blood levels in most patients, and this blood level needs to be monitored closely during therapy.

Bexarotene capsules may cause cataracts. Make sure that you tell your doctor right away if your vision changes during therapy.

If you are taking a vitamin A supplement, DO NOT take more than 15,000 IU/day as this will increase bexarotene (capsule) side effects.

 Tell all the doctors, dentists, and pharmacists you visit that you are taking this drug.
- Most of the following side effects probably will not occur.
- Your doctor or nurse will want to discuss specific care instructions with you.
- They can help you understand these side effects and help you deal with them.

Side Effects:

More Common Side Effects
Increased blood lipid levels (fasting triglycerides, cholesterol)
Decreased blood HDL level
Low thyroid function
Diarrhea

Headache
Itching (gel)
Rash (gel)
Pain at application site (gel)

Less Common Side Effects
Weakness or listlessness
Decreased white blood cells with increased risk of infection
Abdominal pain
Fever and chills
Difficulty sleeping

Flu-like symptoms
Back pain
Rash
Peeling of skin
Hair loss
Swelling of the ankles

Rare Side Effects
Increased blood level of liver function tests
Pancreatitis

Nausea
Vomiting
Loss of appetite

Side Effects / Symptoms of the Drug
You may have to take medicine to decrease your blood lipid levels. Your doctor will monitor your blood values closely. Changes in blood lipid level and thyroid function will go back to normal after the treatment is finished.

Report signs/symptoms of hypothyroidism (weight gain, tiredness, slowed thinking, skin dryness, constipation, or joint pain/stiffness).

Report fever, persistent cough, burning on urination, or other signs/symptoms of infection.

Report rash, severe pain at application site (gel), or peeling of skin right away.

Report nausea, vomiting, or appetite loss.

Other side effects not listed above can also occur in some patients.
Tell your doctor or nurse if you develop any problems.

FDA Approval: This drug is approved for cancer treatment.

bicalutamide

Trade Name:
Casodex

Type of Drug:
Bicalutamide belongs to the general group of drugs known as hormones or hormone antagonists. It is a non-steroidal antiandrogen and is used to treat advanced prostate cancer.

How Drug Works:
Bicalutamide stops the growth of cancer cells that depend on male hormones.

How Drug Is Given:
The bicalutamide tablet should be taken by mouth with a glass of water with or without food. It should be taken about the same time each day. The dose is the same for everyone. Bicalutamide treatment is usually started at the same time as another drug in injection form called a LHRH analogue. This also blocks the action of the hormone testosterone. Keep the pills in a tightly closed container and out of the reach of children and pets.

 Read the following information. If you do not understand it or if any of it causes you special concern, check with your doctor.

Before taking this drug, tell your doctor:
- If you are trying to become pregnant, are pregnant, or breastfeeding. This drug may cause birth defects if either the male or female is taking it at the time of conception or during pregnancy. Men and women who are taking this drug need to use some kind of birth control. However, do not use oral contraceptives ("the pill") without checking with your doctor.
- If you think you may want to have children in the future. Many chemotherapy drugs can cause sterility.
- If you have any of the following medical problems: chickenpox or exposure to chickenpox, gout, heart disease, congestive heart failure, shingles, kidney stones, liver disease, or other forms of cancer.
- If you are taking any other prescription or over-the-counter drugs, including vitamins and herbals.

Should I avoid any other medicines, foods, alcohol, and/or activities?
Your prescription and nonprescription medicines may interact with other drugs, causing harm. Certain foods or alcohol can also interact with drug products. Never begin taking a new medicine—prescription or non-prescription—without asking your doctor or nurse if it will interact with alcohol, food, or other medicines. Some drug products can cause drowsiness and affect activities such as driving.

Precautions:
Bicalutamide is usually given along with another medicine to block testosterone.

Tell all the doctors, dentists, and pharmacists you visit that you are taking this drug.

- Most of the following side effects probably will not occur.
- Your doctor or nurse will want to discuss specific care instructions with you.
- They can help you understand these side effects and help you deal with them.

Side Effects:

More Common Side Effects
Swelling of the breasts
Tenderness of the breasts

Less Common Side Effects
Hot flashes
Constipation

Rare Side Effects
Nausea
Diarrhea
Headache

Other side effects not listed above can also occur in some patients.
Tell your doctor or nurse if you develop any problems.

FDA Approval: This drug is approved for cancer treatment.

bleomycin

Trade Name:
Blenoxane

Type of Drug:
Bleomycin belongs to the general group of chemotherapy drugs known as antibiotics. It is used to treat several types of cancer including testicular cancer and lymphoma.

How Drug Works:
Bleomycin inteferes with cell division, which results in the cell being destroyed.

How Drug Is Given:
Bleomycin is given by a shot into a vein, either over 10 minutes or as a continuous infusion for 24 hours. It can also be given as a shot into the muscle or under the skin. The dose is based on your size. The drug will be given after you have a special breathing test, and the test may be repeated a few times during treatment.

 Read the following information. If you do not understand it or if any of it causes you special concern, check with your doctor.

Before taking this drug, tell your doctor:
- If you are trying to become pregnant, are pregnant, or breastfeeding. This drug may cause birth defects if either the male or female is taking it at the time of conception or during pregnancy. Men and women who are taking this drug need to use some kind of birth control. However, do not use oral contraceptives ("the pill") without checking with your doctor.
- If you think you may want to have children in the future. Many chemotherapy drugs can cause sterility.
- If you have any of the following medical problems: chickenpox or exposure to chickenpox, gout, heart disease, congestive heart failure, shingles, kidney stones, liver disease, or other forms of cancer.
- If you are taking any other prescription or over-the-counter drugs, including vitamins and herbals.

Should I avoid any other medicines, foods, alcohol, and/or activities?
Your prescription and nonprescription medicines may interact with other drugs, causing harm. Certain foods or alcohol can also interact with drug products. Never begin taking a new medicine—prescription or non-prescription—without asking your doctor or nurse if it will interact with alcohol, food, or other medicines. Some drug products can cause drowsiness and affect activities such as driving.

Precautions:
After receiving this drug, it is important not to receive pure oxygen—for example, during surgery.

There is a very small chance that patients with lymphoma will have an allergic reaction when receiving bleomycin. Your doctor may give you a test dose of the medicine before you receive the full dose.

Most patients will have a fever the night after getting the drug. This is caused by the drug, and you will probably get medicine before your next dose to prevent the fever.

Bleomycin can cause lung toxicity. You probably will have a lung test (pulmonary function test) before you get the drug, and this may be repeated several times during treatment. After you have begun receiving the drug, tell your doctor or nurse right away if you notice shortness of breath or difficulty breathing, especially in the cold.

Tell all the doctors, dentists, and pharmacists you visit that you are taking this drug.

- Most of the following side effects probably will not occur.
- Your doctor or nurse will want to discuss specific care instructions with you.
- They can help you understand these side effects and help you deal with them.

Side Effects:

More Common Side Effects
Fever and chills
Nausea
Loss of appetite
Hair loss
Sores in mouth or on lips
Skin changes, such as darkened, thickened areas of skin or nails, rash, or dry skin peeling at the fingertips

Less Common Side Effects
Pain at tumor site
Pain at place of injection
Irritation of vein used for giving the drug
Irritation of lungs

Rare Side Effects
Scarring of lung tissue

Anaphylactic reaction with decreased blood pressure, confusion, rapid heart rate, wheezing, and facial swelling

Other side effects not listed above can also occur in some patients.
Tell your doctor or nurse if you develop any problems.

FDA Approval: This drug is approved for cancer treatment.

buserelin acetate

Trade Names:
Suprefact, Suprefact Depot, Suprefact Nasal Spray

Type of Drug:
Buserelin acetate belongs to the general group of drugs known as hormones or hormone antagonists. It is used to treat advanced prostate and breast cancers.

How Drug Works:
Buserelin acetate is a synthetic version of the body's luteinizing hormone-releasing hormone (LHRH), which regulates the amount of testosterone in men and estrogen in women. Buserelin tells the body to stop making testosterone or estrogen, so the blood levels drop. Cancers that are stimulated by testosterone or estrogen stop dividing.

How Drug Is Given:
Buserelin acetate is given by a shot under the skin (subcutaneous) 3 times a day for the first week of treatment. Then the drug may be given in one of 3 ways: by a nasal spray 3 times, by shot under the skin once a day, or by a shot under the skin once a month. Adults receive the standard dose. If you take buserelin acetate by shot, you or a family member will be taught how to give it. Make sure you understand the directions, and ask your doctor or nurse to review this with you.

It is important to keep the unused syringes in a safe place out of reach of children and pets. After giving the shot, drop the used syringe in a plastic container or glass jar with a cover before discarding it. Make sure you keep taking the drug as directed even when you start feeling better. Talk with your doctor before you stop taking the drug.

How Should I Take This Drug?
Take this drug exactly as directed by your doctor. If you do not understand the instructions, ask your doctor or nurse to explain them to you.

 Read the following information. If you do not understand it or if any of it causes you special concern, check with your doctor.

Before taking this drug, tell your doctor:
- If you are trying to become pregnant, are pregnant, or breastfeeding. This drug may cause birth defects if either the male or female is taking it at the time of conception or during pregnancy. Men and women who are taking this drug need to use some kind of birth control. However, do not use oral contraceptives ("the pill") without checking with your doctor.
- If you think you may want to have children in the future. Many chemotherapy drugs can cause sterility.
- If you have any of the following medical problems: chickenpox or exposure to chickenpox, gout, heart disease, congestive heart failure, shingles, kidney stones, liver disease, or other forms of cancer.
- If you are taking any other prescription or over-the-counter drugs, including vitamins and herbals.

Should I avoid any other medicines, foods, alcohol, and/or activities?
Your prescription and nonprescription medicines may interact with other drugs, causing harm. Certain foods or alcohol can also interact with drug products. Never begin taking a new medicine—prescription or nonprescription—without asking your doctor or nurse if it will interact with alcohol, food, or other medicines. Some drug products can cause drowsiness and affect activities such as driving.

Precautions:
Buserelin acetate may increase testosterone in men when the drug is first started. This causes the symptoms of prostate cancer to get worse for about a week and is called a disease "flare." The prostate gland may also enlarge during this time. The symptoms are increased pain in the bones, blood in the urine, difficulty passing urine, and if prostate cancer is in the bones of the spine, leg weakness. To prevent this, most doctors give drugs that block this testosterone for the first week of treatment. Examples of these drugs are flutamide, nilutamide, or bicalutamide. For men who have prostate cancer in the spine or near the spine, radiation therapy may be given to shrink the tumor.

Men may experience breast swelling and/or soreness.

Hot flashes or sudden feelings of heat and sweating may occur in men and women. These often go away as your body gets used to buserelin acetate.

Men and women may have decreased sexual desire; this will come back when the drug is stopped. Talk with your doctor or nurse about ways to deal with this.

Some men may have difficulty having an erection; this will improve when the drug is stopped. Your doctor or nurse can give you more information about this.

Buserelin acetate nasal spray can irritate the nose. Do not use nasal decongestants before taking buserelin acetate or within 30 minutes after taking it.

 Tell all the doctors, dentists, and pharmacists you visit that you are taking this drug.

- Most of the following side effects probably will not occur.
- Your doctor or nurse will want to discuss specific care instructions with you.
- They can help you understand these side effects and help you deal with them.

Side Effects:

More Common Side Effects
Headache (if drug is taken nasally)   Decreased ability to have an erection
Hot flashes   Decreased sex drive

Less Common Side Effects
Itching
Redness, pain, swelling at the injection site
Irritation of the nose (if drug is taken nasally)
Disease flare when drug is started (increase in bone pain in men and women blood in the urine, weak legs in men)

Rare Side Effects
Swelling of the breasts in men   Allergic reaction with hives
   (gynecomastia)   Weak bones in women (osteoporosis)
Diarrhea   Dry nose (if drug is taken nasally)
Nausea   Difficulty passing urine (men)

Side Effects / Symptoms of the Drug
If women develop vaginal bleeding, it may be caused by not taking enough of the nasal spray. Talk to your doctor or nurse if this occurs. Make sure you do not use a nasal decongestant before or within 30 minutes of taking buserelin acetate spray. Also, check that you are taking the full dose of the drug.

Call your doctor right away if you develop numbness or tingling of the fingers/hands, toes/feet, weakness in the legs, and/or difficulty voiding or moving your bowels. This may happen when buserelin acetate is first started and is a flare reaction. It can be very serious and needs to be evaluated right away. When the flare reaction occurs, you may develop more bone pain. You will need to take more pain medicine during this first week or two of treatment. Call your doctor or nurse right away if the pain medicine is not stopping the pain. They will help you get the right dose or drug for the time that the pain has increased. The pain will go away and you will feel better after the flare reaction is over.

If you are having problems with hot flashes, stop or cut down on tea, coffee, alcohol, and smoking as these often trigger hot flashes. Try to wear layers of clothing; as you feel hot, you can take one layer of clothing off. Drink cool, iced beverages when you feel warm. Ask your doctor or nurse for other suggestions.

> *Other side effects not listed above can also occur in some patients.*
> **Tell your doctor or nurse if you develop any problems.**

FDA Approval: This drug is being studied for cancer treatment.

busulfan

Trade Name:
Myleran

Type of Drug:
Busulfan belongs to the general group of chemotherapy drugs known as alkylating agents. It is used to treat chronic myelogenous leukemia.

How Drug Works:
Busulfan stops the growth of cancer cells, causing them to die.

How Drug Is Given:
Take busulfan tablets by mouth with or without food, at about the same time every day. The dose depends on your blood counts and your size. You will take a higher dose for the first few weeks of treatment then the dose will be lowered for "maintenance." You will have your blood counts checked frequently, and depending upon the white blood cell count, you may be told to stop the medicine for a while. Keep the medicine in a tightly closed container and out of the reach of children and pets. This medicine can also be used to treat other cancers in much higher doses where the medicine is given as a shot in the vein. Make sure that you understand all the instructions from your doctor and that you have the telephone number to call if you have questions.

How Should I Take This Drug?
Take this drug exactly as directed by your doctor. If you do not understand the instructions, ask your doctor or nurse to explain them to you. This drug can be given at different strengths depending on the type of cancer being treated. Dosage may vary depending on your weight and your type of cancer.

 Read the following information. If you do not understand it or if any of it causes you special concern, check with your doctor.

Before taking this drug, tell your doctor:
- If you are trying to become pregnant, are pregnant, or breastfeeding. This drug may cause birth defects if either the male or female is taking it at the time of conception or during pregnancy. Men and women who are taking this drug need to use some kind of birth control. However, do not use oral contraceptives ("the pill") without checking with your doctor.
- If you think you may want to have children in the future. Many chemotherapy drugs can cause sterility.
- If you have any of the following medical problems: chickenpox or exposure to chickenpox, gout, heart disease, congestive heart failure, shingles, kidney stones, liver disease, or other forms of cancer.
- If you are taking any other prescription or over-the-counter drugs, including vitamins and herbals.

Should I avoid any other medicines, foods, alcohol, and/or activities?
Your prescription and nonprescription medicines may interact with other drugs, causing harm. Certain foods or alcohol can also interact with drug products. Never begin taking a new medicine—prescription or nonprescription—without asking your doctor or nurse if it will interact with alcohol, food, or other medicines. Some drug products can cause drowsiness and affect activities such as driving.

Precautions:
Busulfan can lower your blood counts (white blood cells, red blood cells, platelets). Your doctor will check your blood counts before and after each treatment to see how it affects your blood counts. Your doctor or nurse will give you specific instructions if your blood counts are low.

Busulfan can lower your white blood cell count, especially 11 to 30 days after the drug is given. This can increase your chance of getting an infection. Report fever of 100.5°F or higher, or signs of infection such as pain in passing your urine, coughing, and bringing up sputum. The drug will be temporarily stopped if your white blood count falls too fast.

Busulfan can cause a decrease in the platelet count. This can increase your risk of bleeding. DO NOT take any aspirin or aspirin-containing medicines. Report unusual bruising, or bleeding such as nosebleeds, bleeding gums when you brush your teeth, or black, tarry stools.

While you are being treated with busulfan, and after you stop treatment, do not have any immunizations (vaccinations) without your doctor's okay. Try to avoid contact with people who have recently taken the oral polio vaccine. Check with your doctor about this.

Because of the way this drug acts on the body, there is a chance that it can cause other side effects that may not occur until months or years after the drug is used. These very rarely can cause certain types of cancer such as leukemia. Discuss this with your doctor.

Busulfan can cause nausea and vomiting. Ask your doctor or nurse to give you medicines to prevent this or lessen this.

If you develop pain or sores in your mouth, rinse your mouth with a solution of salt and water or a weak bicarbonate (baking soda) solution, after meals and at bedtime as directed by your doctor or nurse. Tell your doctor immediately if you have sores or white patches, or if you cannot eat and/or drink fluids.

 Tell all the doctors, dentists, and pharmacists you visit that you are taking this drug.
- Most of the following side effects probably will not occur.
- Your doctor or nurse will want to discuss specific care instructions with you.
- They can help you understand these side effects and help you deal with them.

Side Effects:

More Common Side Effects
Decreased white blood cell count with increased risk of infection
Decreased platelet count with increased risk of bleeding
Hair loss
Stopping of menstrual periods in women
Reduced or no sperm production (temporary) in men

Less Common Side Effects
Tiredness (fatigue)
Sores in mouth or on lips
Fever
Nausea
Vomiting
Rash
Loss of appetite
Diarrhea

Rare Side Effects
Scarring of lung tissue, with cough, difficulty breathing, and shortness of breath
Changes in liver function blood tests

Other side effects not listed above can also occur in some patients.
Tell your doctor or nurse if you develop any problems.

FDA Approval: This drug is approved for cancer treatment.

capecitabine

Trade Name:
Xeloda

Type of Drug:
Capecitabine belongs to a general group of chemotherapy drugs known as antimetabolites. It is used to treat cancers of the breast or colorectum that have spread (metastasized).

How Drug Works:
Capecitabine prevents cells from making DNA and RNA by interfering with the synthesis of nucleic acids, thus stopping the growth of cancer cells. Capecitabine is converted in your body to the chemotherapy drug 5-fluorouracil (see pages 4–5).

How Drug Is Given:
Take the medicine your doctor orders in 2 doses, once in the morning and once in the evening. Take the pills with a glass of water within 30 minutes after a meal. Try to take the pills at the same time each day. The pills are usually given for 14 days, then no pills for 7 days. The cycle is repeated every 3 weeks if you do not have any problems. The dose depends upon your size, but sometimes the dose needs to be lowered if you have side effects. Your doctor will check your blood counts to see if they are too low. If you have certain side effects, your doctor wil probably stop medicine for a while and may restart the pills at a lower dose. This does not mean the medicine will not work as well; it just means that people need different doses. The medicine should be stored in a closed container, and protected from light. Keep it out of reach of children and pets.

How Should I Take This Drug?
Take this drug exactly as directed by your doctor. If you do not understand the instructions, ask your doctor or nurse to explain them to you.

 Read the following information. If you do not understand it or if any of it causes you special concern, check with your doctor.

Before taking this drug, tell your doctor:
- If you are trying to become pregnant, are pregnant, or breastfeeding. This drug may cause birth defects if either the male or female is taking it at the time of conception or during pregnancy. Men and women who are taking this drug need to use some kind of birth control. However, do not use oral contraceptives ("the pill") without checking with your doctor.
- If you think you may want to have children in the future. Many chemotherapy drugs can cause sterility.
- If you have any of the following medical problems: chickenpox or exposure to chickenpox, gout, heart disease, congestive heart failure, shingles, kidney stones, liver disease, or other forms of cancer.
- If you are taking any other prescription or over-the-counter drugs, including vitamins and herbals.

Should I avoid any other medicines, foods, alcohol, and/or activities?
Your prescription and nonprescription medicines may interact with other drugs, causing harm. Certain foods or alcohol can also interact with drug products. Never begin taking a new medicine—prescription or non-prescription—without asking your doctor or nurse if it will interact with alcohol, food, or other medicines. Some drug products can cause drowsiness and affect activities such as driving.

Precautions:
Tell your doctor if you are taking the vitamin folic acid, or multivitamins that contain folic acid, as this may increase the risk of side effects in your body.

While you are being treated with capecitabine, and after you stop treatment, do not have any immunizations (vaccinations) without your doctor's okay. Try to avoid contact with people who have recently taken the oral polio vaccine. Check with your doctor about this.

Capecitabine can cause a decrease in your white blood cell count. This can increase your risk of getting an infection. Report fever of 100.5°F or higher, or signs of infection such as pain in passing your urine, or coughing and bringing up sputum.

Capecitabine can cause a decrease in the platelet count. This can increase your risk of bleeding. DO NOT take any aspirin or aspirin-containing medicines. Report unusual bruising, or bleeding such as nosebleeds, bleeding gums when you brush your teeth, or black, tarry stools.

 Tell all the doctors, dentists, and pharmacists you visit that you are taking this drug.

- Most of the following side effects probably will not occur.
- Your doctor or nurse will want to discuss specific care instructions with you.
- They can help you understand these side effects and help you deal with them.

Side Effects:

More Common Side Effects
Diarrhea
Nausea
Vomiting
Sores in mouth or on lips
Numbness, tingling, itching of hands or/and feet
Skin redness, rash, dryness
Decreased white blood cell count with increased risk of infection
Decreased platelet count with increased risk of bleeding
Decreased red blood cell count with increased risk of tiredness (fatigue)
Irritation of the skin

Less Common Side Effects
Abdominal pain
Constipation
Heartburn after eating
Fever
Sensation of pins and needles in hands and/or feet
Headache
Dizziness
Difficulty falling asleep
Eye irritation
Increase in blood levels measuring liver function

Rare Side Effects
Swelling of ankles

Side Effects / Symptoms of the Drug
Your doctor or nurse will give you specific instructions if your blood counts are low. Your doctor will check your blood counts before, during, and after receiving the drug to see its effect on you.

Other side effects not listed above can also occur in some patients.
Tell your doctor or nurse if you develop any problems.

FDA Approval: This drug is approved for cancer treatment.

carboplatin

Trade Name:
Paraplatin

Type of Drug:
Carboplatin is a platinum chemotherapy drug that belongs to a general group of drugs known as alkylating agents. It is used to treat ovarian, lungs, and other cancers.

How Drug Works:
Carboplatin stops the growth of cancer cells, causing the cells to die.

How Drug Is Given:
Carboplatin is given as an injection in the vein over 15 to 60 minutes. You will probably get an antinausea drug before receiving this medicine. The dose depends upon your size but may be lowered or not given if your blood counts are low. It can also be given as an infusion into a vein over 24 hours or directly into the peritoneal cavity in advanced ovarian cancer.

 Read the following information. If you do not understand it or if any of it causes you special concern, check with your doctor.

Before taking this drug, tell your doctor:
- If you are trying to become pregnant, are pregnant, or breastfeeding. This drug may cause birth defects if either the male or female is taking it at the time of conception or during pregnancy. Men and women who are taking this drug need to use some kind of birth control. However, do not use oral contraceptives ("the pill") without checking with your doctor.
- If you think you may want to have children in the future. Many chemotherapy drugs can cause sterility.
- If you have any of the following medical problems: chickenpox or exposure to chickenpox, gout, heart disease, congestive heart failure, shingles, kidney stones, liver disease, or other forms of cancer.
- If you are taking any other prescription or over-the-counter drugs, including vitamins and herbals.

Should I avoid any other medicines, foods, alcohol, and/or activities?
Your prescription and nonprescription medicines may interact with other drugs, causing harm. Certain foods or alcohol can also interact with drug products. Never begin taking a new medicine—prescription or non-prescription—without asking your doctor or nurse if it will interact with alcohol, food, or other medicines. Some drug products can cause drowsiness and affect activities such as driving.

Precautions:
While you are being treated with carboplatin, and after you stop treatment, do not have any immunizations (vaccinations) without your doctor's okay. Try to avoid contact with people who have recently taken the oral polio vaccine. Check with your doctor about this.

Carboplatin can lower your blood counts (white blood cells, red blood cells, platelets). Your doctor will check your blood counts before and after each treatment to see its effect on your blood counts. Your doctor or nurse will give you specific instructions if your blood counts are low.

Carboplatin can cause a decrease in your white blood cell count, especially 2 weeks after the drug is given. This can increase your risk of getting an infection. Report fever of 100.5°F or higher, or signs of infection such as pain in passing your urine, coughing and bringing up sputum.

Carboplatin can lower your platelet count. This can increase your risk of bleeding. DO NOT take any aspirin or aspirin-containing medicines. Report unusual bruising, or bleeding such as nosebleeds, bleeding gums when you brush your teeth, or black, tarry stools.

Carboplatin can cause nausea and vomiting. Ask your doctor or nurse to give you medicines to prevent this or lessen it.

Tell all the doctors, dentists, and pharmacists you visit that you are taking this drug.

- Most of the following side effects probably will not occur.
- Your doctor or nurse will want to discuss specific care instructions with you.
- They can help you understand these side effects and help you deal with them.

Side Effects:

More Common Side Effects
Decreased white blood cell count with increased risk of infection
Decreased platelet count with increased risk of bleeding
Brittle hair
Kidney function can be altered at high doses
Fetal abnormalities if pregnant or becoming pregnant while taking this drug

Less Common Side Effects
Nausea
Vomiting
Mild loss of appetite
Mild diarrhea
Constipation
Taste changes
Sensation of pins and needles in hands and/or feet related to nerve irritation

Rare Side Effects
Confusion
Visual changes
Ringing in ears
Rash
Severe allergic reaction
Dizziness

Side Effects / Symptoms of the Drug
You will be monitored closely while receiving the drug to watch for signs or symptoms of an allergic reaction.

Other side effects not listed above can also occur in some patients.
Tell your doctor or nurse if you develop any problems.

FDA Approval: This drug is approved for cancer treatment.

carmustine

Trade Names:
BCNU, BiCNU

Type of Drug:
Carmustine belongs to a special group of alkylating chemotherapy drugs called nitrosoureas. It is used to treat several types of cancer, including brain tumors.

How Drug Works:
Carmustine stops the growth of cancer cells, causing the cells to die.

How Drug Is Given:
Carmustine is given as an injection in the vein over 1 to 2 hours. It can be given based on several different schedules. You will get antinausea medicine before you get the carmustine. The dose depends upon your size but may be lowered or not given if your blood counts are low.

 Read the following information. If you do not understand it or if any of it causes you special concern, check with your doctor.

Before taking this drug, tell your doctor:
- If you are trying to become pregnant, are pregnant, or breastfeeding. This drug may cause birth defects if either the male or female is taking it at the time of conception or during pregnancy. Men and women who are taking this drug need to use some kind of birth control. However, do not use oral contraceptives ("the pill") without checking with your doctor.
- If you think you may want to have children in the future. Many chemotherapy drugs can cause sterility.
- If you have any of the following medical problems: chickenpox or exposure to chickenpox, gout, heart disease, congestive heart failure, shingles, kidney stones, liver disease, or other forms of cancer.
- If you are taking any other prescription or over-the-counter drugs, including vitamins and herbals.

Should I avoid any other medicines, foods, alcohol, and/or activities?
Your prescription and nonprescription medicines may interact with other drugs, causing harm. Certain foods or alcohol can also interact with drug products. Never begin taking a new medicine—prescription or non-prescription—without asking your doctor or nurse if it will interact with alcohol, food, or other medicines. Some drug products can cause drowsiness and affect activities such as driving.

Precautions:
While you are being treated with carmustine, and after you stop treatment, do not have any immunizations (vaccinations) without your doctor's okay. Try to avoid contact with people who have recently taken the oral polio vaccine. Check with your doctor about this.

Carmustine can lower your blood counts (white blood cells, red blood cells, platelets). Your doctor will check your blood counts before and after each treatment to see its effect on your blood counts. Your doctor or nurse will give you specific instructions if your blood counts are low.

Carmustine can lower your white blood cell count, especially 3 to 5 weeks after the drug is given. This can increase your risk of getting an infection. Report fever of 100.5°F or higher, or signs of infection such as pain in passing your urine, coughing, and bringing up sputum.

Carmustine can lower your platelet count. This can increase your risk of bleeding. DO NOT take any aspirin or aspirin-containing medicines. Report unusual bruising, or bleeding such as nosebleeds, bleeding gums when you brush your teeth, or black, tarry stools.

Tell all the doctors, dentists, and pharmacists you visit that you are taking this drug.
- Most of the following side effects probably will not occur.
- Your doctor or nurse will want to discuss specific care instructions with you.
- They can help you understand these side effects and help you deal with them.

Side Effects:

More Common Side Effects
Decreased white blood cell count with increased risk of infection
Decreased platelet count with increased risk of bleeding
Nausea
Vomiting
Irritation of vein used for giving the drug
Loss of appetite
Diarrhea
Headache
Pain along vein during administration
Fetal abnormalities if pregnancy occurs while taking this drug

Less Common Side Effects
Scarring of lung tissue, with cough and shortness of breath
Flushing of skin
Tiredness (fatigue)

Rare Side Effects
Temporary kidney damage
Hardening of vein used for injection
Liver abnormalities, usually reversible

Side Effects / Symptoms of the Drug
Tell your doctor or nurse right away if you develop shortness of breath.

Other side effects not listed above can also occur in some patients.
Tell your doctor or nurse if you develop any problems.

FDA Approval: This drug is approved for cancer treatment.

cetuximab

Trade Name:
C-225

Type of Drug:
Cetuximab is used in molecular targeted therapy to block the cancer cell's communication system. It is being studied in many different cancers, including colon cancer, cancer of the head and neck, pancreatic cancer, nonsmall cell lung cancer, and ovarian cancer.

How Drug Works:
Cetuximab is a monoclonal antibody that fits like a lock and key into receptors on the surface of the cancer cell, blocking an epidermal growth factor receptor (EGFR) from fitting into the receptor. The EGFR is unable to tell the cell to divide. This stops the growth of the cancer cell.

How Drug Is Given:
Cetuximab is given by an injection into the vein over 2 hours during the first treatment, and usually over 1 hour for remaining weekly treatments, per the investigational study. The dose depends upon your size and the investigational study. The first dose is usually larger than the weekly ("maintenance") treatments. You may be given other medicines before cetuximab to lessen the side effects during treatment.

 Read the following information. If you do not understand it or if any of it causes you special concern, check with your doctor.

Before taking this drug, tell your doctor:
• If you are trying to become pregnant, are pregnant, or breastfeeding. This drug may cause birth defects if either the male or female is taking it at the time of conception or during pregnancy. Men and women who are taking this drug need to use some kind of birth control. However, do not use oral contraceptives ("the pill") without checking with your doctor.
• If you think you may want to have children in the future. Many chemotherapy drugs can cause sterility.
• If you have any of the following medical problems: chickenpox or exposure to chickenpox, gout, heart disease, congestive heart failure, shingles, kidney stones, liver disease, or other forms of cancer.
• If you are taking any other prescription or over-the-counter drugs, including vitamins and herbals.

Should I avoid any other medicines, foods, alcohol, and/or activities?
Your prescription and nonprescription medicines may interact with other drugs, causing harm. Certain foods or alcohol can also interact with drug products. Never begin taking a new medicine—prescription or nonprescription—without asking your doctor or nurse if it will interact with alcohol, food, or other medicines. Some drug products can cause drowsiness and affect activities such as driving.

Precautions:
Cetuximab works better when given with chemotherapy or radiotherapy to kill the cancer cells.

While you are being treated with cetuximab and after you stop treatment, do not have any immunizations (vaccinations) without your doctor's okay. Try to avoid contact with people who have recently taken the oral polio vaccine. Check with your doctor about this.

Allergic reactions such as fever and chills may occur but they are not common. Rarely, lower blood pressure, swelling of the face, and coughing can occur. Tell your doctor or nurse right away if you get a fever or chills, hives, nausea, itching, headache, shortness of breath, or swollen tongue or throat during your treatment. Your doctor or nurse will stop your infusion and evaluate you.

Rash on the face, neck, and trunk is very common, beginning during the first 2 weeks of treatment and going away completely when treatment is stopped. The rash may become severe in a few cases, and this should be reported right away.

Tell all the doctors, dentists, and pharmacists you visit that you are taking this drug.
- -
- Most of the following side effects probably will not occur.
- Your doctor or nurse will want to discuss specific care instructions with you.
- They can help you understand these side effects and help you deal with them.

Side Effects:

More Common Side Effects
Acne-like skin rash on face, neck, and trunk

Less Common Side Effects
Fatigue
Fever
Nausea
Diarrhea

Rare Side Effects
Allergic reactions, with fever and chills
Anaphylaxis or life-threatening allergic reaction
Headache
Sore mouth
Vomiting
Weight loss
Loss of appetite
Constipation
Low white blood cell count, with increased risk of infection
Low red blood cell count, with increased risk of anemia and fatigue (tiredness)

Side Effects / Symptoms of the Drug
Call your doctor or nurse right away if you develop a severe rash, fever of 100.5°F or greater, and/or symptoms of infection such as cough with sputum or burning when urinating.

Other side effects not listed above can also occur in some patients.
Tell your doctor or nurse if you develop any problems.

FDA Approval: This drug is being studied for cancer treatment.

chlorambucil

Trade Name:
Leukeran

Type of Drug:
Chlorambucil belongs to the general group of chemotherapy drugs known as alkylating agents. It is used to treat chronic lymphocytic leukemia.

How Drug Works:
Chlorambucil stops the growth of cancer cells, causing the cells to die.

How Drug Is Given:
Chlorambucil is a pill that is given by mouth once a day for a short or long time depending upon the type of cancer being treated. Try to take the pill at about the same time every day. You may need to take an anti-nausea pill 1 hour before taking the medicine if you get sick to your stomach. Remember to drink lots of water during the day to keep your kidneys flushed out. The dose depends on the type of cancer being treated, your size, and your blood counts. Your doctor will check your blood counts frequently, and if your blood counts are low, you may need to stop the medicine for a while until they get higher. It is very important to take your medicine as directed and to keep all your appointments. Call your doctor or nurse if you have any questions. Keep the medicine in a tightly closed container away from heat and moisture and out of the reach of children and pets.

How Should I Take This Drug?
Take this drug exactly as directed by your doctor. If you do not understand the instructions, ask your doctor or nurse to explain them to you. This drug can be given at different strengths depending on the type of cancer being treated. Dosage may vary depending on your weight and the type of cancer.

 Read the following information. If you do not understand it or if any of it causes you special concern, check with your doctor.

Before taking this drug, tell your doctor:
- If you are trying to become pregnant, are pregnant, or breastfeeding. This drug may cause birth defects if either the male or female is taking it at the time of conception or during pregnancy. Men and women who are taking this drug need to use some kind of birth control. However, do not use oral contraceptives ("the pill") without checking with your doctor.
- If you think you may want to have children in the future. Many chemotherapy drugs can cause sterility.
- If you have any of the following medical problems: chickenpox or exposure to chickenpox, gout, heart disease, congestive heart failure, shingles, kidney stones, liver disease, or other forms of cancer.
- If you are taking any other prescription or over-the-counter drugs, including vitamins and herbals.

Should I avoid any other medicines, foods, alcohol, and/or activities?
Your prescription and nonprescription medicines may interact with other drugs, causing harm. Certain foods or alcohol can also interact with drug products. Never begin taking a new medicine—prescription or nonprescription—without asking your doctor or nurse if it will interact with alcohol, food, or other medicines. Some drug products can cause drowsiness and affect activities such as driving.

Precautions:
While you are being treated with chlorambucil, and after you stop treatment, do not have any immunizations (vaccinations) without your doctor's okay. Try to avoid contact with people who have recently taken the oral polio vaccine. Check with your doctor about this.

Chlorambucil can lower your blood counts (white blood cells, red blood cells, and platelets). Your doctor will check your blood counts before and after each treatment to see its effect on your blood counts. Your doctor or nurse will give you specific instructions if your blood counts are low.

Chlorambucil can lower your white blood cell count, especially 3 weeks after the drug is given. This can increase your risk of getting an infection. Report fever of 100.5°F or higher, or signs of infection such as pain in passing your urine, coughing, and bringing up sputum.

Chlorambucil can lower your platelet count. This can increase your risk of bleeding. DO NOT take any aspirin or aspirin-containing medicines. Report unusual bruising or bleeding such as nosebleeds, bleeding gums when you brush your teeth, or black, tarry stools.

 Tell all the doctors, dentists, and pharmacists you visit that you are taking this drug.

- Most of the following side effects probably will not occur.
- Your doctor or nurse will want to discuss specific care instructions with you.
- They can help you understand these side effects and help you deal with them.

Side Effects:

More Common Side Effects
Decreased white blood cell count with increased risk of infection
Decreased platelet count with increased risk of bleeding
Stopping of menstrual periods in women
Reduced sperm production in men
Fetal changes if becoming pregnant while taking chlorambucil

Less Common Side Effects
Loss of appetite
Decreased weight

Rare Side Effects
Nausea
Vomiting
Liver damage
Scarring of lung tissue
Visual disturbances
Confusion
Seizures

Other side effects not listed above can also occur in some patients.
Tell your doctor or nurse if you develop any problems.

FDA Approval: This drug is approved for cancer treatment.

cisplatin

Trade Name:
Platinol

Type of Drug:
Cisplatin is a platinum compound chemotherapy drug that acts like an alkylating agent. It is used to treat testicular and ovarian cancers that have spread. It is also used to treat several other cancers, such as lung cancer.

How Drug Works:
Cisplatin stops the growth of cancer cells, causing the cell to die.

How Drug Is Given:
Cisplatin is given by an injection into the vein over at least 1 hour. Sometimes you will be given other medicines that will help flush the medicine out quickly through the kidneys. You will also get a salt solution by vein and medicine to prevent or stop nausea or vomiting. Before and after the medicine you should drink 2 to 3 quarts of fluid a day (an 8 oz. glass of water or fluid every hour while awake) to protect your kidneys. Your doctor will check your kidney function before giving the medicine. Your dose depends upon the type of cancer being treated, your size, and how well your kidneys are working.

 Read the following information. If you do not understand it or if any of it causes you special concern, check with your doctor.

Before taking this drug, tell your doctor:
- If you are trying to become pregnant, are pregnant, or breastfeeding. This drug may cause birth defects if either the male or female is taking it at the time of conception or during pregnancy. Men and women who are taking this drug need to use some kind of birth control. However, do not use oral contraceptives ("the pill") without checking with your doctor.
- If you think you may want to have children in the future. Many chemotherapy drugs can cause sterility.
- If you have any of the following medical problems: chickenpox or exposure to chickenpox, gout, heart disease, congestive heart failure, shingles, kidney stones, liver disease, or other forms of cancer.
- If you are taking any other prescription or over-the-counter drugs, including vitamins and herbals.

Should I avoid any other medicines, foods, alcohol, and/or activities?
Your prescription and nonprescription medicines may interact with other drugs, causing harm. Certain foods or alcohol can also interact with drug products. Never begin taking a new medicine—prescription or non-prescription—without asking your doctor or nurse if it will interact with alcohol, food, or other medicines. Some drug products can cause drowsiness and affect activities such as driving.

Precautions:
While you are being treated with cisplatin, and after you stop treatment, do not have any immunizations (vaccinations) without your doctor's okay. Try to avoid contact with people who have recently taken the oral polio vaccine. Check with your doctor about this.

Cisplatin can cause kidney damage. This is prevented by checking your kidney function before you receive the drug, giving you extra intravenous fluids, and asking you to drink extra fluid after the drug is given. This extra fluid helps to flush the medicine out of your system and protects your kidneys.

Cisplatin also causes your red blood cell count to decrease over a few months' time. Cisplatin can lower the platelet count, which can increase your risk of bleeding. DO NOT take any aspirin or aspirin-containing medicines. Report unusual bruising, or bleeding such as nosebleeds, bleeding gums when you brush your teeth, or black, tarry stools.

Tell all the doctors, dentists, and pharmacists you visit that you are taking this drug.

- Most of the following side effects probably will not occur.
- Your doctor or nurse will want to discuss specific care instructions with you.
- They can help you understand these side effects and help you deal with them.

Side Effects:

More Common Side Effects
Kidney damage
Decreased blood levels of magnesium, potassium, and calcium
Nausea
Vomiting
Taste changes including metallic taste of foods
Sensation of pins and needles in hands and/or feet caused by irritation of nerves
Fetal changes if becoming pregnant during treatment

Less Common Side Effects
Tiredness (fatigue)
Decreased white blood cell count with increased risk of infection, if given in high doses or with radiation therapy
Decreased platelet count with increased risk of bleeding if given in high doses or with radiation therapy
Loss of appetite
Hair thinning
Diarrhea

Rare Side Effects
Severe allergic reaction
Hearing loss
Difficulty walking
Chest pain and heart attack

Other side effects not listed above can also occur in some patients.
Tell your doctor or nurse if you develop any problems.

FDA Approval: This drug is approved for cancer treatment.

cladribine

Trade Names:
2-CdA, Leustatin

Type of Drug:
Cladribine belongs to the general group of chemotherapy drugs known as antimetabolites. It is used to treat hairy cell leukemia.

How Drug Works:
Cladribine prevents cells from making DNA and RNA by interfering with the synthesis of nucleic acids, thus stopping the growth of cancer cells.

How Drug Is Given:
Cladribine is given as a continuous infusion by vein for 7 days. The dose depends upon your size. You will be assessed for damage to your nerves and kidneys. If either of these happens, the medicine may be delayed or stopped. Also, following treatment, your blood counts will be watched very closely.

 Read the following information. If you do not understand it or if any of it causes you special concern, check with your doctor.

Before taking this drug, tell your doctor:
- If you are trying to become pregnant, are pregnant, or breastfeeding. This drug may cause birth defects if either the male or female is taking it at the time of conception or during pregnancy. Men and women who are taking this drug need to use some kind of birth control. However, do not use oral contraceptives ("the pill") without checking with your doctor.
- If you think you may want to have children in the future. Many chemotherapy drugs can cause sterility.
- If you have any of the following medical problems: chickenpox or exposure to chickenpox, gout, heart disease, congestive heart failure, shingles, kidney stones, liver disease, or other forms of cancer.
- If you are taking any other prescription or over-the-counter drugs, including vitamins and herbals.

Should I avoid any other medicines, foods, alcohol, and/or activities?
Your prescription and nonprescription medicines may interact with other drugs, causing harm. Certain foods or alcohol can also interact with drug products. Never begin taking a new medicine—prescription or non-prescription—without asking your doctor or nurse if it will interact with alcohol, food, or other medicines. Some drug products can cause drowsiness and affect activities such as driving.

Precautions:
While you are being treated with cladribine, and after you stop treatment, do not have any immunizations (vaccinations) without your doctor's okay. Try to avoid contact with people who have recently taken the oral polio vaccine. Check with your doctor about this.

Cladribine can lower your blood counts (white blood cells, red blood cells, platelets). Your doctor will check your blood counts before and after each treatment to see its effect on your blood counts. Your doctor or nurse will give you specific instructions for low blood counts.

Cladribine can lower your white blood cell count, especially 1 to 2 weeks after the drug is given. This can increase your risk of getting an infection. Report fever of 100.5°F or higher, or signs of infection such as pain in passing your urine, coughing, and bringing up sputum.

Cladribine can lower the platelet count, which can increase your risk of bleeding. DO NOT take any aspirin or aspirin-containing medicines. Report unusual bruising or bleeding such as nosebleeds, bleeding gums when you brush your teeth, or black, tarry stools.

Tell all the doctors, dentists, and pharmacists you visit that you are taking this drug.

- Most of the following side effects probably will not occur.
- Your doctor or nurse will want to discuss specific care instructions with you.
- They can help you understand these side effects and help you deal with them.

Side Effects:

More Common Side Effects

Decreased white blood cell count with increased risk of infection
Decreased platelet count with increased risk of bleeding
Mild nausea
Tiredness (fatigue)
Rash
Fever
Headache

Less Common Side Effects

Vomiting
Coughing
Shortness of breath
Redness of skin
Sweating
Dizziness
Muscle and bone aches
Itching

Rare Side Effects

Trouble sleeping
Pain at place of injection
Constipation
Diarrhea
Stomach pain
Swelling of ankles
Fast heart rate

Other side effects not listed above can also occur in some patients.
Tell your doctor or nurse if you develop any problems.

FDA Approval: This drug is approved for cancer treatment.

cyclophosphamide

Trade Name:
Cytoxan

Type of Drug:
Cyclophosphamide belongs to a general group of chemotherapy drugs known as alkylating agents. Cydophosphamide is used for the treatment of lymphoma, leukemias, multiple myeloma, mycosis fungoides, neuroblastoma, retinoblastoma, and cancers of the breast and ovary. It is also used to treat some noncancerous conditions.

How Drug Works:
Cyclophosphamide stops the growth of cancer cells, causing them to die.

How Drug Is Given:
Cyclophosphamide can be given by mouth as a pill or liquid, or as a shot into a vein. The dose depends upon your size and your type of cancer. Cyclophosphamide is given with other anticancer drugs. Antinausea medicines will be given before the shot; if you are taking the pill or liquid, take the antinausea pill 1 hour before your cyclophosphamide dose. If you are taking the liquid, make sure you shake the medicine well before pouring the dose. Also, take the medicine first thing in the morning with at least a full glass of water to lessen bladder problems. Try to drink at least 1 full glass of fluid every hour, and empty your bladder every 1 to 2 hours. If you have stomach problems, your doctor may tell you to take the pill in smaller doses with food during the day. Talk to your doctor or nurse if the antinausea medicine does not stop the nausea or vomiting, so that a better medicine can be given to you. You will have your blood counts checked before each treatment, and if they are too low, your treatment will be delayed. Keep the medicine in a tightly closed container away from heat and moisture and out of the reach of children and pets.

How Should I Take This Drug?
Take this drug exactly as directed by your doctor. If you do not understand the instructions, ask your doctor or nurse to explain them to you.

 Read the following information. If you do not understand it or if any of it causes you special concern, check with your doctor.

Before taking this drug, tell your doctor:
- If you are trying to become pregnant, are pregnant, or breastfeeding. This drug may cause birth defects if either the male or female is taking it at the time of conception or during pregnancy. Men and women who are taking this drug need to use some kind of birth control. However, do not use oral contraceptives ("the pill") without checking with your doctor.
- If you think you may want to have children in the future. Many chemotherapy drugs can cause sterility.
- If you have any of the following medical problems: chickenpox or exposure to chickenpox, gout, heart disease, congestive heart failure, shingles, kidney stones, liver disease, or other forms of cancer.
- If you are taking any other prescription or over-the-counter drugs, including vitamins and herbals.

Should I avoid any other medicines, foods, alcohol, and/or activities?
Your prescription and nonprescription medicines may interact with other drugs, causing harm. Certain foods or alcohol can also interact with drug products. Never begin taking a new medicine—prescription or nonprescription—without asking your doctor or nurse if it will interact with alcohol, food, or other medicines. Some drug products can cause drowsiness and affect activities such as driving.

Precautions:
While you are being treated with cyclophosphamide, and after you stop treatment, do not have any immunizations (vaccinations) without your doctor's okay. Try to avoid contact with people who have recently taken the oral polio vaccine. Check with your doctor about this.

Cyclophosphamide can cause bleeding in your bladder. This is prevented by receiving extra fluid intravenously and drinking extra liquids. Your nurse or doctor will give you specific instructions.

Cyclophosphamide can lower your blood counts (white blood cells, red blood cells, platelets). Your doctor will check your blood counts before and after each treatment to see its effect on your blood counts. Your doctor or nurse will give you specific instructions if your blood counts are low.

Cyclophosphamide can lower your white blood cell count, especially 1 to 2 weeks after the drug is given. This can increase your risk of getting an infection. Report fever of 100.5°F or higher, or signs of infection such as pain in passing your urine, coughing and bringing up sputum.

Cyclophosphamide can lower the platelet count. This can increase your risk of bleeding. DO NOT take any aspirin or aspirin-containing medicines. Report unusual bruising or bleeding such as nosebleeds, bleeding gums when you brush your teeth, or black, tarry stools.

Getting a wig before starting treatment may make it easier to deal with hair loss. Talk to your nurse or doctor about this. If your insurance does not cover it, there may be other resources to help you. Hair loss is temporary, and your hair will grow back after treatment.

 Tell all the doctors, dentists, and pharmacists you visit that you are taking this drug.
- Most of the following side effects probably will not occur.
- Your doctor or nurse will want to discuss specific care instructions with you.
- They can help you understand these side effects and help you deal with them.

Side Effects:

More Common Side Effects
Decreased white blood cell count with increased risk of infection
Hair loss
Nausea
Vomiting
Loss of appetite
Sores in mouth or on lips
Diarrhea
Stopping of menstrual periods in women
Decreased sperm production in men

Less Common Side Effects
Decreased platelet count (mild) with increased risk of bleeding
Blood in urine
Darkening of nail beds
Acne
Tiredness
Fetal changes if you become pregnant while taking cyclophosphamide

Rare Side Effects
Scarring of lung tissue, with cough and shortness of breath
Heart changes with high doses

Side Effects / Symptoms of the Drug
Because of the way this drug acts on the body, there is a chance that after receiving large total doses of the drug, it can cause other side effects that may not occur until months or years after the drug is used. Rarely, a second cancer can occur years after receiving this drug. Discuss this with your doctor.

Other side effects not listed above can also occur in some patients.
Tell your doctor or nurse if you develop any problems.

FDA Approval: This drug is approved for cancer treatment.

cytarabine, cytosine arabinoside

Trade Names:
Ara-C, Cytosar-U

Type of Drug:
Cytarabine belongs to the general group of drugs known as antimetabolites. It is used to treat acute leukemias.

How Drug Works:
Cytarabine prevents cells from making DNA and RNA by interfering with the synthesis of nucleic acids, thus stopping the growth of cancer cells.

How Drug Is Given:
Cytarabine or cytosine arabinoside is given by a shot in a vein over 20 minutes to 2 hours, or as a continuous infusion over 24 hours. It can also be given as a shot under the skin or into the spinal canal. The dose, how long the treatment is, and how often the medicine is given, depends on your size and your type of cancer. If your doctor orders the shot under the skin, you or a family member can be taught to give it at home. If you do, make sure to keep the medicine in its original container in the refrigerator, and the shot equipment in a safe place out of the reach of children and pets. Keep the used needles in a closed needle bucket and take them back to your doctor or nurse.

How Should I Take This Drug?
Take this drug exactly as directed by your doctor. If you do not understand the instructions, ask your doctor or nurse to explain them to you. This drug can be given at different strengths depending on the type of cancer being treated. Dosage may vary depending on your weight and your type of cancer.

 Read the following information. If you do not understand it or if any of it causes you special concern, check with your doctor.

Before taking this drug, tell your doctor:
• If you are trying to become pregnant, are pregnant, or breastfeeding. This drug may cause birth defects if either the male or female is taking it at the time of conception or during pregnancy. Men and women who are taking this drug need to use some kind of birth control. However, do not use oral contraceptives ("the pill") without checking with your doctor.
• If you think you may want to have children in the future. Many chemotherapy drugs can cause sterility.
• If you have any of the following medical problems: chickenpox or exposure to chickenpox, gout, heart disease, congestive heart failure, shingles, kidney stones, liver disease, or other forms of cancer.
• If you are taking any other prescription or over-the-counter drugs, including vitamins and herbals.

Should I avoid any other medicines, foods, alcohol, and/or activities?
Your prescription and nonprescription medicines may interact with other drugs, causing harm. Certain foods or alcohol can also interact with drug products. Never begin taking a new medicine—prescription or nonprescription—without asking your doctor or nurse if it will interact with alcohol, food, or other medicines. Some drug products can cause drowsiness and affect activities such as driving.

Precautions:
While you are being treated with cytarabine, and after you stop treatment, do not have any immunizations (vaccinations) without your doctor's okay. Try to avoid contact with people who have recently taken the oral polio vaccine. Check with your doctor about this.

Cytarabine may be given in many dosage strengths. It can lower your blood counts (white blood cells, red blood cells, platelets). Your doctor will check your blood counts before and after each treatment to see its effect on your blood counts. Your doctor or nurse will give you specific instructions if your blood counts are low.

Cytarabine can decrease your white blood cell count, especially 7 to 9 days after the drug is given. This can increase your risk of getting an infection. Report fever of 100.5°F or higher, or signs of infection such as pain in passing your urine, coughing, and bringing up sputum.

Cytarabine can decrease your platelet count. This can increase your risk of bleeding. DO NOT take any aspirin or aspirin-containing medicines. Report unusual bruising, or bleeding such as nosebleeds, bleeding gums when you brush your teeth, or black, tarry stools.

 Tell all the doctors, dentists, and pharmacists you visit that you are taking this drug.
- -
- Most of the following side effects probably will not occur.
- Your doctor or nurse will want to discuss specific care instructions with you.
- They can help you understand these side effects and help you deal with them.

Side Effects:

More Common Side Effects
Decreased white blood cell count with increased risk of infection
Decreased platelet count with increased risk of bleeding
Nausea
Vomiting
Tiredness (fatigue)
Sores in mouth or on lips

Less Common Side Effects
Mild diarrhea
Decreased appetite
Rash
Hair loss
Fever
Muscle and bone aches
Liver toxicity

Rare Side Effects
Redness of eyes
Sleepiness
Muscle weakness
Difficulty walking
Difficulty writing
Slurred speech
Fetal changes if you become pregnant while taking this drug

Other side effects not listed above can also occur in some patients.
Tell your doctor or nurse if you develop any problems.

FDA Approval: This drug is approved for cancer treatment.

dacarbazine

Trade Names:
DTIC-Dome, dimethyl-triazeno, imidazole carboxamide

Type of Drug:
Dacarbazine is a chemotherapy drug that acts like an alkylating agent. It is used to treat Hodgkin's disease and malignant melanoma.

How Drug Works:
Dacarbazine stops the growth of cancer cells, causing the cells to die.

How Drug Is Given:
Dacarbazine is given as a shot in a vein over 20 minutes or longer. Tell the nurse if you feel pain, burning, or discomfort in the vein when it is given. You will get medicine to stop any nausea or vomiting before the dacarbazine and to take afterward. The dose and how often you get the medicine depends on your size, blood counts, and the type of cancer being treated. You will have your blood counts checked before each treatment; if they are too low, your treatment will be delayed. This medicine may be given in addition to other anticancer medicines.

 Read the following information. If you do not understand it or if any of it causes you special concern, check with your doctor.

Before taking this drug, tell your doctor:
- If you are trying to become pregnant, are pregnant, or breastfeeding. This drug may cause birth defects if either the male or female is taking it at the time of conception or during pregnancy. Men and women who are taking this drug need to use some kind of birth control. However, do not use oral contraceptives ("the pill") without checking with your doctor.
- If you think you may want to have children in the future. Many chemotherapy drugs can cause sterility.
- If you have any of the following medical problems: chickenpox or exposure to chickenpox, gout, heart disease, congestive heart failure, shingles, kidney stones, liver disease, or other forms of cancer.
- If you are taking any other prescription or over-the-counter drugs, including vitamins and herbals.

Should I avoid any other medicines, foods, alcohol, and/or activities?
Your prescription and nonprescription medicines may interact with other drugs, causing harm. Certain foods or alcohol can also interact with drug products. Never begin taking a new medicine—prescription or non-prescription—without asking your doctor or nurse if it will interact with alcohol, food, or other medicines. Some drug products can cause drowsiness and affect activities such as driving.

Precautions:
While you are being treated with dacarbazine, and after you stop treatment, do not have any immunizations (vaccinations) without your doctor's okay. Try to avoid contact with people who have recently taken the oral polio vaccine. Check with your doctor about this.

Dacarbazine can lower your blood counts (white blood cells, red blood cells, platelets). Your doctor will check your blood counts before and after each treatment to see its effect on your blood counts. Your doctor or nurse will give you specific instructions if your blood counts are low.

Dacarbazine can decrease your white blood cell count, especially 14 to 28 days after the drug is given. This can increase your risk of getting an infection. Report fever of 100.5°F or higher, or signs of infection such as pain in passing your urine, coughing, and bringing up sputum.

Dacarbazine can decrease your platelet count. This can increase your risk of bleeding. DO NOT take any aspirin or aspirin-containing medicines. Report unusual bruising, or bleeding such as nosebleeds, bleeding gums when you brush your teeth, or black, tarry stools.

Dacarbazine can make you very sensitive to sunlight or bright ultraviolet light. You can get a very bad sunburn. Wear sunglasses, sunscreen, and protective clothes when out in strong sunlight. Always wear sunscreen when out in the sun.

Getting a wig before starting treatment may make it easier to deal with hair loss. Talk to your nurse or doctor about this. If your insurance does not cover it, there may be other resources to help you. Hair loss is temporary, and your hair will grow back after treatment.

 Tell all the doctors, dentists, and pharmacists you visit that you are taking this drug.

- Most of the following side effects probably will not occur.
- Your doctor or nurse will want to discuss specific care instructions with you.
- They can help you understand these side effects and help you deal with them.

Side Effects:

More Common Side Effects
Decreased white blood cell count with increased risk of infection
Decreased platelet count with increased risk of bleeding
Nausea
Vomiting
Loss of appetite
Irritation of vein used for giving the drug
Flu-like illness up to 7 days after receiving the drug (tiredness, headache, muscle aches, fever, stuffy nose)
Hair loss

Less Common Side Effects
Taste changes, including metallic taste of foods
Hardening of vein used for giving the drug
Tiredness (fatigue)

Rare Side Effects
Diarrhea
Facial flushing
Liver toxicity
Redness and itching at injection site

Other side effects not listed above can also occur in some patients.
Tell your doctor or nurse if you develop any problems.

FDA Approval: This drug is approved for cancer treatment.

dactinomycin

Trade Names:
Actinomycin D, Cosmegen, Act-D

Type of Drug:
Dactinomycin belongs to the general group of chemotherapy drugs known as antibiotics. It is used to treat testicular, ovarian, and germ cell cancers.

How Drug Works:
Dactinomycin stops the growth of cancer cells, causing the cells to die.

How Drug Is Given:
Dactinomycin is given as a shot in a vein over about 15 minutes. Tell the nurse if you feel pain, burning, or discomfort in the vein when the medicine is given. You will get medicine to stop any nausea or vomiting before the dactinomycin and to take afterward. The dose and how often you get the medicine depends upon your size, your blood counts, and the type of cancer being treated. You will have your blood counts checked before each treatment; if they are too low, your treatment will be delayed. This medicine may be given in addition to other anticancer medicines.

 Read the following information. If you do not understand it or if any of it causes you special concern, check with your doctor.

Before taking this drug, tell your doctor:
• If you are trying to become pregnant, are pregnant, or breastfeeding. This drug may cause birth defects if either the male or female is taking it at the time of conception or during pregnancy. Men and women who are taking this drug need to use some kind of birth control. However, do not use oral contraceptives ("the pill") without checking with your doctor.
• If you think you may want to have children in the future. Many chemotherapy drugs can cause sterility.
• If you have any of the following medical problems: chickenpox or exposure to chickenpox, gout, heart disease, congestive heart failure, shingles, kidney stones, liver disease, or other forms of cancer.
• If you are taking any other prescription or over-the-counter drugs, including vitamins and herbals.

Should I avoid any other medicines, foods, alcohol, and/or activities?
Your prescription and nonprescription medicines may interact with other drugs, causing harm. Certain foods or alcohol can also interact with drug products. Never begin taking a new medicine—prescription or non-prescription—without asking your doctor or nurse if it will interact with alcohol, food, or other medicines. Some drug products can cause drowsiness and affect activities such as driving.

Precautions:
While you are being treated with dactinomycin, and after you stop treatment, do not have any immunizations (vaccinations) without your doctor's okay. Try to avoid contact with people who have recently taken the oral polio vaccine. Check with your doctor about this.

Dactinomycin can lower your blood counts (white blood cells, red blood cells, platelets). Your doctor will check your blood counts before and after each treatment to see its effect on your blood counts. Your doctor or nurse will give you specific instructions if your blood counts are low.

Dactinomycin can decrease your white blood cell count, especially 7 to 10 days after the drug is given. This can increase your risk of getting an infection. Report fever of 100.5˚F or higher, or signs of infection such as pain in passing your urine, coughing, and bringing up sputum.

Dactinomycin can decrease your platelet count. This can increase your risk of bleeding. DO NOT take any aspirin or aspirin-containing medicines. Report unusual bruising, or bleeding such as nosebleeds, bleeding gums when you brush your teeth, or black, tarry stools.

Dactinomycin is given intravenously. If the drug accidentally leaks out of the vein where it is given, it may damage the tissue and cause scarring. Tell the nurse right away if you notice redness, pain, or swelling at the place of injection.

Getting a wig before starting treatment may make it easier to deal with hair loss. Talk to your nurse or doctor about this. If your insurance does not cover it, there may be other resources to help you. Hair loss is temporary, and your hair will grow back after treatment.

Dactinomycin can cause radiation recall. When a person has had radiation therapy and then receives this drug, the skin or tissue damage from prior radiation therapy can become red and appear damaged again. Tell your doctor or nurse if your skin gets red in areas where radiation was given.

Dactinomycin can cause severe nausea and vomiting. Ask your doctor or nurse to give you medicines to prevent or lessen this.

Tell all the doctors, dentists, and pharmacists you visit that you are taking this drug.

- Most of the following side effects probably will not occur.
- Your doctor or nurse will want to discuss specific care instructions with you.
- They can help you understand these side effects and help you deal with them.

Side Effects:

More Common Side Effects
Decreased white blood cell count with increased risk of infection
Decreased platelet count with increased risk of bleeding
Darkening of skin along vein used for giving the drug
Hair loss
Nausea
Vomiting
Loss of appetite
Sores in mouth or on lips, esophagus, or rectal area
Diarrhea
Rash
Radiation recall skin changes

Less Common Side Effects
Tiredness (fatigue)
Fever
Muscle and bone aches
Depression
Abdominal pain
Fetal abnormalities if taken while you are pregnant or if you become pregnant while taking this drug

Rare Side Effects
Liver damage
Kidney damage

Other side effects not listed above can also occur in some patients.
Tell your doctor or nurse if you develop any problems.

FDA Approval: This drug is approved for cancer treatment.

daunorubicin

Trade Names:
Cerubidine, Daunomycin, Rubidomycin, DNR

Type of Drug:
Daunorubicin belongs to the general group of chemotherapy drugs known as anthracycline antibiotics. It is used to treat acute lymphocytic and myelocytic leukemias.

How Drug Works:
Daunorubicin stops the growth of cancer cells, causing the cells to die.

How Drug Is Given:
Daunorubicin is given as a shot in a vein over about 15 minutes. Tell the nurse if you feel pain, burning, or discomfort in the vein when it is given. You will get medicine to stop any nausea or vomiting before receiving the daunorubicin and to take afterward. The dose and how often you get the medicine depends on your size, your blood counts, how well your liver is working, and the type of cancer being treated. You will have your blood counts checked before each treatment. If they are too low, your treatment will be delayed. This medicine may be given in addition to other anticancer medicines.

 Read the following information. If you do not understand it or if any of it causes you special concern, check with your doctor.

Before taking this drug, tell your doctor:
- If you are trying to become pregnant, are pregnant, or breastfeeding. This drug may cause birth defects if either the male or female is taking it at the time of conception or during pregnancy. Men and women who are taking this drug need to use some kind of birth control. However, do not use oral contraceptives ("the pill") without checking with your doctor.
- If you think you may want to have children in the future. Many chemotherapy drugs can cause sterility.
- If you have any of the following medical problems: chickenpox or exposure to chickenpox, gout, heart disease, congestive heart failure, shingles, kidney stones, liver disease, or other forms of cancer.
- If you are taking any other prescription or over-the-counter drugs, including vitamins and herbals.

Should I avoid any other medicines, foods, alcohol, and/or activities?
Your prescription and nonprescription medicines may interact with other drugs, causing harm. Certain foods or alcohol can also interact with drug products. Never begin taking a new medicine—prescription or nonprescription—without asking your doctor or nurse if it will interact with alcohol, food, or other medicines. Some drug products can cause drowsiness and affect activities such as driving.

Precautions:
While you are being treated with daunorubicin, and after you stop treatment, do not have any immunizations (vaccinations) without your doctor's okay. Try to avoid contact with people who have recently taken the oral polio vaccine. Check with your doctor about this.

Daunorubicin can lower your blood counts (white blood cells, red blood cells, platelets). Your doctor will check your blood counts before and after each treatment to see how it affects your blood counts. Your doctor or nurse will give you specific instructions if your blood counts are low.

Daunorubicin can lower your white blood cell count, especially 10 to 14 days after the drug is given. This can increase your risk of getting an infection. Report fever of 100.5°F or higher, or signs of infection such as pain in passing your urine, coughing, and bringing up sputum.

Daunorubicin can cause lower your platelet count. This can increase your risk of bleeding. DO NOT take any aspirin or aspirin-containing medicines. Report unusual bruising, or bleeding such as nosebleeds, bleeding gums when you brush your teeth, or black, tarry stools.

Getting a wig before starting treatment may make it easier to deal with hair loss. Talk to your nurse or doctor about this. If your insurance does not cover it, there may be other resources to help you. Hair loss is temporary, and your hair will grow back after treatment.

Daunorubicin can cause radiation recall. When a person has had radiation therapy and then receives this drug, the skin or tissue damage from prior radiation therapy can become red and appear damaged again. Tell your doctor or nurse if your skin gets red in areas where radiation was given.

Daunorubicin can injure the heart muscle when large doses are given. Your doctor will test your heart function before you receive your first treatment, and then during the treatment. This way, any damage can be found early. Talk to your doctor about this.

Daunorubicin can cause severe nausea and vomiting. Ask your doctor or nurse to give you medicines to prevent or lessen this.

Daunorubicin is given intravenously. If the drug accidentally leaks out of the vein where it is given, it may damage the tissue and cause scarring. Tell the nurse right away if you notice redness, pain, or swelling at the place of injection.

Tell all the doctors, dentists, and pharmacists you visit that you are taking this drug.

- Most of the following side effects probably will not occur.
- Your doctor or nurse will want to discuss specific care instructions with you.
- They can help you anticipate and understand these side effects and help you deal with them.

Side Effects:

More Common Side Effects

Decreased white blood cell count
  with increased risk of infection
Decreased platelet count with
  increased risk of bleeding

Nausea
Vomiting
Hair loss
Darkening of nail beds

Less Common Side Effects

Radiation recall skin changes
Rash
Fetal changes if taken while you are pregnant or if you become pregnant while taking this drug

Rare Side Effects

Temporary changes in
  electrocardiogram (EKG)
Irregular heartbeat
Abdominal pain
Sores in mouth or on lips

Loosening of fingernails
Fever
Chills
Heart damage with congestive heart failure

Side Effects / Symptoms of the Drug

Daunorubicin causes the urine to turn reddish, which may stain clothes. This is not blood. It is normal and lasts for 1 to 2 days after each dose is given.

After you stop receiving daunorubicin, the drug may still produce some side effects that need attention. Tell your doctor or nurse if you have any irregular heartbeats, shortness of breath, or swelling of the ankles, feet, or lower legs.

Other side effects not listed above can also occur in some patients.
Tell your doctor or nurse if you develop any problems.

FDA Approval: This drug is approved for cancer treatment.

daunorubicin citrate liposome injection

Trade Name:
DaunoXome

Type of Drug:
Daunorubicin citrate liposome injection belongs to the general group of chemotherapy drugs known as anthracycline antibiotics. It is used to treat Kaposi's sarcoma.

How Drug Works:
Daunorubicin citrate liposome injection is daunorubicin surrounded by a special covering made of fat (liposome) that allows the drug to go directly to the cancer and not be damaged by the body's immune system. Daunorubicin citrate liposome injection stops the growth of cancer cells, causing the cells to die.

How Drug Is Given:
Daunorubicin citrate liposome injection is given by a shot in a vein over 1 hour, usually every 2 weeks. Tell your nurse right away if you get chest pain or tightness, back pain, and/or feel flushed. This can be lessened by slowing or stopping the medicine for a few minutes. You will be given a medicine to stop nausea and/or vomiting. Tell your doctor or nurse if it does not work. Your blood counts will be checked before each treatment. If they are too low, your treatment will be delayed. The dose depends on your size and blood counts, and how well your kidneys and liver are working.

 Read the following information. If you do not understand it or if any of it causes you special concern, check with your doctor.

Before taking this drug, tell your doctor:
- If you are trying to become pregnant, are pregnant, or breastfeeding. This drug may cause birth defects if either the male or female is taking it at the time of conception or during pregnancy. Men and women who are taking this drug need to use some kind of birth control. However, do not use oral contraceptives ("the pill") without checking with your doctor.
- If you think you may want to have children in the future. Many chemotherapy drugs can cause sterility.
- If you have any of the following medical problems: chickenpox or exposure to chickenpox, gout, heart disease, congestive heart failure, shingles, kidney stones, liver disease, or other forms of cancer.
- If you are taking any other prescription or over-the-counter drugs, including vitamins and herbals.

Should I avoid any other medicines, foods, alcohol, and/or activities?
Your prescription and nonprescription medicines may interact with other drugs, causing harm. Certain foods or alcohol can also interact with drug products. Never begin taking a new medicine—prescription or non-prescription—without asking your doctor or nurse if it will interact with alcohol, food, or other medicines. Some drug products can cause drowsiness and affect activities such as driving.

Precautions:
While you are being treated with daunorubicin citrate liposome injection, and after you stop treatment, do not have any immunizations (vaccinations) without your doctor's okay. Try to avoid contact with people who have recently taken the oral polio vaccine. Check with your doctor about this.

Daunorubicin citrate liposome injection can lower your blood counts (white blood cells, red blood cells, platelets). Your doctor will check your blood counts before and after each treatment to see its effect on your blood counts. Your doctor or nurse will give you specific instructions if your blood counts are low.

Daunorubicin citrate liposome injection can cause a decrease in your white blood cell count, especially 7 to 10 days after the drug is given. This may increase your risk of getting an infection. Report fever of 100.5°F or higher, or signs of infection such as pain in passing your urine, coughing, and bringing up sputum.

Daunorubicin citrate liposome injection can lower your platelet count. This may increase your risk of bleeding. DO NOT take any aspirin or aspirin-containing medicines. Report unusual bruising, or bleeding such as nosebleeds, bleeding gums when you brush your teeth, or black, tarry stools.

Daunorubicin citrate liposome injection can injure the heart muscle when large total doses are given. Your doctor will test your heart function before you receive your first treatment, and then during the treatment. This way, any damage can be found early. Talk to your doctor about this.

 Tell all the doctors, dentists, and pharmacists you visit that you are taking this drug.

- Most of the following side effects probably will not occur.
- Your doctor or nurse will want to discuss specific care instructions with you.
- They can help you understand these side effects and help you deal with them.

Side Effects:

More Common Side Effects
Decreased white blood cell count with increased risk of infection
Decreased platelet count with increased risk of bleeding
Mild nausea
Tiredness (fatigue)

Less Common Side Effects
Back pain, flushing, and chest tightness when drug is first given
Vomiting
Loss of appetite
Diarrhea
Moderate nausea

Rare Side Effects
Mild hair loss
Difficulty swallowing
Stomach irritation
Hemorrhoids
Enlarged liver
Dry mouth
Cavities in teeth
Heart damage with congestive heart failure
Dry skin

Other side effects not listed above can also occur in some patients.
Tell your doctor or nurse if you develop any problems.

FDA Approval: This drug is approved for cancer treatment.

denileukin diftitox

Trade Name:
Ontak

Type of Drug:
Denileukin diftitox is a type of molecular targeted therapy called a fusion protein. It is made up of inter-leukin-2 (IL-2) that is fused, or combined, with fragments of diphtheria toxin (a deadly inactive bacteria).

How Drug Works:
Denileukin diftitox attaches to specific cancer cells with receptors for IL-2 and pushes the diphtheria toxin into the cell. This prevents the cell from making protein and kills the cell. It is used to treat T-cell lymphoma of the skin (mycosis fungoides) that has come back.

How Drug Is Given:
Denileukin difitox is given by a shot in a vein over 15 to 80 minutes, once a day, for 5 days. This treatment is usually repeated every 3 weeks for at least 3 treatments. Tell your nurse or doctor right away if you get back pain, flushing, palpitations, itching, or rash, or if you have difficulty speaking or swallowing. If you get any of these symptoms, the medicine will be slowed or stopped for a while, depending upon how you feel. The dose depends on your size and level of a protein (albumin) in your blood. Your blood counts and chemistries will be checked frequently during treatment.

 Read the following information. If you do not understand it or if any of it causes you special concern, check with your doctor.

Before taking this drug, tell your doctor:
- If you are trying to become pregnant, are pregnant, or breastfeeding. This drug may cause birth defects if either the male or female is taking it at the time of conception or during pregnancy. Men and women who are taking this drug need to use some kind of birth control. However, do not use oral contraceptives ("the pill") without checking with your doctor.
- If you think you may want to have children in the future. Many chemotherapy drugs can cause sterility.
- If you have any of the following medical problems: chickenpox or exposure to chickenpox, gout, heart disease, congestive heart failure, shingles, kidney stones, liver disease, or other forms of cancer.
- If you are taking any other prescription or over-the-counter drugs, including vitamins and herbals.

Should I avoid any other medicines, foods, alcohol, and/or activities?
Your prescription and nonprescription medicines may interact with other drugs, causing harm. Certain foods or alcohol can also interact with drug products. Never begin taking a new medicine—prescription or non-prescription—without asking your doctor or nurse if it will interact with alcohol, food, or other medicines. Some drug products can cause drowsiness and affect activities such as driving.

Precautions:
You may develop an allergic reaction to the drug within 24 hours of taking it. Usually it is mild, and you may feel back pain, shortness of breath, flushing, rash, pain or tightness in the chest, and have a lowered blood pressure. Your nurse or doctor will watch you closely during the treatment, and ask you to call right away if you have any problems once you get home.

This drug works by killing cancerous lymphocytes but also kills normal ones. Lymphocytes protect you from certain infections. Thus, you will be at risk for developing infections. Make sure you know how to check your temperature, and call your nurse or doctor if your temperature is over 100.5°F, or if you think you have an infection. Signs or symptoms of infection include a fever, productive cough, or burning when you urinate.

Most patients develop flu-like symptoms, including fever and chills, weakness, nausea with or without vomiting, muscle and/or bone aching. You will receive medicines to prevent these side effects or stop them if they occur. Talk to your nurse or doctor about any questions you may have.

Tell your doctor if you have a heart condition. You will need to be watched closely. This drug may increase or decrease blood pressure, increase your heart rate, or produce an irregular heartbeat. Very rarely, it may cause a heart attack.

The drug may decrease the protein in your blood. This may cause leakage of fluid into the body tissues, causing swelling of the feet, abdomen, or in the lungs. This may lower your blood pressure. Make sure you change position slowly, and hold on to a secure surface when getting up if you are dizzy. Tell your doctor or nurse if you become dizzy and it does not go away.

While you are being treated with denileukin diftitox and after you stop treatment, do not have any immunizations (vaccinations) without your doctor's okay. Try to avoid contact with people who have recently taken the oral polio vaccine, or who have infections.

Although you may have a number of side effects with the first treatment, they usually decrease or disappear with the second.

Because the drug can decrease the protein albumin in your blood, the drug may be withheld until the protein level in your blood is normal.

Tell all the doctors, dentists, and pharmacists you visit that you are taking this drug.

- Most of the following side effects probably will not occur.
- Your doctor or nurse will want to discuss specific care instructions with you.
- They can help you understand these side effects and help you deal with them.

Side Effects:

More Common Side Effects

Decreased blood pressure within 24 hours of drug infusion
Infection
Flu-like symptoms (fever and chills, weakness, aches in muscles)
Nausea and/or vomiting
Back pain within 24 hours of drug infusion

Rash
Shortness of breath within 24 hours of drug infusion
Chest pain or tightness within 24 hours of drug infusion
Low albumin level in the blood and swelling of feet

Less Common Side Effects

Constipation
Loss of appetite
Diarrhea
Weight loss
Increased values on liver function tests of the blood
Decreased calcium level in the blood
Itching of skin

Sweating
Decrease in red blood cell count with risk of anemia and tiredness (fatigue)
Difficulty breathing
Cough
Sore throat
Runny nose

Rare Side Effects

Severe allergic reaction
Difficulty swallowing or talking within 24 hours of drug infusion
Feeling lightheaded within 24 hours of drug infusion
Heartburn
Decreased potassium level in the blood
Blood clots
Increase in blood pressure
Irregular heartbeat

Decreased platelet count with risk of bleeding
Decrease in white blood cell count with risk of infection
Nervousness
Confusion
Difficulty sleeping
Blood in the urine
Protein in the urine
Increased values on kidney function blood test

Side Effects / Symptoms of the Drug

Many patients have a mild reaction during or soon after the drug is given for the first treatment. The side effects are usually much less or absent the next time the treatment is given.

Other side effects not listed above can also occur in some patients.
Tell your doctor or nurse if you develop any problems.

FDA Approval: This drug is approved for cancer treatment.

dexamethasone

Trade Names:
Decadron, Deronil, Dexasone, Dexone, Hexadrol, Mymethasone

Type of Drug:
Dexamethasone is a glucocorticoid steroid. It is similar to the steroid hormone made by the adrenal glands in the body.

How Drug Works:
Dexamethasone is a strong anti-inflammatory agent. This drug works by preventing white blood cells from completing an inflammatory reaction. It is used to reduce swelling of brain tissues during radiation treatments to the brain. This drug can cause lymphocytes, a type of white blood cell, to break apart and die. Thus it is an important drug used in combination with chemotherapy for the treatment of lymphoma, leukemia, and multiple myeloma. The drug is sometimes given to reduce the likelihood that a person will have an allergic reaction to a chemotherapeutic agent, such as paclitaxel. Finally, this medicine is used to prevent nausea and vomiting from chemotherapy, in combination with other drugs.

How Drug Is Given:
Dexamethasone can be given as a pill or as a shot in a vein over 5 minutes. Take the pill with food or milk to protect the stomach from irritation. When given as a shot in the vein, you may be given special medicine to stop the acid in your stomach. The dose and how often you take it depends on the reason you are taking dexamethasone. Make sure you tell your doctor if you have a history of ulcers, as dexamethasone can make them bleed or rupture. Keep the medicine in a tightly closed container away from heat and moisture and out of the reach of children and pets.

How Should I Take This Drug?
Take this drug exactly as directed by your doctor. If you do not understand the instructions, ask your doctor or nurse to explain them to you. This drug can be given at different strengths depending on the type of cancer being treated. Dosage may vary depending on your weight and your type of cancer.

 Read the following information. If you do not understand it or if any of it causes you special concern, check with your doctor.

Before taking this drug, tell your doctor:
- If you are trying to become pregnant, are pregnant, or breastfeeding. This drug may cause birth defects if either the male or female is taking it at the time of conception or during pregnancy. Men and women who are taking this drug need to use some kind of birth control. However, do not use oral contraceptives ("the pill") without checking with your doctor.
- If you think you may want to have children in the future. Many chemotherapy drugs can cause sterility.
- If you have any of the following medical problems: chickenpox or exposure to chickenpox, gout, heart disease, congestive heart failure, shingles, kidney stones, liver disease, or other forms of cancer.
- If you are taking any other prescription or over-the-counter drugs, including vitamins and herbals.

Should I avoid any other medicines, foods, alcohol, and/or activities?
Your prescription and nonprescription medicines may interact with other drugs, causing harm. Certain foods or alcohol can also interact with drug products. Never begin taking a new medicine—prescription or nonprescription—without asking your doctor or nurse if it will interact with alcohol, food, or other medicines. Some drug products can cause drowsiness and affect activities such as driving.

Precautions:
Dexamethasone can irritate the stomach, so the pill form must be taken with food. If you develop stomach pain or vomit any blood, tell your doctor immediately. If you have a stomach ulcer, you may not be able to take this drug without extra protective medicines.

This drug suppresses the immune system so it can increase susceptibility to infections. In addition, the drug may mask the signs of infections, such as fever.

When you are taking dexamethasone, do not have any immunizations (vaccinations) without your doctor's okay. Try to avoid contact with people who have recently taken the oral polio vaccine or who have chickenpox or measles. Check with your doctor about this.

If you take dexamethasone for a long time, do not stop the medicine abruptly as this can cause a decrease in the steroid hormones you body makes (adrenal insufficiency). Symptoms of this are nausea, loss of appetite, tiredness (fatigue), dizziness, difficulty breathing, joint pain, depression, low blood sugar, and low blood pressure.

If you are a diabetic, this medicine will raise your blood sugar levels, and you may need to take extra diabetes medicine. Talk to your doctor about this.

When this drug is taken for a long time, some side effects may not occur until months after the drug is used.

Tell all the doctors, dentists, and pharmacists you visit that you are taking this drug.

- Most of the following side effects probably will not occur.
- Your doctor or nurse will want to discuss specific care instructions with you.
- They can help you understand these side effects and help you deal with them.

Side Effects:

More Common Side Effects

Increased appetite with weight gain
Sodium and fluid retention with swelling of ankles, increased blood pressure, congestive heart failure
Depression
Increased blood sugar

Sleep disturbance
Increased risk of infection
Bruising of the skin
Mood changes
Delayed wound healing

Less Common Side Effects

Decrease in serum potassium (symptoms are loss of appetite, muscle twitching, increased thirst, frequent urination)
Fracture of weak bones
Fungal infections (white patches in mouth, vagina)

Sweating
Diarrhea
Nausea
Headache
Increased heart rate
Loss of calcium from bones

Rare Side Effects

Cataracts
Personality changes
Blurred vision
Stomach ulcer, which may bleed (hemorrhage)

Side Effects / Symptoms of the Drug

Tell your doctor or nurse immediately if you develop any of the following: stomach pain or vomiting blood; new bone pain; signs of infection such as fever, bad cough, and bringing up sputum; or burning when you pass urine. Always take the pill form with food or milk.

Other side effects not listed above can also occur in some patients.
Tell your doctor or nurse if you develop any problems.

FDA Approval: This drug is approved for cancer treatment.

dexrazoxane

Trade Name:
Zinecard

Type of Drug:
Dexrazoxane belongs to the general group of drugs known as cytoprotective agents. It may be used to protect the heart in patients who are receiving chemotherapy medicines such as doxorubicin hydrochloride and daunorubicin that can affect the heart.

How Drug Works:
Dexrazoxane protects the heart from damage caused by high total amounts of chemotherapy that affect the heart. Its exact mechanism is not known.

How Drug Is Given:
Dexrazoxane is given by a shot in a vein before you get the anticancer drug doxorubicin hydrochloride. The dose depends upon the dose of doxorubicin hydrochloride, which depends on your size and blood counts.

 Read the following information. If you do not understand it or if any of it causes you special concern, check with your doctor.

Before taking this drug, tell your doctor:
- If you are trying to become pregnant, are pregnant, or breastfeeding. This drug may cause birth defects if either the male or female is taking it at the time of conception or during pregnancy. Men and women who are taking this drug need to use some kind of birth control. However, do not use oral contraceptives ("the pill") without checking with your doctor.
- If you think you may want to have children in the future. Many chemotherapy drugs can cause sterility.
- If you have any of the following medical problems: chickenpox or exposure to chickenpox, gout, heart disease, congestive heart failure, shingles, kidney stones, liver disease, or other forms of cancer.
- If you are taking any other prescription or over-the-counter drugs, including vitamins and herbals.

Should I avoid any other medicines, foods, alcohol, and/or activities?
Your prescription and nonprescription medicines may interact with other drugs, causing harm. Certain foods or alcohol can also interact with drug products. Never begin taking a new medicine—prescription or nonprescription—without asking your doctor or nurse if it will interact with alcohol, food, or other medicines. Some drug products can cause drowsiness and affect activities such as driving.

Precautions:
Dexrazoxane can increase doxorubicine hydrochloride's effect on your white blood cell count, especially 10 to 14 days after the drug is given. This can increase your risk of getting an infection. Report fever of 100.5°F or higher, or signs of infection such as pain in passing urine, or coughing and bringing up sputum.

Dexrazoxane can increase doxorubicine hydrochloride's effect on your platelet count. This can increase your risk of bleeding. DO NOT take any aspirin or aspirin-containing medicines. Report unusual bruising, or bleeding such as nosebleeds, bleeding gums when you brush your teeth, or black, tarry stools.

Tell all the doctors, dentists, and pharmacists you visit that you are taking this drug.

- Most of the following side effects probably will not occur.
- Your doctor or nurse will want to discuss specific care instructions with you.
- They can help you understand these side effects and help you deal with them.

Side Effects:

More Common Side Effects
Lowered white blood cell count with higher risk of infection
Lowered platelet count with higher risk of bleeding

Less Common Side Effects
Pain at place of injection
Increase in liver and kidney blood tests

Rare Side Effects
Tiredess (fatigue)

Other side effects not listed above can also occur in some patients.
Tell your doctor or nurse if you develop any problems.

FDA Approval: This drug is approved for cancer treatment.

diethylstilbestrol

Trade Names:
DES, Stilbestrol, Stilphostrol

Type of Drug:
Diethylstilbestrol is an estrogen and belongs to the general group of drugs known as hormones or hormone antagonists. It is used to treat advanced prostate cancer and advanced breast cancer in women who are postmenopausal.

How Drug Works:
Diethylstilbestrol stops the growth of cancer cells that depend on the male hormone (androgen) or the female hormone (estrogen) to grow and divide.

How Drug Is Given:
Diethylstilbestrol is a pill taken by mouth, 1 to 3 times a day. The dose, how often, and for how long your doctor tells you to take the pills depends on the stage and type of cancer being treated. Try to take the pill(s) at the same time every day as directed with a glass of water. Keep the medicine in a tightly closed container away from heat and moisture and out of the reach of children and pets.

How Should I Take This Drug?
Take this drug exactly as directed by your doctor. If you do not understand the instructions, ask your doctor or nurse to explain them to you. This drug can be given at different strengths depending on the type of cancer being treated. Dosage may vary depending on your weight and your type of cancer.

 Read the following information. If you do not understand it or if any of it causes you special concern, check with your doctor.

Before taking this drug, tell your doctor:
- If you are trying to become pregnant, are pregnant, or breastfeeding. This drug may cause birth defects if either the male or female is taking it at the time of conception or during pregnancy. Men and women who are taking this drug need to use some kind of birth control. However, do not use oral contraceptives ("the pill") without checking with your doctor.
- If you think you may want to have children in the future. Many chemotherapy drugs can cause sterility.
- If you have any of the following medical problems: chickenpox or exposure to chickenpox, gout, heart disease, congestive heart failure, shingles, kidney stones, liver disease, or other forms of cancer.
- If you are taking any other prescription or over-the-counter drugs, including vitamins and herbals.

Should I avoid any other medicines, foods, alcohol, and/or activities?
Your prescription and nonprescription medicines may interact with other drugs, causing harm. Certain foods or alcohol can also interact with drug products. Never begin taking a new medicine—prescription or nonprescription—without asking your doctor or nurse if it will interact with alcohol, food, or other medicines. Some drug products can cause drowsiness and affect activities such as driving.

Precautions:
Patients with heart, kidney, or liver damage should use diethylstilbestrol cautiously.

In rare cases, diethylstilbestrol may cause blood clots to form in the legs or in the lungs.

Tell your doctor right away if you develop any of the following: pain, redness or swelling in the calf of your leg, shortness of breath, sudden severe headache, changes in vision, weakness or sensation of pins and needles in your arm or leg, chest pain, coughing up blood, or feeling faint.

Tell all the doctors, dentists, and pharmacists you visit that you are taking this drug.

- Most of the following side effects probably will not occur.
- Your doctor or nurse will want to discuss specific care instructions with you.
- They can help you understand these side effects and help you deal with them.

Side Effects:

More Common Side Effects
Increase in breast size
Decreased sexual desire
Change in voice
Breast tenderness

Less Common Side Effects
Nausea and vomiting, which go away after a few weeks of treatment
Uterine bleeding
Loss of bladder control

Rare Side Effects
Blood clot in leg or lungs
Increased calcium blood level for a short time after the drug is started

Other side effects not listed above can also occur in some patients.
Tell your doctor or nurse if you develop any problems.

FDA Approval: This drug is approved for cancer treatment.

docetaxel

Trade Name:
Taxotere

Type of Drug:
Docetaxel belongs to the general group of chemotherapy drugs known as taxanes. It is also called a mitotic inhibitor because of its effect on the cell during mitosis. It is used to treat locally advanced or metastatic breast and lung cancers.

How Drug Works:
Docetaxel stops the growth of cancer cells, causing the cells to die.

How Drug Is Given:
Docetaxel is given by a shot in a vein over 1 hour, every 3 weeks, or in lower doses, weekly. You will probably get another medicine, dexamethasone, to take the day before and for 2 days after to lessen the chance you will get swelling in your body. Also, you will probably get an antinausea medicine before the docetaxel, especially if the medicine is given every 3 weeks. The dose depends on your size, how well your liver is working, and how often the medicine is given. Your blood counts will be checked before treatment; if they are too low, the dose may be lowered or the treatment delayed.

 Read the following information. If you do not understand it or if any of it causes you special concern, check with your doctor.

Before taking this drug, tell your doctor:
• If you are trying to become pregnant, are pregnant, or breastfeeding. This drug may cause birth defects if either the male or female is taking it at the time of conception or during pregnancy. Men and women who are taking this drug need to use some kind of birth control. However, do not use oral contraceptives ("the pill") without checking with your doctor.
• If you think you may want to have children in the future. Many chemotherapy drugs can cause sterility.
• If you have any of the following medical problems: chickenpox or exposure to chickenpox, gout, heart disease, congestive heart failure, shingles, kidney stones, liver disease, or other forms of cancer.
• If you are taking any other prescription or over-the-counter drugs, including vitamins and herbals.

Should I avoid any other medicines, foods, alcohol, and/or activities?
Your prescription and nonprescription medicines may interact with other drugs, causing harm. Certain foods or alcohol can also interact with drug products. Never begin taking a new medicine—prescription or non-prescription—without asking your doctor or nurse if it will interact with alcohol, food, or other medicines. Some drug products can cause drowsiness and affect activities such as driving.

Precautions:
While you are being treated with docetaxel, and after you stop treatment, do not have any immunizations (vaccinations) without your doctor's okay. Try to avoid contact with people who have recently taken the oral polio vaccine. Check with your doctor about this.

Docetaxel can lower your blood counts (white blood cells, red blood cells, platelets). Your doctor will check your blood counts before and after each treatment to see how it affects your blood counts. Your doctor or nurse will give you specific instructions if your blood counts are low.

Docetaxel can lower your white blood cell count, especially 9 days after the drug is given. This can increase your risk of getting an infection. Report fever of 100.5°F or higher, or signs of infection such as pain in passing your urine, coughing, and bringing up sputum.

Docetaxel can lower your platelet count. This can increase your risk of bleeding. DO NOT take any aspirin or aspirin-containing medicines. Report unusual bruising, or bleeding such as nosebleeds, bleeding gums when you brush your teeth, or black, tarry stools.

Getting a wig before starting treatment may make it easier to deal with hair loss. Talk to your nurse or doctor about this. If your insurance does not cover it, there may be other resources to help you. Hair loss is temporary, and your hair will grow back after treatment.

Rarely, it is possible to have an allergic reaction when docetaxel is given. You may receive medicines to prevent this.

 Tell all the doctors, dentists, and pharmacists you visit that you are taking this drug.
- -
- Most of the following side effects probably will not occur.
- Your doctor or nurse will want to discuss specific care instructions with you.
- They can help you understand these side effects and help you deal with them.

Side Effects:

More Common Side Effects
Decreased white blood cell count with increased risk of infection
Decreased platelet count with increased risk of bleeding
Hair thinning or loss
Diarrhea
Loss of appetite
Nausea
Vomiting
Rash
Numbness and tingling in hands and/or feet related to peripheral nerve irritation or damage

Less Common Side Effects
Sores in mouth or on lips
Swelling of ankles or hands
Increased weight due to fluid retention
Tiredness (fatigue)
Muscle aches

Rare Side Effects
Severe allergic reaction
Redness, swelling and pain in hands and/or feet

Side Effects / Symptoms of the Drug
Tell your doctor or nurse if you develop swelling of the ankles, shortness of breath, weight gain, or your clothes feel too tight at the waist.

Other side effects not listed above can also occur in some patients.
Tell your doctor or nurse if you develop any problems.

FDA Approval: This drug is approved for cancer treatment.

doxorubicin hydrochloride

Trade Name:
Adriamycin

Type of Drug:
Doxorubicin hydrochloride belongs to the general group of chemotherapy drugs known as anthracycline antibiotics. It is used to treat non-Hodgkin's lymphoma, multiple myeloma, acute leukemias, and cancers of the breast, adrenal cortex, endometrium, lung, and ovary.

How Drug Works:
Doxorubicin stops the growth of cancer cells, causing the cells to die.

How Drug Is Given:
Doxorubicin hydrochloride is given as a shot in a vein over about 15 minutes. Tell the nurse right away if you feel pain, burning, or discomfort in the vein when it is given. You will get medicine to stop any nausea or vomiting before the doxorubicin hydrochloride and to take afterward. The dose and how often you get the medicine depends on your size, your blood counts, how well your liver is working, and the type of cancer being treated. You will have your blood counts checked before each treatment; if they are too low, your treatment will be delayed. This medicine may be given in addition to other anticancer medicines.

 Read the following information. If you do not understand it or if any of it causes you special concern, check with your doctor.

Before taking this drug, tell your doctor:
- If you are trying to become pregnant, are pregnant, or breastfeeding. This drug may cause birth defects if either the male or female is taking it at the time of conception or during pregnancy. Men and women who are taking this drug need to use some kind of birth control. However, do not use oral contraceptives ("the pill") without checking with your doctor.
- If you think you may want to have children in the future. Many chemotherapy drugs can cause sterility.
- If you have any of the following medical problems: chickenpox or exposure to chickenpox, gout, heart disease, congestive heart failure, shingles, kidney stones, liver disease, or other forms of cancer.
- If you are taking any other prescription or over-the-counter drugs, including vitamins and herbals.

Should I avoid any other medicines, foods, alcohol, and/or activities?
Your prescription and nonprescription medicines may interact with other drugs, causing harm. Certain foods or alcohol can also interact with drug products. Never begin taking a new medicine—prescription or non-prescription—without asking your doctor or nurse if it will interact with alcohol, food, or other medicines. Some drug products can cause drowsiness and affect activities such as driving.

Precautions:
While you are being treated with doxorubicin hydrochloride, and after you stop treatment, do not have any immunizations (vaccinations) without your doctor's okay. Try to avoid contact with people who have recently taken the oral polio vaccine. Check with your doctor about this.

Doxorubicin hydrochloride can lower your blood counts (white blood cells, red blood cells, platelets). Your doctor will check your blood counts before and after each treatment to see how it affects your blood counts. Your doctor or nurse will give you specific instructions if your blood counts are low.

Doxorubicin hydrochloride can cause a decrease in your white blood cell count, especially 10 to 14 days after the drug is given. This can increase your risk of getting an infection. Report fever of 100.5°F or higher, or signs of infection such as pain in passing your urine, coughing, and bringing up sputum.

Doxorubicin hydrochloride can cause a decrease in the platelet count. This can increase your risk of bleeding. DO NOT take any aspirin or aspirin-containing medicines. Report unusual bruising, or bleeding such as nosebleeds, bleeding gums when you brush your teeth, or black, tarry stools.

Getting a wig before starting treatment may make it easier to deal with hair loss. Talk to your nurse or doctor about this. If your insurance does not cover it, there may be other resources to help you. Hair loss is temporary, and your hair will grow back after treatment.

Doxorubicin hydrochloride is given intravenously. If the drug accidentally leaks out of the vein where it is given, it may damage the tissue and cause scarring. Tell the nurse right away if you notice redness, pain, or swelling at the place of injection.

Doxorubicin hydrochloride can injure the heart muscle when large total doses are given. Your doctor will test your heart function test before you receive your first treatment, and then during the treatment. This way, any damage can be found early. Talk to your doctor about this.

Doxorubicin hydrochloride can cause radiation recall. When a person has had radiation therapy and then receives this drug, the skin or tissue damage from the prior radiation therapy can become red and appear damaged again. Tell your doctor if your skin gets red in areas where radiation was given.

Doxorubicin hydrochloride can cause severe nausea and vomiting. Ask your doctor or nurse to give you medicines to prevent or lessen this.

Tell all the doctors, dentists, and pharmacists you visit that you are taking this drug.
- Most of the following side effects probably will not occur.
- Your doctor or nurse will want to discuss specific care instructions with you.
- They can help you understand these side effects and help you deal with them.

Side Effects:

More Common Side Effects
Decreased white blood cell count with increased risk of infection
Decreased platelet count with increased risk of bleeding
Loss of appetite
Darkening of nail beds and skin creases of hands
Hair loss
Nausea
Vomiting

Less Common Side Effects
Sores in mouth or on lips
Radiation recall skin changes
Fetal abnormalities if taken while pregnant or if becoming pregnant while on this drug

Rare Side Effects
Temporary changes in electrocardiogram (EKG)
Irregular heartbeat
Heart damage with congestive heart failure

Side Effects / Symptoms of the Drug
Doxorubicin causes the urine to turn a reddish color, which may stain clothes. This is not blood. It is normal and lasts for 1 to 2 days after each dose is given.

After you stop receiving doxorubicin, the drug may still produce some side effects that need attention. Tell your doctor or nurse if you get any irregular heartbeats, shortness of breath, or swelling of the ankles, feet, or lower legs.

Other side effects not listed above can also occur in some patients.
Tell your doctor or nurse if you develop any problems.

FDA Approval: This drug is approved for cancer treatment.

doxorubicin hydrochloride liposome injection

Trade Name:
Doxil

Type of Drug:
Doxorubicin hydrochloride liposome injection belongs to the general group of chemotherapy drugs known as anthracycline antibiotics that are lipid encapsulated. It is used to treat Kaposi's sarcoma and metastatic ovarian cancer.

How Drug Works:
Doxorubicin hydrochloride liposome injection is doxorubicin surrounded by a special covering made of fat (liposome) that allows the drug to go directly to the cancer and not be damaged by the body's immune system. Doxorubicin hydrochloride liposome injection stops the growth of cancer cells, causing them to die.

How Drug Is Given:
Doxorubicin hydrochloride liposome injection is given by a shot in a vein over 1 hour, usually every 4 weeks. Tell your nurse right away if you get chest pain or tightness, back pain, and/or feel flushed. The medicine may need to be stopped until you feel better. You will be given a medicine to stop nausea and/or vomiting. Make sure to tell your doctor or nurse if it does not work. Your blood counts will be checked before each treatment; if they are too low, your treatment will be delayed. The dose depends upon your size and blood counts and how well your liver is working.

 Read the following information. If you do not understand it or if any of it causes you special concern, check with your doctor.

Before taking this drug, tell your doctor:
- If you are trying to become pregnant, are pregnant, or breastfeeding. This drug may cause birth defects if either the male or female is taking it at the time of conception or during pregnancy. Men and women who are taking this drug need to use some kind of birth control. However, do not use oral contraceptives ("the pill") without checking with your doctor.
- If you think you may want to have children in the future. Many chemotherapy drugs can cause sterility.
- If you have any of the following medical problems: chickenpox or exposure to chickenpox, gout, heart disease, congestive heart failure, shingles, kidney stones, liver disease, or other forms of cancer.
- If you are taking any other prescription or over-the-counter drugs, including vitamins and herbals.

Should I avoid any other medicines, foods, alcohol, and/or activities?
Your prescription and nonprescription medicines may interact with other drugs, causing harm. Certain foods or alcohol can also interact with drug products. Never begin taking a new medicine—prescription or non-prescription—without asking your doctor or nurse if it will interact with alcohol, food, or other medicines. Some drug products can cause drowsiness and affect activities such as driving.

Precautions:
While you are being treated with doxorubicin hydrochloride liposome injection, and after you stop treatment, do not have any immunizations (vaccinations) without your doctor's okay. Try to avoid contact with people who have recently taken the oral polio vaccine. Check with your doctor about this.

Doxorubicin hydrochloride liposome injection can lower your blood counts (white blood cells, red blood cells, platelets). Your doctor will check your blood counts before and after each treatment to see how it affects your blood counts. Your doctor or nurse will give you specific instructions if your blood counts are low.

Doxorubicin hydrochloride liposome injection can decrease your white blood cell count, especially 10 to 14 days after the drug is given. This can increase your risk of getting an infection. Report fever of 100.5°F or higher, or signs of infection such as pain in passing your urine, coughing, and bringing up sputum.

Doxorubicin hydrochloride liposome injection can decrease the platelet count. This can increase your risk of bleeding. DO NOT take any aspirin or aspirin-containing medicines. Report unusual bruising, or bleeding such as nosebleeds, bleeding gums when you brush your teeth, or black, tarry stools.

Doxorubicin hydrochloride liposome injection can cause swelling, redness, and/or pain on the palms of the hands and/or soles of the feet. Tell your doctor or nurse if this occurs.

Rarely, doxorubicin hydrochloride liposome injection can cause a reaction when the infusion starts. Tell your nurse if you feel flushed or short of breath, or if you have chest tightness, chills, back pain, headache, or swelling of your face.

Doxorubicin hydrochloride liposome injection can injure your heart muscle if large total doses are given. Your doctor will test your heart function before you receive your first treatment, and then during the treatment. This way, any damage can be found early. Talk to your doctor about this.

Doxorubicin hydrochloride liposome injection can cause radiation recall. When a person has had radiation therapy and then receives this drug, the skin or tissue damage from prior radiation therapy can become red and appear damaged again. Tell your doctor or nurse if your skin gets red in areas where radiation was given.

Tell all the doctors, dentists, and pharmacists you visit that you are taking this drug.

- Most of the following side effects probably will not occur.
- Your doctor or nurse will want to discuss specific care instructions with you.
- They can help you understand these side effects and help you deal with them.

Side Effects:

More Common Side Effects

Decreased white blood cell count with increased risk of infection

Decreased platelet count with increased risk of bleeding

Less Common Side Effects

Swelling, pain, redness of hands and/or feet
Mild nausea
Mild vomiting
Diarrhea

Sores in mouth and on legs
Hair loss
Fetal abnormalities if taken while pregnant or if pregnancy occurs while taking this drug

Rare Side Effects

Flushing, shortness of breath, swelling of the face, chills, back pain, headache, and/or chest tightness during the infusion
Irregular heartbeat

Loss of appetite
Radiation recall skin changes
Rash
Itching
Heart damage with congestive heart failure

Side Effects / Symptoms of the Drug

After you stop receiving doxorubicin hydrochloride liposome injections, the drug may still produce some side effects that need attention.

Tell your doctor or nurse if you get any irregular heartbeats, shortness of breath, or swelling of the ankles, feet or lower legs.

Other side effects not listed above can also occur in some patients.
Tell your doctor or nurse if you develop any problems.

FDA Approval: This drug is approved for cancer treatment.

epirubicin hydrochloride

Trade Names:
Ellence, Farmorubicin(e), Farmorubicina, Pharmorubicin

Type of Drug:
Epirubicin hydrochloride belongs to the general group of chemotherapy drugs known as anthracycline antibiotics. It is used together with other drugs to treat breast cancer after surgery to prevent any breast cancer cells from coming back.

How Drug Works:
Epirubicin hydrochloride stops the growth of cancer cells, causing the cells to die.

How Drug Is Given:
Epirubicin hydrochloride is given as a shot in a vein over about 15 minutes. Tell the nurse right away if you feel pain, burning, or discomfort in the vein when it is given. You will get medicine to stop any nausea or vomiting before the epirubicin, and to take afterward. The dose and how often you get epirubicin hydrochloride depends upon your size, your blood counts, how well your liver is working, and the type of cancer being treated. You will have your blood counts checked before each treatment; if they are too low, your treatment will be delayed. This medicine may be given in addition to other chemotherapy medicines.

 Read the following information. If you do not understand it or if any of it causes you special concern, check with your doctor.

Before taking this drug, tell your doctor:
- If you are trying to become pregnant, are pregnant, or breastfeeding. This drug may cause birth defects if either the male or female is taking it at the time of conception or during pregnancy. Men and women who are taking this drug need to use some kind of birth control. However, do not use oral contraceptives ("the pill") without checking with your doctor.
- If you think you may want to have children in the future. Many chemotherapy drugs can cause sterility.
- If you have any of the following medical problems: chickenpox or exposure to chickenpox, gout, heart disease, congestive heart failure, shingles, kidney stones, liver disease, or other forms of cancer.
- If you are taking any other prescription or over-the-counter drugs, including vitamins and herbals.

Should I avoid any other medicines, foods, alcohol, and/or activities?
Your prescription and nonprescription medicines may interact with other drugs, causing harm. Certain foods or alcohol can also interact with drug products. Never begin taking a new medicine—prescription or nonprescription—without asking your doctor or nurse if it will interact with alcohol, food, or other medicines. Some drug products can cause drowsiness and affect activities such as driving.

Precautions:
Tell your doctor if you are taking cimetidine (Tagamet). You should not take this drug during epirubicin hydrochloride therapy because it increases levels of chemotherapy in your blood.

You should not take this medicine if you have had a recent heart attack, have severe heart problems, have had an allergic reaction to other anthracycline chemotherapy medicines, or have received large doses of another anthracycline drug.

Doses of epirubicin will be reduced if you have any liver problems.

While you are being treated with epirubicin hydrochloride, and after you stop treatment, do not have any immunizations (vaccinations) without your doctor's okay. Try to avoid contact with people who have recently taken the oral polio vaccine or who have infections.

Epirubicin hydrochloride can lower your blood counts (white blood cells, red blood cells, platelets). Your doctor will check your blood counts before and after each treatment to see how it affects your blood counts.

Epirubicin can lower your white blood cell count, especially 10 to 14 days after the drug is given. This can increase your risk of getting an infection. Report fever, of 100.5°F or higher, or signs of infection such as a sore throat, productive cough, or burning on urination.

Epirubicin hydrochloride can lower your platelet count. This can increase your risk of bleeding. DO NOT take any aspirin or aspirin-containing medicines. Report unusual bruising, bleeding such as nosebleeds or bleeding gums when you brush your teeth, or black, tarry stools.

Epirubicin hydrochloride is given intravenously. If the drug accidentally leaks out of the vein where it is given, it may damage the tissue and cause scarring. Tell the nurse right away if you notice redness, pain, or swelling at the injection site during the treatment or afterward.

Epirubicin hydrochloride can injure the heart muscle when large total doses are given. Your doctor will test your heart function before you receive your first treatment, and then during treatment. This way, any changes in heart function can be found early, and the drug can be stopped before any serious injury occurs.

Epirubicin hydrochloride can cause radiation recall. When a person has had radiation therapy and then receives this drug, the skin or tissue damage from prior radiation therapy can become red and appear damaged again. Tell your doctor or nurse if your skin gets red in areas where radiation was given.

Epirubicin hydrochloride can cause severe nausea and vomiting. Ask your doctor or nurse to give you medicines to prevent or lessen this.

Getting a wig before starting treatment may make it easier to deal with hair loss. Talk to your nurse or doctor about this. If your insurance does not cover it, there may be other resources to help you. Hair loss is temporary, and your hair will grow back after treatment.

 Tell all the doctors, dentists, and pharmacists you visit that you are taking this drug.

- Most of the following side effects probably will not occur.
- Your doctor or nurse will want to discuss specific care instructions with you.
- They can help you understand these side effects and help you deal with them.

Side Effects:

More Common Side Effects

Decreased white blood cell count with increased risk of infection
Decreased platelet count with increased risk of bleeding
Decreased red blood cell count with increased risk of anemia and tiredness (fatigue)
Stopping of menstrual periods in women

Tiredness (fatigue)
Nausea
Vomiting
Sores in mouth
Diarrhea
Hair loss

Less Common Side Effects
Irritation of the eyes (conjunctivitis)

Rare Side Effects
Loss of appetite
Fever
Darkening of nails and skin
Radiation recall skin changes

Facial flushing
Heart damage with congestive heart failure

Side Effects / Symptoms of the Drug
Epirubicin hydrochloride causes the urine to turn pink for 1 to 2 days after treatment, so do not be alarmed.

After you stop receiving epirubicin hydrochloride, the drug may still cause later changes in your heart. It is important to make sure any new doctor, such as your primary care doctor, knows that you have received this medicine.

Rarely, people who have received this drug develop long-term side effects. Report any changes in your condition, even if it is months or years after you receive the drug.

Rarely, people can develop a second cancer. Discuss this with your doctor.

Other side effects not listed above can also occur in some patients.
Tell your doctor or nurse if you develop any problems.

FDA Approval: This drug is approved for cancer treatment.

epoetin alfa

Trade Names:
Epogen, Procrit

Type of Drug:
Epoetin alfa belongs to a general class of synthetic substances called biologic response modifiers. This drug is made by recombinant DNA techniques. It is used to prevent or treat anemia (low red blood cell count) after chemotherapy.

How Drug Works:
Epoetin alfa is similar to a hormone in your body that makes the body's bone marrow produce more red blood cells. Thus, this drug can make the body produce more red blood cells.

How Drug Is Given:
Epoetin alfa is given by a shot under the skin once a week. You or a family member can learn how to give the shot at home. Make sure to keep the medicine in its original container in the refrigerator, and the shot equipment in a safe place out of reach of children and pets. Keep used needles in a closed needle bucket and bring them back to your doctor or nurse.

How Should I Take This Drug?
Take this drug exactly as directed by your doctor. If you do not understand the instructions, ask your doctor or nurse to explain them to you.

 Read the following information. If you do not understand it or if any of it causes you special concern, check with your doctor.

Before taking this drug, tell your doctor:
- If you are trying to become pregnant, are pregnant, or breastfeeding. This drug may cause birth defects if either the male or female is taking it at the time of conception or during pregnancy. Men and women who are taking this drug need to use some kind of birth control. However, do not use oral contraceptives ("the pill") without checking with your doctor.
- If you think you may want to have children in the future. Many chemotherapy drugs can cause sterility.
- If you have any of the following medical problems: chickenpox or exposure to chickenpox, gout, heart disease, congestive heart failure, shingles, kidney stones, liver disease, or other forms of cancer.
- If you are taking any other prescription or over-the-counter drugs, including vitamins and herbals.

Should I avoid any other medicines, foods, alcohol, and/or activities?
Your prescription and nonprescription medicines may interact with other drugs, causing harm. Certain foods or alcohol can also interact with drug products. Never begin taking a new medicine—prescription or non-prescription—without asking your doctor or nurse if it will interact with alcohol, food, or other medicines. Some drug products can cause drowsiness and affect activities such as driving.

Precautions:
Symptoms of anemia (tiredness, low energy level, headache) will go away once your red blood count increases.

Tell all the doctors, dentists, and pharmacists you visit that you are taking this drug.
- Most of the following side effects probably will not occur.
- Your doctor or nurse will want to discuss specific care instructions with you.
- They can help you understand these side effects and help you deal with them.

Side Effects:

Less Common Side Effects
Fever
Tiredness (fatigue)
Headache
Hives

Other side effects not listed above can also occur in some patients.
Tell your doctor or nurse if you develop any problems.

FDA Approval: This drug is approved for cancer treatment.

erlotinib

Trade Names:
Tarceva, OSI-774

Type of Drug:
Erlotinib is an epidermal growth factor receptor (EGFR) tyrosine kinase inhibitor used in molecular targeted therapy. It is one of a new group of drugs that targets tiny flaws in the cell's communication machinery. It is being studied in many different cancers including breast cancer.

How Drug Works:
Erlotinib blocks the tyrosene kinase protein in the cancer cell from getting a message that tells the cell to grow and divide. This causes the cells to stop growing.

How Drug Is Given:
Erlotinib is a pill taken by mouth. Take the dose each morning as directed with a large glass of water, with or without food. The dose depends on your size and the investigational study. Keep the medicine in a tightly closed container away from heat and moisture and out of the reach of children and pets.

How Should I Take This Drug?
Take this drug exactly as directed by your doctor. If you do not understand the instructions, ask your doctor or nurse to explain them to you. This drug can be given at different strengths depending on the type of cancer being treated. Dosage may vary depending on your weight and your type of cancer.

 Read the following information. If you do not understand it or if any of it causes you special concern, check with your doctor.

Before taking this drug, tell your doctor:
- If you are trying to become pregnant, are pregnant, or breastfeeding. This drug may cause birth defects if either the male or female is taking it at the time of conception or during pregnancy. Men and women who are taking this drug need to use some kind of birth control. However, do not use oral contraceptives ("the pill") without checking with your doctor.
- If you think you may want to have children in the future. Many chemotherapy drugs can cause sterility.
- If you have any of the following medical problems: chickenpox or exposure to chickenpox, gout, heart disease, congestive heart failure, shingles, kidney stones, liver disease, or other forms of cancer.
- If you are taking any other prescription or over-the-counter drugs, including vitamins and herbals.

Should I avoid any other medicines, foods, alcohol, and/or activities?
Your prescription and nonprescription medicines may interact with other drugs, causing harm. Certain foods or alcohol can also interact with drug products. Never begin taking a new medicine—prescription or nonprescription—without asking your doctor or nurse if it will interact with alcohol, food, or other medicines. Some drug products can cause drowsiness and affect activities such as driving.

Precautions:
Erlotinib may injure the corneas in your eyes so you should have a full eye exam by an eye doctor (ophthalmologist) before starting treatment. You should not wear contact lenses while taking the drug.

Erlotinib can cause heart damage so a special heart study is done to test heart function before you start the drug.

If you develop eye problems, diarrhea, or a severe rash, the drug dose must be modified. Your nurse or doctor will teach you how to manage diarrhea if it develops. Make sure that you understand the instructions, and when and who to call if needed.

You might develop a rash on face, neck, chest, back, and arms, beginning on days 8 to 10 of treatment, peaking at 2 weeks, and then getting better by the fourth week.

While you are being treated with erlotinib and after you stop treatment, do not have any immunizations (vaccinations) without your doctor's okay. Try to avoid contact with people who have recently taken the oral polio vaccine. Check with your doctor about this.

Tell all the doctors, dentists, and pharmacists you visit that you are taking this drug.
- -
- Most of the following side effects probably will not occur.
- Your doctor or nurse will want to discuss specific care instructions with you.
- They can help you understand these side effects and help you deal with them.

Side Effects:

More Common Side Effects
Rash on face, neck, chest, back, and arms
Diarrhea

Less Common Side Effects
Mild headache
Sore mouth

Rare Side Effects
Inflammation of the cornea in the eye
Puncture of the cornea

Side Effects / Symptoms of the Drug
Call your doctor or nurse right away if you develop any changes in your vision, eye pain, severe rash, or diarrhea that lasts for more than 1 day.

Other side effects not listed above can also occur in some patients.
Tell your doctor or nurse if you develop any problems.

FDA Approval: This drug is being studied for cancer treatment.

estramustine

Trade Names:
Emcyt, Estracyte

Type of Drug:
Estramustine is a chemotherapy drug used as an alkylating chemotherapy agent. It is a combination of nitrogen mustard and estradiol phosphate. It is used to treat advanced prostate cancer.

How Drug Works:
Estramustine enters cells with estrogen receptors and causes the cell to die.

How Drug Is Given:
Estramustine usually taken as a capsule by mouth in 3 to 4 divided doses. Take each dose 1 hour before or 2 hours after eating with a glass of water. Do not take with milk, milk products, or foods high in calcium as dairy products can lessen its effect. Take your antinausea medicine 1 hour before taking your dose. If you still feel sick to your stomach, talk to your doctor about a stronger antinausea medicine. Keep the medicine in a tightly closed container in the refrigerator, away from heat and moisture, and out of the the reach of children and pets. Estramustine can also be given by an injection in a vein. The dose depends on your size and the type of cancer being treated.

How Should I Take This Drug?
Take this drug exactly as directed by your doctor. If you do not understand the instructions, ask your doctor or nurse to explain them to you. This drug can be given at different strengths depending on the type of cancer being treated. Dosage may vary depending on your weight and your type of cancer.

 Read the following information. If you do not understand it or if any of it causes you special concern, check with your doctor.

Before taking this drug, tell your doctor:
- If you are trying to become pregnant, are pregnant, or breastfeeding. This drug may cause birth defects if either the male or female is taking it at the time of conception or during pregnancy. Men and women who are taking this drug need to use some kind of birth control. However, do not use oral contraceptives ("the pill") without checking with your doctor.
- If you think you may want to have children in the future. Many chemotherapy drugs can cause sterility.
- If you have any of the following medical problems: chickenpox or exposure to chickenpox, gout, heart disease, congestive heart failure, shingles, kidney stones, liver disease, or other forms of cancer.
- If you are taking any other prescription or over-the-counter drugs, including vitamins and herbals.

Should I avoid any other medicines, foods, alcohol, and/or activities?
Your prescription and nonprescription medicines may interact with other drugs, causing harm. Certain foods or alcohol can also interact with drug products. Never begin taking a new medicine—prescription or nonprescription—without asking your doctor or nurse if it will interact with alcohol, food, or other medicines. Some drug products can cause drowsiness and affect activities such as driving.

Precautions:
Tell your doctor if you have or have had blood clots in your legs or elsewhere in the body, peptic ulcers, liver problems, heart attack, hypertension, or diabetes.

Estramustine may be given intravenously. If the drug accidentally leaks out of the vein where it is given, it can damage the tissue and cause scarring. Tell the nurse right away if you notice redness, pain, or swelling at the place of injection.

While you are being treated with estramustine, and after you stop treatment, do not have any immunizations (vaccinations) without your doctor's okay. Try to avoid contact with people who have recently taken the oral polio vaccine. Check with your doctor about this.

Tell all the doctors, dentists, and pharmacists you visit that you are taking this drug.

- Most of the following side effects probably will not occur.
- Your doctor or nurse will want to discuss specific care instructions with you.
- They can help you understand these side effects and help you deal with them.

Side Effects:

More Common Side Effects
Breast enlargement
Nipple tenderness
Itching
Dry skin
Night sweats

Less Common Side Effects
Itching and pain in the genital area
Numbness of mouth
Rash
Peeling skin of fingertips
Thinning hair
Tiredness (fatigue)
Pain in eyes
Nausea
Vomiting

Rare Side Effects
Blood clots in legs, lungs, heart, or brain

Side Effects / Symptoms of the Drug
Stop the drug and tell your doctor or nurse right away if you have pain in your leg (calf) or chest, difficulty breathing, changes in your thinking, or headache.

Other side effects not listed above can also occur in some patients.
Tell your doctor or nurse if you develop any problems.

FDA Approval: This drug is approved for cancer treatment.

etanidazole

Trade Name:
Nitrolmidazole

Type of Drug:
Etanidazole belongs to a general group of drugs known as hypoxic radiosensitizers. These are drugs that increase the effect of radiation on cancer cells by pretending to be oxygen, which cancer cells without oxygen (hypoxic) need.

How Drug Works:
Cancer cells are injured by radiation more effectively when they have adequate oxygen. Etanidazole mimics oxygen, thus increasing the damaging effects of radiation therapy. This drug also makes it harder for cancer cells to repair themselves, so they die.

How Drug Is Given:
Etanidazole is given by a shot in a vein before radiation therapy. The dose depends on the investigational study.

 Read the following information. If you do not understand it or if any of it causes you special concern, check with your doctor.

Before taking this drug, tell your doctor:
- If you are trying to become pregnant, are pregnant, or breastfeeding. This drug may cause birth defects if either the male or female is taking it at the time of conception or during pregnancy. Men and women who are taking this drug need to use some kind of birth control. However, do not use oral contraceptives ("the pill") without checking with your doctor.
- If you think you may want to have children in the future. Many chemotherapy drugs can cause sterility.
- If you have any of the following medical problems: chickenpox or exposure to chickenpox, gout, heart disease, congestive heart failure, shingles, kidney stones, liver disease, or other forms of cancer.
- If you are taking any other prescription or over-the-counter drugs, including vitamins and herbals.

Should I avoid any other medicines, foods, alcohol, and/or activities?
Your prescription and nonprescription medicines may interact with other drugs, causing harm. Certain foods or alcohol can also interact with drug products. Never begin taking a new medicine—prescription or nonprescription—without asking your doctor or nurse if it will interact with alcohol, food, or other medicines. Some drug products can cause drowsiness and affect activities such as driving.

Precautions:
Report numbness, burning, or decreased feeling in your hands and/or feet right away.

Tell all the doctors, dentists, and pharmacists you visit that you are taking this drug.
- Most of the following side effects probably will not occur.
- Your doctor or nurse will want to discuss specific care instructions with you.
- They can help you understand these side effects and help you deal with them.

Side Effects:

More Common Side Effects
Feeling of pins and needles in hands and/or feet
Decreased feeling in hands and feet

Less Common Side Effects
Nausea
Vomiting

Rare Side Effects
Rash
Muscle aches

Other side effects not listed above can also occur in some patients.
Tell your doctor or nurse if you develop any problems.

FDA Approval: This drug is being studied for cancer treatment.

etoposide

Trade Names:
VePesid, VP-16, Etophophos

Type of Drug:
Etoposide belongs to the general class of chemotherapy drugs known as plant alkaloids. It is used to treat small cell lung and testicular cancers.

How Drug Works:
Etoposide stops cell division, causing the cells to die.

How Drug Is Given:
Etoposide can be given as an injection in a vein over 30 to 60 minutes, or at higher doses over 1 to 4 hours. Etoposide can also be given by mouth as a capsule once a day, or in divided doses. Take antinausea medicine 1 hour before the dose of etoposide. Take the capsule with a glass of water. The dose depends on your size and the type of cancer being treated. Keep the medicine in a tightly closed container away from heat and moisture and out of the reach of children and pets.

How Should I Take This Drug?
Take this drug exactly as directed by your doctor. If you do not understand the instructions, ask your doctor or nurse to explain them to you. This drug can be given at different strengths depending on the type of cancer being treated. Dosage may vary depending on your weight and your type of cancer.

 Read the following information. If you do not understand it or if any of it causes you special concern, check with your doctor.

Before taking this drug, tell your doctor:
- If you are trying to become pregnant, are pregnant, or breastfeeding. This drug may cause birth defects if either the male or female is taking it at the time of conception or during pregnancy. Men and women who are taking this drug need to use some kind of birth control. However, do not use oral contraceptives ("the pill") without checking with your doctor.
- If you think you may want to have children in the future. Many chemotherapy drugs can cause sterility.
- If you have any of the following medical problems: chickenpox or exposure to chickenpox, gout, heart disease, congestive heart failure, shingles, kidney stones, liver disease, or other forms of cancer.
- If you are taking any other prescription or over-the-counter drugs, including vitamins and herbals.

Should I avoid any other medicines, foods, alcohol, and/or activities?
Your prescription and nonprescription medicines may interact with other drugs, causing harm. Certain foods or alcohol can also interact with drug products. Never begin taking a new medicine—prescription or nonprescription—without asking your doctor or nurse if it will interact with alcohol, food, or other medicines. Some drug products can cause drowsiness and affect activities such as driving.

Precautions:
While you are being treated with etoposide, and after you stop treatment, do not have any immunizations (vaccinations) without your doctor's okay. Try to avoid contact with people who have recently taken the oral polio vaccine. Check with your doctor about this.

Etoposide can lower your blood counts (white blood cells, red blood cells, platelets). Your doctor will check your blood counts before and after each treatment to see how it affects your blood counts. Your doctor or nurse will give you specific instructions if your blood counts are low.

Etoposide can lower your white blood cell count, especially 10 to 14 days after the drug is given. This can increase your risk of getting an infection. Report fever of 100.5°F or higher, or signs of infection such as pain in passing your urine, coughing, and bringing up sputum.

Etoposide can cause a decrease in the platelet count. This can increase your risk of bleeding. DO NOT take any aspirin or aspirin-containing medicines. Report unusual bruising, or bleeding such as nosebleeds, bleeding gums when you brush your teeth, or black, tarry stools.

Etoposide capsules can cause nausea and vomiting. Ask your doctor or nurse to give you medicines to prevent or lessen this.

Getting a wig before starting treatment may make it easier to deal with hair loss. Talk to your nurse or doctor about this. If your insurance does not cover it, there may be other resources to help you. Hair loss is temporary, and your hair will grow back after treatment.

Tell all the doctors, dentists, and pharmacists you visit that you are taking this drug.
- Most of the following side effects probably will not occur.
- Your doctor or nurse will want to discuss specific care instructions with you.
- They can help you understand these side effects and help you deal with them.

Side Effects:

More Common Side Effects
Decreased white blood cell count with increased risk of infection
Decreased platelet count with increased risk of bleeding
Mild nausea
Mild vomiting
Loss of appetite
Changes in taste including metallic taste of foods
Hair loss
Fetal damage if pregnancy occurs while taking this drug

Less Common Side Effects
Constipation
Diarrhea
Pain in stomach
Radiation recall skin changes

Rare Side Effects
Decrease in blood pressure
Difficulty breathing during drug infusion
Rash
Itching
Heart changes
Numbness and tingling in hands and/or feet related to nerve irritation or damage
Fever
Chills
Allergic reactions

Side Effects / Symptoms of the Drug
After you stop receiving etoposide, the drug may still produce some side effects that need attention. Tell your doctor or nurse if you get any irregular heartbeats, shortness of breath, or swelling of the ankles, feet, or lower legs.

Other side effects not listed above can also occur in some patients.
Tell your doctor or nurse if you develop any problems.

FDA Approval: This drug is approved for cancer treatment.

exemestane

Trade Name:
Aromasin

Type of Drug:
Exemestane belongs to a general group of drugs called hormone or hormone antagonists. An antagonist blocks the effect of a hormone. It is used to treat advanced breast cancer in postmenopausal women whose cancer no longer responds to tamoxifen therapy.

How Drug Works:
Exemestane prevents the body's adrenal glands and ovaries from making estrogen. Other steroid hormones are not affected.

How Drug Is Given:
Exemestane is given as a pill once a day after eating a meal. The dose is standard for everyone. Keep the pills in a tightly closed container away from heat and moisture and out of the reach of children and pets.

How Should I Take This Drug?
Take this drug exactly as directed by your doctor. If you do not understand the instructions, ask your doctor or nurse to explain them to you. This drug can be given at different strengths depending on the type of cancer being treated. Dosage may vary depending on your weight and your type of cancer.

 Read the following information. If you do not understand it or if any of it causes you special concern, check with your doctor.

Before taking this drug, tell your doctor:
- If you are trying to become pregnant, are pregnant, or breastfeeding. This drug may cause birth defects if either the male or female is taking it at the time of conception or during pregnancy. Men and women who are taking this drug need to use some kind of birth control. However, do not use oral contraceptives ("the pill") without checking with your doctor.
- If you think you may want to have children in the future. Many chemotherapy drugs can cause sterility.
- If you have any of the following medical problems: chickenpox or exposure to chickenpox, gout, heart disease, congestive heart failure, shingles, kidney stones, liver disease, or other forms of cancer.
- If you are taking any other prescription or over-the-counter drugs, including vitamins and herbals.

Should I avoid any other medicines, foods, alcohol, and/or activities?
Your prescription and nonprescription medicines may interact with other drugs, causing harm. Certain foods or alcohol can also interact with drug products. Never begin taking a new medicine—prescription or non-prescription—without asking your doctor or nurse if it will interact with alcohol, food, or other medicines. Some drug products can cause drowsiness and affect activities such as driving.

Precautions:
It is important to keep taking the drug even though you are feeling well.

You may feel depressed or have difficulty sleeping while taking this medicine. Talk to your doctor or nurse about ways to manage these side effects to make you feel better.

Tell all the doctors, dentists, and pharmacists you visit that you are taking this drug.
- -
- Most of the following side effects probably will not occur.
- Your doctor or nurse will want to discuss specific care instructions with you.
- They can help you understand these side effects and help you deal with them.

Side Effects:

More Common Side Effects
Tiredness (fatigue)

Less Common Side Effects
Hot flashes
Pain at tumor site
Nausea
Depression
Difficulty sleeping

Rare Side Effects
Increased appetite
Weight gain
Pain
Increased sweating

Side Effects / Symptoms of the Drug
Tell your doctor or nurse if you have severe hot flashes, difficulty sleeping, or feel depressed. There is much that can be done.

Other side effects not listed above can also occur in some patients.
Tell your doctor or nurse if you develop any problems.

FDA Approval: This drug is approved for cancer treatment.

filgrastim

Trade Names:
G-CSF, Neupogen

Type of Drug:
Filgrastim is a protein cytokine that belongs to the general class of synthetic drugs called biologic response modifiers. It is used to increase the neutrophils (white blood cells) in the blood after chemotherapy.

How Drug Works:
Filgrastim is similar to a substance made by the body's immune system. It stimulates the body's bone marrow to make more neutrophils, a type of white blood cell involved in fighting infections. It also makes them work better.

How Drug Is Given:
Filgrastim is given as a shot under the skin or as an injection in a vein. You or a family member can be taught to give the shot under the skin once a day. Keep the syringes, needles, and supplies in a safe place, out of the reach of children and pets. The medicine should be kept in its original container in the refrigerator. The dose depends on your weight, and the number of doses depends on your white blood cell count (neutrophil count), and can vary from 5 to 10 doses. Keep the used syringes and needles in a special container. Ask your nurse or doctor about this, and when you should bring the filled container back to the office.

How Should I Take This Drug?
Take this drug exactly as directed by your doctor. If you do not understand the instructions, ask your doctor or nurse to explain them to you.

 Read the following information. If you do not understand it or if any of it causes you special concern, check with your doctor.

Before taking this drug, tell your doctor:
- If you are trying to become pregnant, are pregnant, or breastfeeding. This drug may cause birth defects if either the male or female is taking it at the time of conception or during pregnancy. Men and women who are taking this drug need to use some kind of birth control. However, do not use oral contraceptives ("the pill") without checking with your doctor.
- If you think you may want to have children in the future. Many chemotherapy drugs can cause sterility.
- If you have any of the following medical problems: chickenpox or exposure to chickenpox, gout, heart disease, congestive heart failure, shingles, kidney stones, liver disease, or other forms of cancer.
- If you are taking any other prescription or over-the-counter drugs, including vitamins and herbals.

Should I avoid any other medicines, foods, alcohol, and/or activities?
Your prescription and nonprescription medicines may interact with other drugs, causing harm. Certain foods or alcohol can also interact with drug products. Never begin taking a new medicine—prescription or nonprescription—without asking your doctor or nurse if it will interact with alcohol, food, or other medicines. Some drug products can cause drowsiness and affect activities such as driving.

Precautions:
Filgrastim is given at least 24 hours after chemotherapy and is continued for up to 2 weeks or until the neutrophils in the blood have reached a certain level.

You may get pain in your bones that is easily controlled. Talk to your nurse or doctor about ways to lessen this side effect.

Also, you or your family member can learn how to give this medicine at home.

Tell all the doctors, dentists, and pharmacists you visit that you are taking this drug.

- Most of the following side effects probably will not occur.
- Your doctor or nurse will want to discuss specific care instructions with you.
- They can help you understand these side effects and help you deal with them.

Side Effects:

More Common Side Effects
Bone pain

Side Effects / Symptoms of the Drug
Your blood counts will be monitored twice weekly during treatment to determine the drugs' effect on your neutrophil count.

Other side effects not listed above can also occur in some patients.
Tell your doctor or nurse if you develop any problems.

FDA Approval: This drug is approved for cancer treatment.

floxuridine

Trade Names:
Fluorodeoxyuridine, FUDR

Type of Drug:
Floxuridine belongs to the general group of chemotherapy drugs known as antimetabolites. It is used to treat some cancers involving the liver.

How Drug Works:
Floxuridine prevents cells from making DNA and RNA by interfering with the synthesis of nucleic acids, thus stopping the growth of cancer cells.

How Drug Is Given:
Floxuridine is given by a special pump into an artery in the liver. It is usually given as a continuous infusion for 14 to 21 days. You will probably also get a medicine to decrease the stomach acid to prevent ulcers. Sometimes it can be given as an injection into a vein by specially trained doctors or nurses. The dose depends on your size.

 Read the following information. If you do not understand it or if any of it causes you special concern, check with your doctor.

Before taking this drug, tell your doctor:
- If you are trying to become pregnant, are pregnant, or breastfeeding. This drug may cause birth defects if either the male or female is taking it at the time of conception or during pregnancy. Men and women who are taking this drug need to use some kind of birth control. However, do not use oral contraceptives ("the pill") without checking with your doctor.
- If you think you may want to have children in the future. Many chemotherapy drugs can cause sterility.
- If you have any of the following medical problems: chickenpox or exposure to chickenpox, gout, heart disease, congestive heart failure, shingles, kidney stones, liver disease, or other forms of cancer.
- If you are taking any other prescription or over-the-counter drugs, including vitamins and herbals.

Should I avoid any other medicines, foods, alcohol, and/or activities?
Your prescription and nonprescription medicines may interact with other drugs, causing harm. Certain foods or alcohol can also interact with drug products. Never begin taking a new medicine—prescription or non-prescription—without asking your doctor or nurse if it will interact with alcohol, food, or other medicines. Some drug products can cause drowsiness and affect activities such as driving.

Precautions:
While you are being treated with floxuridine, and after you stop treatment, do not have any immunizations (vaccinations) without your doctor's okay. Try to avoid contact with people who have recently taken the oral polio vaccine. Check with your doctor about this.

Floxuridine is given through an artery directly into the liver. Injection into a vein is being studied and is still investigational. Your doctor or nurse will explain the problems that can happen when the drug is given through an artery and what you should do if they occur.

Tell all the doctors, dentists, and pharmacists you visit that you are taking this drug.
- -
- Most of the following side effects probably will not occur.
- Your doctor or nurse will want to discuss specific care instructions with you.
- They can help you understand these side effects and help you deal with them.

Side Effects:

More Common Side Effects
Loss of appetite
Diarrhea
Numbness or tingling in hands and/or feet

Less Common Side Effects
Stomach cramping and pain
Sores in mouth or on lips
Bleeding at catheter site
Catheter infection
Catheter occlusion

Rare Side Effects
Nausea
Vomiting
Sore throat
Difficulty swallowing
Rash
Itching
Seizures
Depression
Hiccups
Blurred vision
Decreased white blood cell count with increased risk of infection
Decreased platelet count with increased risk of bleeding
Difficulty walking

Other side effects not listed above can also occur in some patients.
Tell your doctor or nurse if you develop any problems.

FDA Approval: This drug is approved for cancer treatment.

fludarabine phosphate

Trade Names:
Fludara, 2-fluoro-ara-AMP

Type of Drug:
Fludarabine phosphate belongs to the general group of chemotherapy drugs known as antimetabolites. It is used to treat chronic lymphocytic leukemia that no longer responds to at least 1 standard treatment with an alkylating agent.

How Drug Works:
Fludarabine phosphate prevents cells from making DNA and RNA by interfering with the synthesis of nucleic acids, thus stopping the growth of cancer cells.

How Drug Is Given:
Fludarabine phosphate is usually given as an injection in a vein over 30 minutes once a day for 5 days. A pill form is being studied. The dose depends on your size, how well your kidneys are working, and your blood counts.

 Read the following information. If you do not understand it or if any of it causes you special concern, check with your doctor.

Before taking this drug, tell your doctor:
- If you are trying to become pregnant, are pregnant, or breastfeeding. This drug may cause birth defects if either the male or female is taking it at the time of conception or during pregnancy. Men and women who are taking this drug need to use some kind of birth control. However, do not use oral contraceptives ("the pill") without checking with your doctor.
- If you think you may want to have children in the future. Many chemotherapy drugs can cause sterility.
- If you have any of the following medical problems: chickenpox or exposure to chickenpox, gout, heart disease, congestive heart failure, shingles, kidney stones, liver disease, or other forms of cancer.
- If you are taking any other prescription or over-the-counter drugs, including vitamins and herbals.

Should I avoid any other medicines, foods, alcohol, and/or activities?
Your prescription and nonprescription medicines may interact with other drugs, causing harm. Certain foods or alcohol can also interact with drug products. Never begin taking a new medicine—prescription or nonprescription—without asking your doctor or nurse if it will interact with alcohol, food, or other medicines. Some drug products can cause drowsiness and affect activities such as driving.

Precautions:
While you are being treated with fludarabine, and after you stop treatment, do not have any immunizations (vaccinations) without your doctor's okay. Try to avoid contact with people who have recently taken the oral polio vaccine. Check with your doctor about this.

Fludarabine can lower your blood counts (white blood cells, red blood cells, platelets). Your doctor will check your blood counts before and after each treatment, to see how it affects your blood counts. Your doctor or nurse will give you specific instructions if your blood counts are low.

Fludarabine can decrease your white blood cell count, especially 13 days after the drug is given. This can increase your risk of getting an infection. Report fever of 100.5°F or higher, or signs of infection such as pain in passing your urine, coughing, and bringing up sputum.

Fludarabine can decrease your platelet count. This can increase your risk of bleeding. DO NOT take any aspirin or aspirin-containing medicines. Report unusual bruising, or bleeding such as nosebleeds, bleeding gums when you brush your teeth, or black, tarry stools.

Rarely, fludarabine can cause an allergic reaction in the lungs or pneumonia. Tell your doctor right away if you develop shortness of breath or chest pain.

Tell all the doctors, dentists, and pharmacists you visit that you are taking this drug.

- Most of the following side effects probably will not occur.
- Your doctor or nurse will want to discuss specific care instructions with you.
- They can help you understand these side effects and help you deal with them.

Side Effects:

More Common Side Effects
Decreased white blood cell count with increased risk of infection
Decreased platelet count with increased risk of bleeding
Tiredness (fatigue)
Nausea
Vomiting

Less Common Side Effects
Pneumonia
Diarrhea

Rare Side Effects
Numbness and tingling in hands and/or feet related to irritation of nerves in the extremities
Changes in vision
Agitation
Confusion
Cough
Difficulty breathing
Weakness

Other side effects not listed above can also occur in some patients.
Tell your doctor or nurse if you develop any problems.

FDA Approval: This drug is approved for cancer treatment.

fluosol DA (20%)

Trade Name:
Investigational

Type of Drug:
Fluosol DA belongs to a general group of drugs known as hypoxic radiosensitizers. These are drugs that increase the effect of radiation on cancer cells by pretending to be oxygen, which the hypoxic (without oxygen) cancer cells need.

How Drug Works:
Cancer cells are injured more effectively when they have adequate oxygen. Fluosol DA acts as an artificial oxygen carrier, thus increasing the damaging effects of radiation therapy. This drug also makes it harder for cancer cells to repair themselves, so they die.

How Drug Is Given:
Fluosol DA (20%) is given as an injection in a vein before radiation therapy. You will be asked to breathe 100% oxygen before, during, and after treatment. The dose depends on the investigational treatment protocol.

 Read the following information. If you do not understand it or if any of it causes you special concern, check with your doctor.

Before taking this drug, tell your doctor:
• If you are trying to become pregnant, are pregnant, or breastfeeding. This drug may cause birth defects if either the male or female is taking it at the time of conception or during pregnancy. Men and women who are taking this drug need to use some kind of birth control. However, do not use oral contraceptives ("the pill") without checking with your doctor.
• If you think you may want to have children in the future. Many chemotherapy drugs can cause sterility.
• If you have any of the following medical problems: chickenpox or exposure to chickenpox, gout, heart disease, congestive heart failure, shingles, kidney stones, liver disease, or other forms of cancer.
• If you are taking any other prescription or over-the-counter drugs, including vitamins and herbals.

Should I avoid any other medicines, foods, alcohol, and/or activities?
Your prescription and nonprescription medicines may interact with other drugs, causing harm. Certain foods or alcohol can also interact with drug products. Never begin taking a new medicine—prescription or nonprescription—without asking your doctor or nurse if it will interact with alcohol, food, or other medicines. Some drug products can cause drowsiness and affect activities such as driving.

Precautions:
Allergic reactions can occur during the first treatment. Tell your nurse or doctor right away if you feel your face flush, or you have chills, fever, or chest pressure.

Tell all the doctors, dentists, and pharmacists you visit that you are taking this drug.

- Most of the following side effects probably will not occur.
- Your doctor or nurse will want to discuss specific care instructions with you.
- They can help you understand these side effects and help you deal with them.

Side Effects:

More Common Side Effects
Facial flushing immediately after first dose
Chest pressure immediately after first dose
Chills immediately after first dose
Fever immediately after first dose

Less Common Side Effects
Abnormal blood liver function tests

Other side effects not listed above can also occur in some patients.
Tell your doctor or nurse if you develop any problems.

FDA Approval: This drug is being studied for cancer treatment.

flutamide

Trade Name:
Eulexin

Type of Drug:
Flutamide belongs to the general group of drugs known as hormones or hormone antagonists. It is used to treat advanced prostate cancer.

How Drug Works:
Flutamide, an antiandrogen, stops the growth of cancer cells that depend on the male hormone (androgen) to grow and divide.

How Drug Is Given:
Flutamide is a pill given by mouth 3 times a day. When used to treat prostate cancer, it is usually given with another medicine to stop all the hormones that stimulate the cancer. The dose of flutamide is standard. Take with a glass of water. Keep the medicine in a tightly closed container away from heat and moisture and out of the reach of children and pets.

How Should I Take This Drug?
Take this drug exactly as directed by your doctor. If you do not understand the instructions, ask your doctor or nurse to explain them to you.

 Read the following information. If you do not understand it or if any of it causes you special concern, check with your doctor.

Before taking this drug, tell your doctor:
• If you are trying to become pregnant, are pregnant, or breastfeeding. This drug may cause birth defects if either the male or female is taking it at the time of conception or during pregnancy. Men and women who are taking this drug need to use some kind of birth control. However, do not use oral contraceptives ("the pill") without checking with your doctor.
• If you think you may want to have children in the future. Many chemotherapy drugs can cause sterility.
• If you have any of the following medical problems: chickenpox or exposure to chickenpox, gout, heart disease, congestive heart failure, shingles, kidney stones, liver disease, or other forms of cancer.
• If you are taking any other prescription or over-the-counter drugs, including vitamins and herbals.

Should I avoid any other medicines, foods, alcohol, and/or activities?
Your prescription and nonprescription medicines may interact with other drugs, causing harm. Certain foods or alcohol can also interact with drug products. Never begin taking a new medicine—prescription or nonprescription—without asking your doctor or nurse if it will interact with alcohol, food, or other medicines. Some drug products can cause drowsiness and affect activities such as driving.

Precautions:
It is important to continue taking flutamide, even if you feel well or if you have side effects. Talk to your doctor or nurse about ways to lessen the side effects.

Tell all the doctors, dentists, and pharmacists you visit that you are taking this drug.

- Most of the following side effects probably will not occur.
- Your doctor or nurse will want to discuss specific care instructions with you.
- They can help you understand these side effects and help you deal with them.

Side Effects:

More Common Side Effects
Hot flashes or sweating

Less Common Side Effects
Decreased sexual interest
Decreased sexual ability
Swelling of breasts
Diarrhea
Nausea

Other side effects not listed above can also occur in some patients.
Tell your doctor or nurse if you develop any problems.

FDA Approval: This drug is approved for cancer treatment.

fulvestrant

Trade Name:
Faslodex

Type of Drug:
Fulvestrant belongs to a new group of drugs called estrogen receptor downregulators. It is used to treat post-menopausal women with advanced breast cancer that no longer responds to antiestrogens like tamoxifen.

How Drug Works:
Breast cancer cells often have estrogen receptors on their cell surface. Estrogen stimulates cells with estrogen receptors to divide without regard to the body's needs. This is called estrogen receptor positive breast cancer. Fulvestrant binds to the estrogen receptor in the cell so that estrogen cannot bind to it and destroys the receptor. This "down regulates," or decreases, the expression of the estrogen receptor in the cell so that the cell acts like a normal cell.

How Drug Is Given:
Fulvestrant is given by injection into the muscle of your buttock, once a month. It can be a single shot, or can be divided into 2 shots. The dose is standard for all women.

 Read the following information. If you do not understand it or if any of it causes you special concern, check with your doctor.

Before taking this drug, tell your doctor:
- If you are trying to become pregnant, are pregnant, or breastfeeding. This drug may cause birth defects if either the male or female is taking it at the time of conception or during pregnancy. Men and women who are taking this drug need to use some kind of birth control. However, do not use oral contraceptives ("the pill") without checking with your doctor.
- If you think you may want to have children in the future. Many chemotherapy drugs can cause sterility.
- If you have any of the following medical problems: chickenpox or exposure to chickenpox, gout, heart disease, congestive heart failure, shingles, kidney stones, liver disease, or other forms of cancer.
- If you are taking any other prescription or over-the-counter drugs, including vitamins and herbals.

Should I avoid any other medicines, foods, alcohol, and/or activities?
Your prescription and nonprescription medicines may interact with other drugs, causing harm. Certain foods or alcohol can also interact with drug products. Never begin taking a new medicine—prescription or non-prescription—without asking your doctor or nurse if it will interact with alcohol, food, or other medicines. Some drug products can cause drowsiness and affect activities such as driving.

Precautions:
Fulvestrant should not be taken by pregnant or premenopausal women.

Fulvestrant should not be taken by women who have bleeding problems or who are on drugs like Coumadin to stop blood clots.

Tell all the doctors, dentists, and pharmacists you visit that you are taking this drug.

- Most of the following side effects probably will not occur.
- Your doctor or nurse will want to discuss specific care instructions with you.
- They can help you understand these side effects and help you deal with them.

Side Effects:

More Common Side Effects
Nausea
Feeling listless or tired

Less Common Side Effects
Vomiting
Constipation
Diarrhea
Abdominal pain
Headache
Back pain
Hot flashes
Sore throat
Pain at the site where the shot is given

Rare Side Effects
Pain in the chest or pelvis
Flu-like syndrome with fever, chills, and muscle and joint aches
Swelling of the hands and feet

Side Effects / Symptoms of the Drug
It is very important to keep your doctor's appointments for the monthly injection. Fulvestrant has few side effects. Call your doctor or nurse if you have an unusual or different reaction.

Other side effects not listed above can also occur in some patients.
Tell your doctor or nurse if you develop any problems.

FDA Approval: This drug is approved for cancer treatment.

gemcitabine

Trade Name:
Gemzar

Type of Drug:
Gemcitabine belongs to a general group of chemotherapy drugs known as antimetabolites. It is used to treat pancreatic cancer and lung cancer (with cisplatin).

How Drug Works:
Gemcitabine prevents cells from making DNA and RNA by interfering with the synthesis of nucleic acids. This stops the growth of cancer cells, causing the cells to die.

How Drug Is Given:
Gemcitabine is given as an injection in a vein over 30 minutes. For pancreatic cancer, gemcitabine is given once a week for up to 7 weeks to start. Then it is given once a week for 3 weeks, and 1 week without treatment. This is repeated every 4 weeks. When given for lung cancer or other cancers, it usually is given weekly for 3 weeks, then 1 week off. The dose depends on your size, your blood counts, and the cancer being treated.

 Read the following information. If you do not understand it or if any of it causes you special concern, check with your doctor.

Before taking this drug, tell your doctor:
- If you are trying to become pregnant, are pregnant, or breastfeeding. This drug may cause birth defects if either the male or female is taking it at the time of conception or during pregnancy. Men and women who are taking this drug need to use some kind of birth control. However, do not use oral contraceptives ("the pill") without checking with your doctor.
- If you think you may want to have children in the future. Many chemotherapy drugs can cause sterility.
- If you have any of the following medical problems: chickenpox or exposure to chickenpox, gout, heart disease, congestive heart failure, shingles, kidney stones, liver disease, or other forms of cancer.
- If you are taking any other prescription or over-the-counter drugs, including vitamins and herbals.

Should I avoid any other medicines, foods, alcohol, and/or activities?
Your prescription and nonprescription medicines may interact with other drugs, causing harm. Certain foods or alcohol can also interact with drug products. Never begin taking a new medicine—prescription or non-prescription—without asking your doctor or nurse if it will interact with alcohol, food, or other medicines. Some drug products can cause drowsiness and affect activities such as driving.

Precautions:
While you are being treated with gemcitabine, and after you stop treatment, do not have any immunizations (vaccinations) without your doctor's okay. Try to avoid contact with people who have recently taken the oral polio vaccine. Check with your doctor about this.

Gemcitabine can lower your blood counts (white blood cells, red blood cells, platelets). Your doctor will check your blood counts before and after each treatment to see how it affects your blood counts. Your doctor or nurse will give you specific instructions if your blood counts are low.

Gemcitabine can decrease your white blood cell count, especially 10 to 14 days after the drug is given. This can increase your risk of getting an infection. Report fever of 100.5°F or higher, or signs of infection such as pain in passing your urine, coughing, and bringing up sputum.

Gemcitabine can decrease the platelet count. This can increase your risk of bleeding. DO NOT take any aspirin or aspirin-containing medicines. Report unusual bruising, or bleeding such as nosebleeds, bleeding gums when you brush your teeth, or black, tarry stools.

Tell all the doctors, dentists, and pharmacists you visit that you are taking this drug.
- -
- Most of the following side effects probably will not occur.
- Your doctor or nurse will want to discuss specific care instructions with you.
- They can help you understand these side effects and help you deal with them.

Side Effects:

More Common Side Effects
Decreased white blood cell count with increased risk of infection
Decreased platelet count with increased risk of bleeding
Nausea
Vomiting
Increased liver function blood tests
Tiredness (fatigue)

Less Common Side Effects
Diarrhea
Sores in mouth or on lips
Flu-like symptoms with first treatment (headache, muscle aches, fever, stuffy nose)
Skin rash
Swelling of hands, ankles, or face
Hair thinning
Itching

Rare Side Effects
Sedation

Other side effects not listed above can also occur in some patients.
Tell your doctor or nurse if you develop any problems.

FDA Approval: This drug is approved for cancer treatment.

gemtuzumab ozogamicin

Trade Name:
Mylotarg

Type of Drug:
Gemtuzumab ozogamicin is a monoclonal antibody attached to chemotherapy. It belongs to the class called chemoimmunotherapy agents, meaning that it is both a chemotherapy and an immunotherapy agent. It is used to treat some leukemias.

How Drug Works:
Gemtuzumab ozogamicin is like a "smart bomb." The monoclonal antibody part of gemtuzumab ozogamicin is directed against a certain receptor (CD33) located on leukemic cells. This receptor is found on the leukemia white blood cells in 80% of people with acute myelocytic leukemia (AML). The antibody attaches to the CD33 receptor and is taken into the cell, along with the chemotherapy. This kills the leukemic cell.

How Drug Is Given:
Gemtuzumab ozogamicin is given by an injection in a vein over 2 hours, every 14 days for 2 cycles. You will get medicine before taking gemtuzumab ozogamicin to lessen the chance you will have an allergic reaction. The dose depends on your size.

 Read the following information. If you do not understand it or if any of it causes you special concern, check with your doctor.

Before taking this drug, tell your doctor:
- If you are trying to become pregnant, are pregnant, or breastfeeding. This drug may cause birth defects if either the male or female is taking it at the time of conception or during pregnancy. Men and women who are taking this drug need to use some kind of birth control. However, do not use oral contraceptives ("the pill") without checking with your doctor.
- If you think you may want to have children in the future. Many chemotherapy drugs can cause sterility.
- If you have any of the following medical problems: chickenpox or exposure to chickenpox, gout, heart disease, congestive heart failure, shingles, kidney stones, liver disease, or other forms of cancer.
- If you are taking any other prescription or over-the-counter drugs, including vitamins and herbals.

Should I avoid any other medicines, foods, alcohol, and/or activities?
Your prescription and nonprescription medicines may interact with other drugs, causing harm. Certain foods or alcohol can also interact with drug products. Never begin taking a new medicine—prescription or nonprescription—without asking your doctor or nurse if it will interact with alcohol, food, or other medicines. Some drug products can cause drowsiness and affect activities such as driving.

Precautions:
Your blood cells will be examined to make sure they have the CD33 receptor before the treatment is started. This treatment only works when your white blood cells have this receptor.

This drug may cause chills, fever, nausea, vomiting, headache, or low blood pressure after the first treatment. Thus, 1 hour before the treatment, your doctor will probably give you medicine to prevent this.

Gemtuzumab ozogamicin can lower your blood counts (white blood cells, red blood cells, platelets). Your doctor will check your blood counts before and after each treatment to see how it affects your blood counts. The blood counts reach their lowest level in about 6 to 7 weeks after treatment. Your doctor or nurse will give you specific instructions if your blood counts are low.

Gemtuzumab ozogamicin can lower your white blood cell count. This can increase your risk of getting an infection. Report fever, of 100.5°F or higher, or signs of infection such as pain in passing your urine or a cough that produces sputum.

Gemtuzumab ozogamicin can lower your platelet count. This can increase your risk of bleeding. DO NOT take any aspirin or aspirin-containing medicines. Report unusual bruising, bleeding such as nosebleeds, bleeding gums when you brush your teeth, or black, tarry stools.

Rarely, you can have a severe allergic reaction to the monoclonal antibody. Your nurse or doctor will watch you very closely during the treatment.

Nausea and vomiting are common side effects. Talk with your doctor or nurse about taking medicine to prevent nausea and vomiting.

Gemtuzumab ozogamicin can kill large numbers of leukemic cells. Your doctor and nurse may give you special intravenous fluids and medicine to prevent uric acid from forming, which might hurt your kidneys. Also, they will test your blood frequently to make sure your electrolytes are normal; if the level is not normal, they will give you medicine to fix it.

Patients with kidney or liver disease should use this drug cautiously.

 Tell all the doctors, dentists, and pharmacists you visit that you are taking this drug.
- • Most of the following side effects probably will not occur.
- • Your doctor or nurse will want to discuss specific care instructions with you.
- • They can help you understand these side effects and help you deal with them.

Side Effects:

More Common Side Effects
Severe decrease in white blood cell count with increased risk of infection
Severe decrease in platelet count with increased risk of bleeding
Decreased red blood cell count with increased risk of anemia and tiredness (fatigue)
Nausea
Vomiting
Syndrome of chills, fever, nausea, vomiting, headache, low blood pressure or high blood pressure, breathing difficulty, and high blood sugar within 24 hours of treatment
Tiredness (fatigue)
Mouth sores
Temporary increase in level of liver function enzymes in the blood
Diarrhea
Constipation
Rash
Swelling of the hands or feet

Rare Side Effects
Liver problems
Liver failure

Side Effects / Symptoms of the Drug
Make sure you have the name of a doctor or nurse and telephone number to call if you have any questions or problems after the treatment.

Other side effects not listed above can also occur in some patients.
Tell your doctor or nurse if you develop any problems.

FDA Approval: This drug is approved for cancer treatment.

goserelin acetate

Trade Name:
Zoladex

Type of Drug:
Goserelin acetate belongs to the general group of drugs known as hormones or hormone antagonists. It is used to treat advanced prostate and breast cancers.

How Drug Works:
Goserelin acetate is a synthetic version of the body's luteinizing hormone-releasing hormone (LHRH). It blocks the release of sex hormones—testosterone in men and estrogen in women. Cancers that are stimulated to grow by these hormones stop growing.

How Drug Is Given:
Goserelin acetate is given by a shot under the skin once a month. The dose is standard for all adults. The medicine is slowly released over 1 month.

 Read the following information. If you do not understand it or if any of it causes you special concern, check with your doctor.

Before taking this drug, tell your doctor:
• If you are trying to become pregnant, are pregnant, or breastfeeding. This drug may cause birth defects if either the male or female is taking it at the time of conception or during pregnancy. Men and women who are taking this drug need to use some kind of birth control. However, do not use oral contraceptives ("the pill") without checking with your doctor.
• If you think you may want to have children in the future. Many chemotherapy drugs can cause sterility.
• If you have any of the following medical problems: chickenpox or exposure to chickenpox, gout, heart disease, congestive heart failure, shingles, kidney stones, liver disease, or other forms of cancer.
• If you are taking any other prescription or over-the-counter drugs, including vitamins and herbals.

Should I avoid any other medicines, foods, alcohol, and/or activities?
Your prescription and nonprescription medicines may interact with other drugs, causing harm. Certain foods or alcohol can also interact with drug products. Never begin taking a new medicine—prescription or nonprescription—without asking your doctor or nurse if it will interact with alcohol, food, or other medicines. Some drug products can cause drowsiness and affect activities such as driving.

Precautions:
After the first injection, there may be a "flare" of symptoms, such as bone pain. This will go away in a few days.

Tell all the doctors, dentists, and pharmacists you visit that you are taking this drug.
- -
- Most of the following side effects probably will not occur.
- Your doctor or nurse will want to discuss specific care instructions with you.
- They can help you understand these side effects and help you deal with them.

Side Effects:

More Common Side Effects
Hot flashes
Decrease in sexual desire
Menstrual periods will stop in women
Vaginal dryness
Swelling of breasts
Decrease in ability to have erections

Less Common Side Effects
Breast tenderness

Rare Side Effects
Irregular heartbeat
Increased blood pressure
Chest pain
Depression
Chills
Fever
Anxiety
Vomiting
Increased weight
Constipation
Diarrhea
Stroke
Heart attack
Headache
Increased blood sugar
Urinary tract infection
Kidney damage
Decreased blood flow in extremeties

Side Effects / Symptoms of the Drug
Tell your doctor or nurse right away if you get pain in your chest, shortness of breath, painful urination, or leg pain.

Other side effects not listed above can also occur in some patients.
Tell your doctor or nurse if you develop any problems.

FDA Approval: This drug is approved for cancer treatment.

hydroxyurea

Trade Name:
Hydrea

Type of Drug:
Hydroxyurea belongs to a general group of chemotherapy drugs called antimetabolites. It is used to treat chronic myeloid leukemia and blood disorders including polycythemia vera and sickle cell anemia.

How Drug Works:
Hydroxyurea prevents cells from making DNA and RNA by interfering with the synthesis of nucleic acids, thus stopping the growth of cancer cells.

How Drug Is Given:
Hydroxyurea is taken by mouth as a capsule or pill. Take the medicine with a full glass of water. If the medicine makes you feel sick to your stomach, take an antinausea pill 1 hour before the hydroxyurea. The dose depends on the reason you are taking it, how well your kidneys are working, and your blood counts. Keep the medicine in a tightly closed container away from heat and moisture and out of the reach of children and pets.

How Should I Take This Drug?
Take this drug exactly as directed by your doctor. If you do not understand the instructions, ask your doctor or nurse to explain them to you. This drug can be given at different strengths depending on the type of cancer being treated. Dosage may vary depending on your weight and your type of cancer.

Read the following information. If you do not understand it or if any of it causes you special concern, check with your doctor.

Before taking this drug, tell your doctor:
- If you are trying to become pregnant, are pregnant, or breastfeeding. This drug may cause birth defects if either the male or female is taking it at the time of conception or during pregnancy. Men and women who are taking this drug need to use some kind of birth control. However, do not use oral contraceptives ("the pill") without checking with your doctor.
- If you think you may want to have children in the future. Many chemotherapy drugs can cause sterility.
- If you have any of the following medical problems: chickenpox or exposure to chickenpox, gout, heart disease, congestive heart failure, shingles, kidney stones, liver disease, or other forms of cancer.
- If you are taking any other prescription or over-the-counter drugs, including vitamins and herbals.

Should I avoid any other medicines, foods, alcohol, and/or activities?
Your prescription and nonprescription medicines may interact with other drugs, causing harm. Certain foods or alcohol can also interact with drug products. Never begin taking a new medicine—prescription or nonprescription—without asking your doctor or nurse if it will interact with alcohol, food, or other medicines. Some drug products can cause drowsiness and affect activities such as driving.

Precautions:
While you are being treated with hydroxyurea, and after you stop treatment, do not have any immunizations (vaccinations) without your doctor's okay. Try to avoid contact with people who have recently taken the oral polio vaccine. Check with your doctor about this.

Hydroxyurea can lower your blood counts (white blood cells, red blood cells, platelets). Your doctor will check your blood counts before and after each treatment to see how it affects your blood counts. Your doctor or nurse will give you specific instructions for low blood counts.

Hydroxyurea can cause a dramatic decrease in your white blood cell count, especially 24 to 48 hours after the drug is given. This can increase your risk of getting an infection. Report fever of 100.5°F or higher, or signs of infection such as pain in passing your urine, coughing, and bringing up sputum.

Hydroxyurea can cause a decrease in the platelet count. This can increase your risk of bleeding. DO NOT take any aspirin or aspirin-containing medicines. Report unusual bruising, or bleeding such as nosebleeds, bleeding of gums when you brush your teeth, or black, tarry stools.

 Tell all the doctors, dentists, and pharmacists you visit that you are taking this drug.

- Most of the following side effects probably will not occur.
- Your doctor or nurse will want to discuss specific care instructions with you.
- They can help you understand these side effects and help you deal with them.

Side Effects:

More Common Side Effects
Decreased white blood cell count with increased risk of infection

Less Common Side Effects
Decreased platelet count with increased risk of bleeding
Tiredness (fatigue)
Fetal abnormalities if becoming pregnant while taking the drug

Rare Side Effects
Nausea
Vomiting
Sores in mouth or on lips
Diarrhea
Confusion
Disorientation
Headache
Drowsiness
Loss of appetite
Increased liver function tests

Other side effects not listed above can also occur in some patients.
Tell your doctor or nurse if you develop any problems.

FDA Approval: This drug is approved for cancer treatment.

idarubicin

Trade Name:
Idamycin

Type of Drug:
Idarubicin belongs to a general group of chemotherapy drugs known as anthracycline antibiotics. It is used to treat nonlymphocytic leukemia in combination with other drugs.

How Drug Works:
Idarubicin prevents cells from making DNA and/or RNA, thus altering cell growth.

How Drug Is Given:
Idarubicin is given as an injection in the vein over about 15 minutes. Tell the nurse if you feel pain, burning, or discomfort in the vein when it is given. You will get medicine to stop any nausea or vomiting before the idarubicin and to take afterward. The dose and how often you get the medicine depends upon your size, your blood counts, how well your liver is working, and the type of cancer being treated. You will have your blood counts checked before each treatment. If they are too low, your treatment will be delayed. This medicine may be given in addition to other chemotherapy medicines.

 Read the following information. If you do not understand it or if any of it causes you special concern, check with your doctor.

Before taking this drug, tell your doctor:
- If you are trying to become pregnant, are pregnant, or breastfeeding. This drug may cause birth defects if either the male or female is taking it at the time of conception or during pregnancy. Men and women who are taking this drug need to use some kind of birth control. However, do not use oral contraceptives ("the pill") without checking with your doctor.
- If you think you may want to have children in the future. Many chemotherapy drugs can cause sterility.
- If you have any of the following medical problems: chickenpox or exposure to chickenpox, gout, heart disease, congestive heart failure, shingles, kidney stones, liver disease, or other forms of cancer.
- If you are taking any other prescription or over-the-counter drugs, including vitamins and herbals.

Should I avoid any other medicines, foods, alcohol, and/or activities?
Your prescription and nonprescription medicines may interact with other drugs, causing harm. Certain foods or alcohol can also interact with drug products. Never begin taking a new medicine—prescription or nonprescription—without asking your doctor or nurse if it will interact with alcohol, food, or other medicines. Some drug products can cause drowsiness and affect activities such as driving.

Precautions:
While you are being treated with idarubicin, and after you stop treatment, do not have any immunizations (vaccinations) without your doctor's okay. Try to avoid contact with people who have recently taken the oral polio vaccine. Check with your doctor about this.

Idarubicin can lower your blood counts (white blood cells, red blood cells, platelets). Your doctor will check your blood counts before and after each treatment to see how it affects your blood counts. Your doctor or nurse will give you specific instructions if your blood counts are low.

Idarubicin can decrease your white blood cell count, especially 10 to 20 days after the drug is given. This can increase your risk of getting an infection. Report fever of 100.5°F or higher, or signs of infection such as pain in passing your urine, coughing, and bringing up sputum. Idarubicin can decrease the platelet count. This can increase your risk of bleeding. DO NOT take any aspirin or aspirin-containing medicines. Report unusual bruising, or bleeding such as nosebleeds, bleeding gums when you brush your teeth, or black, tarry stools.

Idarubicin is given in a vein. If the drug accidentally leaks out of the vein where it is given, it can damage the tissue and cause scarring. Tell the nurse right away if you notice redness, pain, or swelling at the place of injection.

Idarubicin can injure the heart muscle when large doses are given. Your doctor will test your heart function before you receive your first treatment, and then during the treatment. This way, any damage can be found early. Talk to your doctor about this.

Getting a wig before starting treatment may make it easier to deal with hair loss. Talk to your nurse or doctor about this. If your insurance does not cover it, there may be other resources to help you. Hair loss is temporary, and your hair will grow back after treatment.

Idarubicin can cause severe nausea and vomiting. Ask your doctor or nurse to give you medicines to prevent or lessen this.

 Tell all the doctors, dentists, and pharmacists you visit that you are taking this drug.
- Most of the following side effects probably will not occur.
- Your doctor or nurse will want to discuss specific care instructions with you.
- They can help you understand these side effects and help you deal with them.

Side Effects:

More Common Side Effects

Decreased white blood cell count with increased risk of infection
Decreased platelet count with increased risk of bleeding
Nausea
Vomiting
Decreased appetite
Sores in mouth or on lips
Hair loss
Skin Rash

Less Common Side Effects

Darkening of nail beds
Abnormal liver function blood tests
Diarrhea

Rare Side Effects

Inflammation of the liver
Heart damage with congestive heart failure

Side Effects / Symptoms of the Drug

Idarubicin causes the urine to turn reddish, which may stain clothes. This is not blood. It is normal and lasts for 1 to 2 days after each dose is given.

After you stop taking idarubicin, the drug may still produce some side effects that need attention. Tell your doctor if you have irregular heartbeats, shortness of breath, or swelling of the ankles, feet, or lower legs.

Other side effects not listed above can also occur in some patients.
Tell your doctor or nurse if you develop any problems.

FDA Approval: This drug is approved for cancer treatment.

idoxifene

Trade Name:
(Investigational)

Type of Drug:
Idoxifene is a synthetic antiestrogen. It belongs to the general group of drugs known as hormones or hormone antagonists. It is being studied in several types of cancer including breast cancer.

How Drug Works:
Idoxifene blocks estrogen. The cancer cells, which depend on estrogen to divide, stop growing and die.

How Drug Is Given:
Idoxifene is a pill, taken by mouth with a glass of water, with or without meals. The dose depends on the investigational study. Keep the medicine in a tightly closed container away from heat and moisture and out of the reach of children and pets.

How Should I Take This Drug?
Take this drug exactly as directed by your doctor. If you do not understand the instructions, ask your doctor or nurse to explain them to you. This drug can be given at different strengths depending on the type of cancer being treated. Dosage may vary depending on your weight and your type of cancer.

 Read the following information. If you do not understand it or if any of it causes you special concern, check with your doctor.

Before taking this drug, tell your doctor:
- If you are trying to become pregnant, are pregnant, or breastfeeding. This drug may cause birth defects if either the male or female is taking it at the time of conception or during pregnancy. Men and women who are taking this drug need to use some kind of birth control. However, do not use oral contraceptives ("the pill") without checking with your doctor.
- If you think you may want to have children in the future. Many chemotherapy drugs can cause sterility.
- If you have any of the following medical problems: chickenpox or exposure to chickenpox, gout, heart disease, congestive heart failure, shingles, kidney stones, liver disease, or other forms of cancer.
- If you are taking any other prescription or over-the-counter drugs, including vitamins and herbals.

Should I avoid any other medicines, foods, alcohol, and/or activities?
Your prescription and nonprescription medicines may interact with other drugs, causing harm. Certain foods or alcohol can also interact with drug products. Never begin taking a new medicine—prescription or nonprescription—without asking your doctor or nurse if it will interact with alcohol, food, or other medicines. Some drug products can cause drowsiness and affect activities such as driving.

Precautions:
There are few side effects with this medicine. It is important to continue to take this medicine even though you feel well.

Tell all the doctors, dentists, and pharmacists you visit that you are taking this drug.

- Most of the following side effects probably will not occur.
- Your doctor or nurse will want to discuss specific care instructions with you.
- They can help you understand these side effects and help you deal with them.

Side Effects:

More Common Side Effects
Mild nausea

Less Common Side Effects
Mild vomiting
Tiredness (fatigue)
Loss of appetite

Rare Side Effects
Lethargy
Weakness

Side Effects / Symptoms of the Drug
The investigational study will give additional information, side effects, and what to report.

Other side effects not listed above can also occur in some patients.
Tell your doctor or nurse if you develop any problems.

FDA Approval: This drug is being studied for cancer treatment.

ifosfamide

Trade Names:
Ifex, Isophosphamide

Type of Drug:
Ifosfamide belongs to a general group of chemotherapy drugs known as alkylating agents. It is used to treat lymphoma, leukemia, testicular, and bladder cancers.

How Drug Works:
Ifosfamide stops the growth of cancer cells, causing them to die.

How Drug Is Given:
Ifosfamide is given as an injection in a vein over a period of time from 1 hour to 24 hours for a few days. Because ifosfamide can hurt your bladder, you will need to get a salt or sugar solution by vein. You will also get the medicine mesna, which will protect your bladder. If you take mesna by mouth, make sure you take it exactly like your doctor told you. It is also very important to drink 3 or more quarts of fluid a day: at least one 12 oz glass of juice, water, or Gatorade while awake (no alcohol). This will flush your kidneys, and make you pass your urine frequently. The dose of ifosfamide depends on your size, how well your kidneys are working, your blood counts, and the type of cancer being treated.

 Read the following information. If you do not understand it or if any of it causes you special concern, check with your doctor.

Before taking this drug, tell your doctor:
- If you are trying to become pregnant, are pregnant, or breastfeeding. This drug may cause birth defects if either the male or female is taking it at the time of conception or during pregnancy. Men and women who are taking this drug need to use some kind of birth control. However, do not use oral contraceptives ("the pill") without checking with your doctor.
- If you think you may want to have children in the future. Many chemotherapy drugs can cause sterility.
- If you have any of the following medical problems: chickenpox or exposure to chickenpox, gout, heart disease, congestive heart failure, shingles, kidney stones, liver disease, or other forms of cancer.
- If you are taking any other prescription or over-the-counter drugs, including vitamins and herbals.

Should I avoid any other medicines, foods, alcohol, and/or activities?
Your prescription and nonprescription medicines may interact with other drugs, causing harm. Certain foods or alcohol can also interact with drug products. Never begin taking a new medicine—prescription or non-prescription—without asking your doctor or nurse if it will interact with alcohol, food, or other medicines. Some drug products can cause drowsiness and affect activities such as driving.

Precautions:
While you are being treated with ifosfamide, and after you stop treatment, do not have any immunizations (vaccinations) without your doctor's okay. Try to avoid contact with people who have recently taken the oral polio vaccine. Check with your doctor about this.

Ifosfamide can cause serious bleeding in the bladder, so it is ALWAYS given with fluids in the vein and mesna, a drug that protects the bladder. Your doctor will discuss how best to give you the fluids you will need.

Ifosfamide can lower your blood counts (white blood cells, red blood cells, platelets). Your doctor will check your blood counts before and after each treatment to see the treatment's effect on your blood counts. Your doctor or nurse will give you specific instructions if your blood counts are low.

Ifosfamide can decrease your white blood cell count, especially 10 to 14 days after the drug is given. This can increase your risk of getting an infection. Report fever of 100.5°F or higher, or signs of infection such as pain in passing your urine, coughing, and bringing up sputum.

Ifosfamide can decrease the platelet count. This can increase your risk of bleeding. DO NOT take any aspirin or aspirin-containing medicines. Report unusual bruising, or bleeding such as nosebleeds, bleeding gums when you brush your teeth, or black, tarry stools.

Getting a wig before starting treatment may make it easier to deal with hair loss. Talk to your nurse or doctor about this. If your insurance does not cover it, there may be other resources to help you. Hair loss is temporary, and your hair will grow back after treatment.

Ifosfamide can cause nausea and vomiting. Ask your doctor or nurse to give you medicines to prevent or lessen this.

 Tell all the doctors, dentists, and pharmacists you visit that you are taking this drug.
- -
- Most of the following side effects probably will not occur.
- Your doctor or nurse will want to discuss specific care instructions with you.
- They can help you understand these side effects and help you deal with them.

Side Effects:

More Common Side Effects
Nausea

Vomiting

Hair loss

Bladder irritation, blood in the urine

Kidney function abnormalities

Fetal abnormalities if pregnancy occurs
while taking ifosfamide

Less Common Side Effects
Decreased white blood cell count with increased risk of infection

Pain at place of injection

Rare Side Effects
Decreased platelet count with
increased risk of bleeding

Tiredness (fatigue)

Confusion

Sleepiness

Dizziness

Side Effects / Symptoms of the Drug
Call your doctor or nurse right away if you have painful urination or if your urine is red.

Other side effects not listed above can also occur in some patients.
Tell your doctor or nurse if you develop any problems.

FDA Approval: This drug is approved for cancer treatment.

imatinib mesylate

Trade Names:
Gleevec, STI 571

Type of Drug:
Imatinib mesylate is a protein-tyrosine kinase inhibitor used in molecular targeted therapy to treat patients with chronic myeloid leukemia (CML). It has been approved by the FDA to treat gastrointestinal stromal tumors (GIST).

How Drug Works:
Imatinib mesylate inhibits (blocks) the Bcr-Abl protein tyrosine kinase, which is made by the abnormal Philadelphia chromosome in chronic myeloid leukemia. The protein tyrosine kinase carries messages to the cell telling it to divide and grow. By blocking this message, imatinib mesylate prevents the cancer cells from making more cells and causes them to die (apoptosis). Imatinib mesylate also blocks the receptor tyrosine kinase for c-kit, which carries the message for the cancer cells in GIST telling them to divide, causing the cells to stop dividing and to die. The drug is used to treat patients with chronic myeloid leukemia (CML) and GIST when the tumor cannot be removed.

How Drug Is Given:
Imatinib mesylate is a capsule taken by mouth once a day with a full glass of water. If your doctor increases your dose, you may need to split the dose and take it once in the morning and once later in the day. The dose depends on the type of cancer being treated, how well your liver is working, and your blood counts. Keep the medicine in a tightly closed container away from heat and moisture and out of the reach of children and pets.

How Should I Take This Drug?
Take this drug exactly as directed by your doctor. If you do not understand the instructions, ask your doctor or nurse to explain them to you. This drug can be given at different strengths depending on the type of cancer being treated. Dosage may vary depending on your weight and your type of cancer.

 Read the following information. If you do not understand it or if any of it causes you special concern, check with your doctor.

Before taking this drug, tell your doctor:
- If you are trying to become pregnant, are pregnant, or breastfeeding. This drug may cause birth defects if either the male or female is taking it at the time of conception or during pregnancy. Men and women who are taking this drug need to use some kind of birth control. However, do not use oral contraceptives ("the pill") without checking with your doctor.
- If you think you may want to have children in the future. Many chemotherapy drugs can cause sterility.
- If you have any of the following medical problems: chickenpox or exposure to chickenpox, gout, heart disease, congestive heart failure, shingles, kidney stones, liver disease, or other forms of cancer.
- If you are taking any other prescription or over-the-counter drugs, including vitamins and herbals.

Should I avoid any other medicines, foods, alcohol, and/or activities?
Your prescription and nonprescription medicines may interact with other drugs, causing harm. Certain foods or alcohol can also interact with drug products. Never begin taking a new medicine—prescription or nonprescription—without asking your doctor or nurse if it will interact with alcohol, food, or other medicines. Some drug products can cause drowsiness and affect activities such as driving.

Precautions:
Imatinib mesylate may interact with other drugs. Tell your doctor if you are also taking ketoconazole, itraconazole, erythromycin, clarithromycin, dexamethasone, phenytoin, carbamazapine, rifampicin, phenobarbital, St. John's wort, cyclosporine, pimozide, triazino-benzodiazepines, dihydropyridine calcium channel blockers, HMG-CoA reductase inhibitors, or Coumadin.

DO NOT take Coumadin while taking imatinib mesylate. If you need to take an anticoagulant, your doctor will give you a different drug to take (heparin or low molecular weight heparin).

Imatinib mesylate may cause fluid retention and swelling around the eyes or feet (edema). Tell your doctor or nurse if you are gaining weight, develop swelling around your eyes or in your hands or feet, notice swelling in your abdomen, or have difficulty breathing (shortness of breath).

Imatinib mesylate can irritate your stomach. It is important to take your dose with food and a large glass of water.

Imatinib mesylate can lower your blood counts, especially if you have CML in blast or accelerated phases. Your doctor will tell you when to have your blood counts checked depending on your condition. This is often every week for the first month, then every other week for the second month, then every 2 to 3 months or as needed. Your drug dose may need to be reduced or interrupted if your blood counts get too low. Your doctor or nurse will give you specific instructions about this, and how to care for yourself if your blood counts are low.

Imatinib mesylate can lower your white blood cells, which can last for 2 to 3 weeks. During this time, you are at high risk for getting an infection. Report fever of 100.5°F or higher, or signs of infection such as pain in passing your urine, coughing, and bringing up sputum.

Imatinib mesylate can lower your platelets, which can last for 3 to 4 weeks. This can increase your risk of bleeding. DO NOT take any aspirin or aspirin-containing medicines. Report unusual bruising, or bleeding such as nosebleeds, bleeding gums when you brush your teeth, or black, tarry stools.

Your doctor will check your liver function tests regularly. If you have any liver problems before starting this drug, you will be watched very closely. If the tests are elevated, your doctor may reduce the dose or interrupt therapy for a short while until the tests come back to normal.

 Tell all the doctors, dentists, and pharmacists you visit that you are taking this drug.

- Most of the following side effects probably will not occur.
- Your doctor or nurse will want to discuss specific care instructions with you.
- They can help you understand these side effects and help you deal with them.

Side Effects:

More Common Side Effects

Nausea
Vomiting
Swelling around the eyes or feet (edema)
Muscle cramps
Diarrhea
Low platelet count with increased risk for bleeding

Low white blood cell count with increased risk for infection
Muscle aches and pains
Skin rash
Tiredness (fatigue)
Headache
Joint and bone pain
Abdominal pain

Less Common Side Effects

Heartburn
Weight increase
Itching
Shortness of breath
Constipation

Low blood level of potassium
Fluid in the lining of the lungs (pleural effusion), heart (pericardial effusion), or abdomen (ascites)

Rare Side Effects

Liver damage

Side Effects / Symptoms of the Drug

Call your doctor or nurse right away if you have a fever, signs or symptoms of infection such as sore throat, bad cough, or burning when you pass urine; if you have any bleeding; if you have any trouble breathing; or any other problem you are unsure about.

Other side effects not listed above can also occur in some patients.
Tell your doctor or nurse if you develop any problems.

FDA Approval: This drug is approved for cancer treatment.

interferon alpha

Trade Names:
Actimmune, Alferon N, Avonex, Intron A, Roferon A, IFN-α, Interferon-α 2b, Interferon-α 2a, α-interferon

Type of Drug:
Interferon alpha is a protein cytokine that belongs to a general class of synthetic substances called biological response modifiers. It is used to treat several cancers including hairy cell leukemia and Kaposi's sarcoma. Other forms of interferon, such as Interferon beta, are investigational.

How Drug Works:
Interferon alpha is similar to a substance made by the body's immune system. This drug fights viruses and cancer cells and stimulates the body's immune system to work better.

How Drug Is Given:
Interferon alpha is given by an injection under the skin, in a vein, or in a muscle. You or a family member can be taught how to give the medicine under the skin. The medicine should be kept in its original container in the refrigerator. The dose and the number of doses depend on your weight and the cancer being treated. Keep the syringes, needles, and supplies in a safe place, out of the reach of children and pets. Keep the used syringes and needles in a special sharps container. Ask your nurse or doctor about this, and when you should bring the filled container back to the office.

How Should I Take This Drug?
Take this drug exactly as directed by your doctor. If you do not understand the instructions, ask your doctor or nurse to explain them to you.

 Read the following information. If you do not understand it or if any of it causes you special concern, check with your doctor.

Before taking this drug, tell your doctor:
- f you are trying to become pregnant, are pregnant or breastfeeding. This drug may cause birth defects if either the male or female is taking it at the time of conception or during pregnancy. Men and women who are taking this drug need to use some kind of birth control. However, do not use oral contraceptives ("the pill") without checking with your doctor.
- If you think you may want to have children in the future. Many chemotherapy drugs can cause sterility.
- If you have any of the following medical problems: chickenpox or exposure to chickenpox, gout, heart disease, congestive heart failure, shingles, kidney stones, liver disease, or other forms of cancer.
- If you are taking any other prescription or over-the-counter drugs, including vitamins and herbals.

Should I avoid any other medicines, foods, alcohol, and/or activities?
Your prescription and nonprescription medicines may interact with other drugs, causing harm. Certain foods or alcohol can also interact with drug products. Never begin taking a new medicine—prescription or nonprescription—without asking your doctor or nurse if it will interact with alcohol, food, or other medicines. Some drug products can cause drowsiness and affect activities such as driving.

Precautions:
While you are being treated with interferon alpha, and after you stop treatment, do not have any immunizations (vaccinations) without your doctor's okay. Try to avoid contact with people who have recently taken the oral polio vaccine. Check with your doctor about this.

Interferon alpha often causes flu-like symptoms 3 to 6 hours after it is given. The fever, chills, and tiredness will decrease as you continue to take the drug. Talk to your doctor or nurse about ways to lessen these side effects.

Tell all the doctors, dentists, and pharmacists you visit that you are taking this drug.

- Most of the following side effects probably will not occur.
- Your doctor or nurse will want to discuss specific care instructions with you.
- They can help you understand these side effects and help you deal with them.

Side Effects:

More Common Side Effects

Flu-like syndrome with fever, chills, tiredness, headache, muscle and bone aches
Decreased appetite
Mild nausea
Mild diarrhea
Seizures
Irritability
Poor mental concentration
Sleepiness

Less Common Side Effects

Changes in taste and dry mouth
Dizziness
Abnormal results on kidney function blood tests

Rare Side Effects

Decreased white blood cell count with increased risk of infection
Decreased platelet count with increased risk of bleeding
Vomiting
Confusion
Depression
Increased heart rate
Chest pain
Change in blood pressure
Partial hair loss
Rash
Dry throat
Irritation at the place of injection
Congestive heart failure
Impotence
Menstrual irregularities

Side Effects / Symptoms of the Drug

Tell your doctor or nurse right away if you have fever above 100.5°F, symptoms of infection such as a cough with sputum or burning when urinating, unusual bruising, or bleeding such as nosebleeds, bleeding gums when you brush your teeth, or black, tarry stools.

Other side effects not listed above can also occur in some patients.
Tell your doctor or nurse if you develop any problems.

FDA Approval: This drug is approved for cancer treatment.

interleukin-2

Trade Names:
Aldesleukin, Proleukin

Type of Drug:
Interleukin-2 is a protein cytokine that belongs to a general class of synthetic substances called biologic response modifiers. It is used to treat advanced renal cell cancer and malignant melanoma.

How Drug Works:
Interleukin-2 is similar to a substance made naturally by the body's immune system. This drug fights against cancer cells, and stimulates the body's immune system to work better.

How Drug Is Given:
Interleukin-2 is given by an injection under the skin, in the vein over 15 minutes, or as a continuous infusion for 24 hours. The dose depends on your weight, the type of cancer being treated, and how well you tolerate it.

 Read the following information. If you do not understand it or if any of it causes you special concern, check with your doctor.

Before taking this drug, tell your doctor:
• If you are trying to become pregnant, are pregnant, or breastfeeding. This drug may cause birth defects if either the male or female is taking it at the time of conception or during pregnancy. Men and women who are taking this drug need to use some kind of birth control. However, do not use oral contraceptives ("the pill") without checking with your doctor.
• If you think you may want to have children in the future. Many chemotherapy drugs can cause sterility.
• If you have any of the following medical problems: chickenpox or exposure to chickenpox, gout, heart disease, congestive heart failure, shingles, kidney stones, liver disease, or other forms of cancer.
• If you are taking any other prescription or over-the-counter drugs, including vitamins and herbals.

Should I avoid any other medicines, foods, alcohol, and/or activities?
Your prescription and nonprescription medicines may interact with other drugs, causing harm. Certain foods or alcohol can also interact with drug products. Never begin taking a new medicine—prescription or nonprescription—without asking your doctor or nurse if it will interact with alcohol, food, or other medicines. Some drug products can cause drowsiness and affect activities such as driving.

Precautions:
Interleukin-2 can lower your blood counts (red blood cells and platelets). Your doctor will check your blood counts before and after each treatment to see how it affects your blood counts. Your doctor or nurse will give you specific instructions if your blood counts are low.

Interleukin-2 can decrease your red blood cell count. This can increase your risk of anemia. If severe, this can cause shortness of breath and chest pain.

Interleukin-2 can decrease your platelet count. This can increase your risk of bleeding. DO NOT take any aspirin or aspirin-containing medicines. Report unusual bruising, or bleeding such as nosebleeds, bleeding gums when you brush your teeth, or black, tarry stools.

A syndrome can occur where fluid leaks out of the small blood vessels in the body. This may lead to decreased blood pressure, swelling in abdomen or lungs, and difficulty breathing. Tell your nurse or doctor right away if you get shortness of breath, cough up pink and frothy sputum, stop urinating, or have confusion or irritability. Your doctor will give you medicine to help decrease the chance that these side effects will happen. Also, your doctor or nurse will give you more instructions and watch you closely.

While you are being treated with interleukin-2, and after you stop treatment, do not have any immunizations (vaccinations) without your doctor's okay. Try to avoid contact with people who have recently taken the oral polio vaccine. Check with your doctor about this.

Tell all the doctors, dentists, and pharmacists you visit that you are taking this drug.

- Most of the following side effects probably will not occur.
- Your doctor or nurse will want to discuss specific care instructions with you.
- They can help you understand these side effects and help you deal with them.

Side Effects:

More Common Side Effects

Fever and chills
Decreased red blood cell count with increased risk of anemia and tiredness (fatigue)
Decreased platelet count with increased risk of bleeding
Confusion
Depression
Abnormal results on kidney function blood tests
Abnormal results on liver function blood tests
Irritability
Low blood pressure
Increased heart rate
Difficulty breathing
Nausea and vomiting
Diarrhea
Decreased urine output
Itching
Rash
Headache
Tiredness
Chest pain
Heart attack

Less Common Side Effects

Decreased white blood cell count with increased risk of infection
Disorientation
Sleeping problems
Sores in mouth or on lips
Impaired memory
Difficulty talking
Kidney damage

Rare Side Effects

Severe difficulty breathing
Irregular heartbeat
Fluid in the lungs
Peeling of skin on hands and/or feet

Side Effects / Symptoms of the Drug

Most patients get fever and chills 1 to 4 hours after the drug is given. Talk to your doctor or nurse for ways to lessen this side effect.

Tell your doctor or nurse right away if you have breathing difficulties, cough up blood or pink sputum, vomit blood, have blood when you move your bowels, or have black, tarry stools.

Other side effects not listed above can also occur in some patients.
Tell your doctor or nurse if you develop any problems.

FDA Approval: This drug is approved for cancer treatment.

interleukin-3

Trade Name:
(Investigational)

Type of Drug:
Interleukin-3 is a protein cytokine that is part of the immune system. It belongs to a general class of synthetic substances called biologic response modifiers.

How Drug Works:
Interleukin-3 helps the (pluripotent) bone marrow stem cells grow and stimulates the growth and release of white blood cells and platelets. It is a growth factor for mast cells that help remove debris from tissues and can bind to invading microorganisms. This drug also stimulates histamine secretion when there is tissue injury. All this helps the immune system to work better and more effectively.

How Drug Is Given:
Interleukin-3 is given as an injection under the skin or in a vein. The dose, how often it is given, and how it is given depends on the investigational study and your weight.

 Read the following information. If you do not understand it or if any of it causes you special concern, check with your doctor.

Before taking this drug, tell your doctor:
• If you are trying to become pregnant, are pregnant, or breastfeeding. This drug may cause birth defects if either the male or female is taking it at the time of conception or during pregnancy. Men and women who are taking this drug need to use some kind of birth control. However, do not use oral contraceptives ("the pill") without checking with your doctor.
• If you think you may want to have children in the future. Many chemotherapy drugs can cause sterility.
• If you have any of the following medical problems: chickenpox or exposure to chickenpox, gout, heart disease, congestive heart failure, shingles, kidney stones, liver disease, or other forms of cancer.
• If you are taking any other prescription or over-the-counter drugs, including vitamins and herbals.

Should I avoid any other medicines, foods, alcohol, and/or activities?
Your prescription and nonprescription medicines may interact with other drugs, causing harm. Certain foods or alcohol can also interact with drug products. Never begin taking a new medicine—prescription or non-prescription—without asking your doctor or nurse if it will interact with alcohol, food, or other medicines. Some drug products can cause drowsiness and affect activities such as driving.

Precautions:
A flu-like syndrome is common after the drug is given. Fever often begins on the first day of therapy and lasts 2 to 16 hours.

While you are being treated with interleukin-3, and after you stop treatment, do not have any immunizations (vaccinations) without your doctor's okay. Try to avoid contact with people who have recently taken the oral polio vaccine. Check with your doctor about this.

Tell all the doctors, dentists, and pharmacists you visit that you are taking this drug.

- Most of the following side effects probably will not occur.
- Your doctor or nurse will want to discuss specific care instructions with you.
- They can help you understand these side effects and help you deal with them.

Side Effects:

More Common Side Effects
Fever
Headache
Stiff neck
Facial flushing

Less Common Side Effects
Redness at place of injection
Mild bone pain
Swelling of feet

Rare Side Effects
Decrease in blood pressure
Rash

Other side effects not listed above can also occur in some patients.
Tell your doctor or nurse if you develop any problems.

FDA Approval: This drug is being studied for cancer treatment.

interleukin-6

Trade Name:
(Investigational)

Type of Drug:
Interleukin-6 is a protein cytokine that is part of the immune system. It belongs to a general class of synthetic substances called biologic response modifiers.

How Drug Works:
Interleukin-6 tells the plasma cells to make more antibodies. It works with interleukin-1 (IL-1) to stimulate T-cell activation and helps myeloid stem cells differentiate so they can make white blood cells. This drug also helps make more plasma cells. All this helps the immune system to work better and more effectively.

How Drug Is Given:
Interleukin-6 is given as an injection under the skin. The dose, how often it is given, and how it is given depends on the investigational study and your weight.

 Read the following information. If you do not understand it or if any of it causes you special concern, check with your doctor.

Before taking this drug, tell your doctor:
- If you are trying to become pregnant, are pregnant, or breastfeeding. This drug may cause birth defects if either the male or female is taking it at the time of conception or during pregnancy. Men and women who are taking this drug need to use some kind of birth control. However, do not use oral contraceptives ("the pill") without checking with your doctor.
- If you think you may want to have children in the future. Many chemotherapy drugs can cause sterility.
- If you have any of the following medical problems: chickenpox or exposure to chickenpox, gout, heart disease, congestive heart failure, shingles, kidney stones, liver disease, or other forms of cancer.
- If you are taking any other prescription or over-the-counter drugs, including vitamins and herbals.

Should I avoid any other medicines, foods, alcohol, and/or activities?
Your prescription and nonprescription medicines may interact with other drugs, causing harm. Certain foods or alcohol can also interact with drug products. Never begin taking a new medicine—prescription or nonprescription—without asking your doctor or nurse if it will interact with alcohol, food, or other medicines. Some drug products can cause drowsiness and affect activities such as driving.

Precautions:
A flu-like syndrome is common after the drug is given. Fever and chills occur commonly with headaches that can be severe within 1 to 4 hours after the drug is given. Ask your doctor or nurse about medicines that can prevent these side effects.

While you are being treated with interleukin-6, and after you stop treatment, do not have any immunizations (vaccinations) without your doctor's okay. Try to avoid contact with people who have recently taken the oral polio vaccine. Check with your doctor about this.

Tell all the doctors, dentists, and pharmacists you visit that you are taking this drug.
- Most of the following side effects probably will not occur.
- Your doctor or nurse will want to discuss specific care instructions with you.
- They can help you understand these side effects and help you deal with them.

Side Effects:

More Common Side Effects
Fever
Chills
Headache
Decreased red blood cell counts with increased risk of anemia and tiredness (fatigue)

Less Common Side Effects
Decreased appetite
Joint aches

Rare Side Effects
Abnormal results on liver function blood tests

Other side effects not listed above can also occur in some patients.
Tell your doctor or nurse if you develop any problems.

FDA Approval: This drug is being studied for cancer treatment.

irinotecan

Trade Names:
Camptosar, Camptothecan-11, CPT-11

Type of Drug:
Irinotecan belongs to a general group of chemotherapy drugs known as topoisomerase inhibitors. It is used to treat colon and rectal cancers.

How Drug Works:
Irinotecan stops the growth of cancer cells by preventing the development of elements necessary for cell division.

How Drug Is Given:
Irinotecan is given by an injection in a vein over 90 minutes weekly for 3 weeks and then 1 off, or once every 3 weeks. The dose depends on your size, your age, whether you have had radiation to your abdomen/pelvis, how well your liver is working, your blood counts, and whether you have had any side effects such as diarrhea.

 Read the following information. If you do not understand it or if any of it causes you special concern, check with your doctor.

Before taking this drug, tell your doctor:
• If you are trying to become pregnant, are pregnant, or breastfeeding. This drug may cause birth defects if either the male or female is taking it at the time of conception or during pregnancy. Men and women who are taking this drug need to use some kind of birth control. However, do not use oral contraceptives ("the pill") without checking with your doctor.
• If you think you may want to have children in the future. Many chemotherapy drugs can cause sterility.
• If you have any of the following medical problems: chickenpox or exposure to chickenpox, gout, heart disease, congestive heart failure, shingles, kidney stones, liver disease, or other forms of cancer.
• If you are taking any other prescription or over-the-counter drugs, including vitamins and herbals.

Should I avoid any other medicines, foods, alcohol, and/or activities?
Your prescription and nonprescription medicines may interact with other drugs, causing harm. Certain foods or alcohol can also interact with drug products. Never begin taking a new medicine—prescription or non-prescription—without asking your doctor or nurse if it will interact with alcohol, food, or other medicines. Some drug products can cause drowsiness and affect activities such as driving.

Precautions:
While you are being treated with irinotecan, and after you stop treatment, do not have any immunizations (vaccinations) without your doctor's okay. Try to avoid contact with people who have recently taken the oral polio vaccine. Check with your doctor about this.

Irinotecan may lower your blood counts (white blood cells, red blood cells, platelets). Your doctor will check your blood counts before and after each treatment to see how it affects your blood counts. Your doctor or nurse will give you specific instructions if your blood counts are low.

Irinotecan can decrease your white blood cell count, especially 21 days after the drug is given. This can increase your risk of getting an infection. Report fever of 100.5°F or higher, or signs of infection such as pain in passing your urine, or coughing, and bringing up sputum.

Irinotecan can decrease your platelet count. This can increase your risk of bleeding. DO NOT take any aspirin or aspirin-containing medicines. Report unusual bruising, or bleeding such as nosebleeds, bleeding gums when you brush your teeth, or black, tarry stools.

During the drug infusion, tell your nurse if you start sweating, have abdominal cramping, or diarrhea. Your nurse will give you a special medicine to stop this reaction.

Irinotecan can cause nausea and vomiting. Ask your doctor or nurse to give you medicines to prevent or lessen this.

Irinotecan can cause severe diarrhea. It is very important to understand how to give yourself medicine to stop the diarrhea. Your doctor or nurse will give you instructions. Make sure you get the medicine right away, so that you will have it at home to stop the diarrhea immediately.

 Tell all the doctors, dentists, and pharmacists you visit that you are taking this drug.

- Most of the following side effects probably will not occur.
- Your doctor or nurse will want to discuss specific care instructions with you.
- They can help you understand these side effects and help you deal with them.

Side Effects:

More Common Side Effects
Nausea
Vomiting
Decreased white blood cell count with increased risk of infection
Sweating, abdominal cramping, or diarrhea during infusion
Diarrhea occurring the day after treatment, which can be severe
Tiredness (fatigue)
Anemia

Less Common Side Effects
Flushing during infusion

Rare Side Effects
Decreased platelet count with increased risk of bleeding

**Other side effects not listed above can also occur in some patients.
Tell your doctor or nurse if you develop any problems.**

FDA Approval: This drug is approved for cancer treatment.

letrozole

Trade Name:
Femara

Type of Drug:
Letrozole belongs to the general class of hormones or hormone antagonists. It is used to treat locally advanced and advanced breast cancer in postmenopausal women.

How Drug Works:
Letrozole blocks estrogen. Cancer cells that need estrogen are stopped from growing.

How Drug Is Given:
Letrozole is a pill taken by mouth once a day. The dose is the same for all patients. Take with water, with or without food. Keep the medicine in a tightly closed container away from heat and moisture and out of the reach of children and pets.

How Should I Take This Drug?
Take this drug exactly as directed by your doctor. If you do not understand the instructions, ask your doctor or nurse to explain them to you. This drug can be given at different strengths depending on the type of cancer being treated. Dosage may vary depending on your weight and your type of cancer.

 Read the following information. If you do not understand it or if any of it causes you special concern, check with your doctor.

Before taking this drug, tell your doctor:
- If you are trying to become pregnant, are pregnant, or breastfeeding. This drug may cause birth defects if either the male or female is taking it at the time of conception or during pregnancy. Men and women who are taking this drug need to use some kind of birth control. However, do not use oral contraceptives ("the pill") without checking with your doctor.
- If you think you may want to have children in the future. Many chemotherapy drugs can cause sterility.
- If you have any of the following medical problems: chickenpox or exposure to chickenpox, gout, heart disease, congestive heart failure, shingles, kidney stones, liver disease, or other forms of cancer.
- If you are taking any other prescription or over-the-counter drugs, including vitamins and herbals.

Should I avoid any other medicines, foods, alcohol, and/or activities?
Your prescription and nonprescription medicines may interact with other drugs, causing harm. Certain foods or alcohol can also interact with drug products. Never begin taking a new medicine—prescription or non-prescription—without asking your doctor or nurse if it will interact with alcohol, food, or other medicines. Some drug products can cause drowsiness and affect activities such as driving.

Precautions:
There are few side effects. If you develop side effects, talk to your doctor or nurse to find out how the side effects can be lessened.

Tell all the doctors, dentists, and pharmacists you visit that you are taking this drug.

- Most of the following side effects probably will not occur.
- Your doctor or nurse will want to discuss specific care instructions with you.
- They can help you understand these side effects and help you deal with them.

Side Effects:

More Common Side Effects
Pain in bone and muscle

Less Common Side Effects
Headache
Tiredness (fatigue)
Nausea

Rare Side Effects
Hot flashes
Vomiting
Loss of appetite
Diarrhea
Constipation
Chest pain

Side Effects / Symptoms of the Drug
It is important to continue to take this drug even if you feel well.

Other side effects not listed above can also occur in some patients.
Tell your doctor or nurse if you develop any problems.

FDA Approval: This drug is approved for cancer treatment.

leucovorin calcium

Trade Names:
Citrovorum Factor, Folinic acid

Type of Drug:
Leucovorin calcium is a water soluble vitamin in the folate group (folinic acid).

How Drug Works:
Leucovorin calcium can do 2 things. First, it helps drugs such as 5-fluorouracil work better than they can work alone (potentiates). This makes the 5-fluorouracil kill cancer cells more effectively. Second, it can rescue normal cells from the action of methotrexate. This allows cells lining the mouth and gastrointestinal tract as well as the cells in the bone marrow to be less affected by the methotrexate. It is an antidote when used this way, and MUST be taken exactly as directed. Otherwise, you can have severe side effects from the methotrexate.

How Drug Is Given:
Leucovorin calcium is a pill or liquid taken by mouth, or it can be given as an injection in the vein over 5 minutes. When used to "rescue" normal cells after high-dose methotrexate, it must be given exactly on time, usually starting 24 hours after high-dose methotrexate, and taken every 6 hours as directed by your doctor. When given together with 5-fluorouracil, it is given by vein over 5 to 20 minutes to 2 hours. The dose depends on your size and the reason you are taking it. If taking the medicine at home, keep it in a tightly closed container away from heat and moisture and out of the reach of children and pets.

How Should I Take This Drug?
Take this drug exactly as directed by your doctor. If you do not understand the instructions, ask your doctor or nurse to explain them to you. This drug can be given at different strengths depending on the type of cancer being treated. Dosage may vary depending on your weight and your type of cancer.

 Read the following information. If you do not understand it or if any of it causes you special concern, check with your doctor.

Before taking this drug, tell your doctor:
- If you are trying to become pregnant, are pregnant, or breastfeeding. This drug may cause birth defects if either the male or female is taking it at the time of conception or during pregnancy. Men and women who are taking this drug need to use some kind of birth control. However, do not use oral contraceptives ("the pill") without checking with your doctor.
- If you think you may want to have children in the future. Many chemotherapy drugs can cause sterility.
- If you have any of the following medical problems: chickenpox or exposure to chickenpox, gout, heart disease, congestive heart failure, shingles, kidney stones, liver disease, or other forms of cancer.
- If you are taking any other prescription or over-the-counter drugs, including vitamins and herbals.

Should I avoid any other medicines, foods, alcohol, and/or activities?
Your prescription and nonprescription medicines may interact with other drugs, causing harm. Certain foods or alcohol can also interact with drug products. Never begin taking a new medicine—prescription or nonprescription—without asking your doctor or nurse if it will interact with alcohol, food, or other medicines. Some drug products can cause drowsiness and affect activities such as driving.

Precautions:

Tell your doctor if you are taking seizure medicines. If you receive high doses of leucovorin calcium, this may decrease the antiseizure action of your medicine.

Tell your doctor if you are taking folic acid or multivitamins that contain folic acid.

Leucovorin calcium has very few side effects.

 Tell all the doctors, dentists, and pharmacists you visit that you are taking this drug.
- Most of the following side effects probably will not occur.
- Your doctor or nurse will want to discuss specific care instructions with you.
- They can help you understand these side effects and help you deal with them.

Side Effects:

Rare Side Effects
Allergic reaction with flushing of face and itching
Nausea
Vomiting

Other side effects not listed above can also occur in some patients.
Tell your doctor or nurse if you develop any problems.

FDA Approval: This drug is approved for cancer treatment.

leuprolide acetate

Trade Names:
Viadur, Lupron

Type of Drug:
Leuprolide acetate belongs to the general class of drugs known as hormones or hormone antagonists. It is used to treat advanced prostate cancer. It is also used to treat uterine fibroids and endometriosis.

How Drug Works:
Leuprolide acetate is a hormone similar to the hormone LHRH (luteininzing hormone-releasing hormone) that regulates the production of FSH (follicle-stimulating hormone) and LH (luteinizing hormone) produced by the pituitary gland. It reduces the production of FSH and LH. The decrease in LH causes the reduction in testosterone. This prevents cancer cells that depend on testosterone from growing.

How Drug Is Given:
Leuprolide acetate is given as an injection into a muscle or under the skin. It can be given monthly, every 3 months, or once a year, depending on how stable the cancer is. The dose is the same for all patients.

 Read the following information. If you do not understand it or if any of it causes you special concern, check with your doctor.

Before taking this drug, tell your doctor:
- If you are trying to become pregnant, are pregnant, or breastfeeding. This drug may cause birth defects if either the male or female is taking it at the time of conception or during pregnancy. Men and women who are taking this drug need to use some kind of birth control. However, do not use oral contraceptives ("the pill") without checking with your doctor.
- If you think you may want to have children in the future. Many chemotherapy drugs can cause sterility.
- If you have any of the following medical problems: chickenpox or exposure to chickenpox, gout, heart disease, congestive heart failure, shingles, kidney stones, liver disease, or other forms of cancer.
- If you are taking any other prescription or over-the-counter drugs, including vitamins and herbals.

Should I avoid any other medicines, foods, alcohol, and/or activities?
Your prescription and nonprescription medicines may interact with other drugs, causing harm. Certain foods or alcohol can also interact with drug products. Never begin taking a new medicine—prescription or non-prescription—without asking your doctor or nurse if it will interact with alcohol, food, or other medicines. Some drug products can cause drowsiness and affect activities such as driving.

Precautions:
Leuprolide acetate can cause a "flare" reaction after you start taking the drug. You will feel increased pain in bone and/or the tumor site, and men may have difficulty urinating. This will last about 2 weeks. Tell your doctor right away if the flare reaction lasts longer than this.

Tell all the doctors, dentists, and pharmacists you visit that you are taking this drug.
- -
- Most of the following side effects probably will not occur.
- Your doctor or nurse will want to discuss specific care instructions with you.
- They can help you understand these side effects and help you deal with them.

Side Effects:

More Common Side Effects
Hot flashes
Headache
Dizziness
Menstrual periods will stop in females
"Flare" reaction with initial dose

Less Common Side Effects
Breast tenderness
Decreased sexual desire
Decreased sexual ability

Rare Side Effects
Swelling of the hands and feet
Increased breast size
Loss of appetite
Nausea
Vomiting

Side Effects / Symptoms of the Drug
It is important to continue taking the medicine even if you feel well.

Other side effects not listed above can also occur in some patients.
Tell your doctor or nurse if you develop any problems.

FDA Approval: This drug is approved for cancer treatment.

leuprolide acetate implant

Trade Name:
Viadur Implant

Type of Drug:
Leuprolide acetate implant belongs to the general class of drugs known as hormones or hormone antagonists. It is used to treat advanced prostate cancer.

How Drug Works:
Leuprolide acetate is a hormone similar to the hormone LHRH (luteinizing hormone-releasing hormone) that regulates the production of FSH (follicle-stimulating hormone) and LH (luteinizing hormone) from the pituitary gland. It reduces the production of FSH and LH. The decrease in LH causes a reduction in testosterone. This prevents cancer cells that depend on testosterone from growing.

How Drug Is Given:
Leuprolide acetate implant is a drug-delivery system that contains the drug leuprolide acetate and is placed under the skin. It looks like a small, thin metal tube. After it is placed under the skin, it delivers leuprolide acetate to the body continuously for 12 months. Your doctor numbs your arm, makes a small incision, and then places the leuprolide acetate implant under your skin. The incision is closed with special surgical tape and covered with a bandage. The incision should heal in a few days. After 12 months, the implant is removed and may be replaced by your doctor.

 Read the following information. If you do not understand it or if any of it causes you special concern, check with your doctor.

Before taking this drug, tell your doctor:
- If you are trying to become pregnant, are pregnant, or breastfeeding. This drug may cause birth defects if either the male or female is taking it at the time of conception or during pregnancy. Men and women who are taking this drug need to use some kind of birth control. However, do not use oral contraceptives ("the pill") without checking with your doctor.
- If you think you may want to have children in the future. Many chemotherapy drugs can cause sterility.
- If you have any of the following medical problems: chickenpox or exposure to chickenpox, gout, heart disease, congestive heart failure, shingles, kidney stones, liver disease, or other forms of cancer.
- If you are taking any other prescription or over-the-counter drugs, including vitamins and herbals.

Should I avoid any other medicines, foods, alcohol, and/or activities?
Your prescription and nonprescription medicines may interact with other drugs, causing harm. Certain foods or alcohol can also interact with drug products. Never begin taking a new medicine—prescription or nonprescription—without asking your doctor or nurse if it will interact with alcohol, food, or other medicines. Some drugs can cause drowsiness and affect activities such as driving.

Precautions:
Leuprolide acetate implant can cause a "flare" reaction after you start taking the drug. You will feel increased pain in bone and/or the tumor site, and men may have difficulty urinating. This will last about 2 weeks. Tell your doctor right away if the flare reaction lasts longer than this.

Tell all the doctors, dentists, and pharmacists you visit that you are taking this drug.
- Most of the following side effects probably will not occur.
- Your doctor or nurse will want to discuss specific care instructions with you.
- They can help you understand these side effects and help you deal with them.

Side Effects:

More Common Side Effects
Hot flashes
Lack of energy
Headache
Dizziness
Sweating
Bruising
Breast enlargement
"Flare" reaction with initial dose
Local reaction to implantation: bruising, burning

Less Common Side Effects
Breast tenderness
Decreased sexual desire
Decreased sexual ability

Rare Side Effects
Swelling of the hands and feet
Loss of appetite
Nausea
Diarrhea

Side Effects/Symptoms of the Drug
It is important to continue taking the medicine even if you feel well.

Some patients may experience other side effects that are not listed above. Discuss any problems with your doctor or nurse.

Other side effects not listed above can also occur in some patients.
Tell your doctor or nurse if you develop any problems.

FDA Approval: This drug is approved for cancer treatment in men only.

levamisole hydrochloride

Trade Name:
Ergamisol

Type of Drug:
Levamisole hydrochloride belongs to a general class of agents called biologic response modifiers. It is used together with 5-Fluorouracil to treat Duke's Stage C colon cancer.

How Drug Works:
Levasmisole hydrochloride appears to stimulate the immune system to help it work better and prevent metastases when given after surgical removal of colon cancer. It is combined with the chemotherapy drug 5-fluorouracil. It may be used to treat other cancers along with other chemotherapy drugs.

How Drug Is Given:
Levamisole hydrochloride is a pill taken by mouth 3 times a day every 2 weeks, together with 5-fluorouracil, for 1 year. The dose is the same for all patients. Make sure not to drink alcohol when taking this medicine. Keep the medicine in a tightly closed container away from heat and moisture and out of the reach of children and pets.

How Should I Take This Drug?
Take this drug exactly as directed by your doctor. If you do not understand the instructions, ask your doctor or nurse to explain them to you. This drug can be given at different strengths depending on your weight and other factors.

 Read the following information. If you do not understand it or if any of it causes you special concern, check with your doctor.

Before taking this drug, tell your doctor:
- If you are trying to become pregnant, are pregnant, or breastfeeding. This drug may cause birth defects if either the male or female is taking it at the time of conception or during pregnancy. Men and women who are taking this drug need to use some kind of birth control. However, do not use oral contraceptives ("the pill") without checking with your doctor.
- If you think you may want to have children in the future. Many chemotherapy drugs can cause sterility.
- If you have any of the following medical problems: chickenpox or exposure to chickenpox, gout, heart disease, congestive heart failure, shingles, kidney stones, liver disease, or other forms of cancer.
- If you are taking any other prescription or over-the-counter drugs, including vitamins and herbals.

Should I avoid any other medicines, foods, alcohol, and/or activities?
Your prescription and nonprescription medicines may interact with other drugs, causing harm. Certain foods or alcohol can also interact with drug products. Never begin taking a new medicine—prescription or nonprescription—without asking your doctor or nurse if it will interact with alcohol, food, or other medicines. Some drug products can cause drowsiness and affect activities such as driving.

Precautions:
When given with 5-Fluorouracil, levamisole hydrochloride can lower your white blood cell count. This can increase your risk of getting an infection. Report fever of 100.5°F or higher, or signs of infection such as pain in passing your urine, or coughing and bringing up sputum.

Tell your doctor or nurse right away if you develop sores in your mouth or have diarrhea. Your doctor may tell you to stop taking your pills, and/or reduce the dose of the pills you are taking.

While you are being treated with levamisole hydrochloride, and after you stop treatment, do not have any immunizations (vaccinations) without your doctor's okay. Try to avoid contact with people who have recently taken the oral polio vaccine. Check with your doctor about this.

Avoid alcohol when taking levamisole hydrochloride. Severe side effects may result if you drink alcohol, including flushing, throbbing in head and neck, throbbing headaches, nausea and vomiting, sweating, chest pain, difficulty breathing, low blood pressure, weakness, blurred vision, confusion, coma, and death.

Tell all the doctors, dentists, and pharmacists you visit that you are taking this drug.

- Most of the following side effects probably will not occur.
- Your doctor or nurse will want to discuss specific care instructions with you.
- They can help you understand these side effects and help you deal with them.

Side Effects:

More Common Side Effects
Decreased white blood cell count with increased risk of infection
Nausea

Less Common Side Effects
Flu-like symptoms (fever, chills)
Vomiting
Diarrhea
Itching
Hair loss
Skin changes

Rare Side Effects
Dizziness
Headache
Numbness and tingling in hands and/or feet
Changes in taste
Changes in sense of smell
Sleepiness
Depression
Nervousness
Difficulty sleeping
Anxiety
Tiredness (fatigue)
Chest pain

Other side effects not listed above can also occur in some patients.
Tell your doctor or nurse if you develop any problems.

FDA Approval: This drug is approved for cancer treatment.

liposomal tretinoin

Trade Names:
Atragen, Lipo ATRA, Tretinoin Liposomal, AR-623, All-Trans-Retinoic Acid Liposomal

Type of Drug:
Tretinoin is a retinoid used in molecular targeted therapy. A retinoid is a naturally occuring substance in the body that helps to regulate, or control, the work of genes to help cells grow (mature) and divide (reproduce). Liposomal tretinoin is the same drug in a fat molecule. The drug is being studied in patients newly diagnosed with APL, Kaposi's sarcoma, and other types of cancer.

How Drug Works:
Tretinoin causes acute promyelocytic leukemia (APL) cells to mature, thus stopping them from dividing. Giving the drug in a liposome (a fat molecule) allows it to be given intravenously so that the blood levels of the drug may be higher for a longer time than when taken in pill form. This may reduce side effects and overcome resistance that sometimes occurs with the pill form of the drug.

How Drug Is Given:
Liposomal tretinoin is given by an injection in a vein every other day in the beginning of treatment (induction) then 3 times a week for 9 months (maintenance) for promyelocytic leukemia, per clinical trial. It is given 3 times a week for 4 weeks for Kaposi's sarcoma, per clinical trial. The dose depends on your weight, how well you do with the therapy, and certain blood test results (for example, complete blood count, kidney and liver function tests, and cholesterol levels).

 Read the following information. If you do not understand it or if any of it causes you special concern, check with your doctor.

Before taking this drug, tell your doctor:
- If you are trying to become pregnant, are pregnant, or breastfeeding. This drug may cause birth defects if either the male or female is taking it at the time of conception or during pregnancy. Men and women who are taking this drug need to use some kind of birth control. However, do not use oral contraceptives ("the pill") without checking with your doctor.
- If you think you may want to have children in the future. Many chemotherapy drugs can cause sterility.
- If you have any of the following medical problems: chickenpox or exposure to chickenpox, gout, heart disease, congestive heart failure, shingles, kidney stones, liver disease, or other forms of cancer.
- If you are taking any other prescription or over-the-counter drugs, including vitamins and herbals.

Should I avoid any other medicines, foods, alcohol, and/or activities?
Your prescription and nonprescription medicines may interact with other drugs, causing harm. Certain foods or alcohol can also interact with drug products. Never begin taking a new medicine—prescription or nonprescription—without asking your doctor or nurse if it will interact with alcohol, food, or other medicines. Some drug products can cause drowsiness and affect activities such as driving.

Precautions:
Liposomal tretinoin may cause an increase in the following: cholesterol, triglycerides, liver function tests, and kidney function tests. These will all be tested before you begin the drug and monitored during your therapy.

Side effects are less severe than they are with oral tretinoin.

Liposomal tretinoin should not be used by women who are pregnant or breastfeeding, or by patients who are allergic to tretinoin or to any of the liposome components.

Although not common, liposomal tretinoin can cause a syndrome of symptoms. This is called retinoic acid-acute promyelocytic leukemic (RA-APL) syndrome, similar to what can occur with the oral form of tretinoin. You will be watched for and should report fever, difficulty breathing, or joint pain as soon as possible.

Vitamin A toxicity may occur but is less severe than it is with oral tretinoin. This includes headache usually starting the first week of therapy and then fading, fever, dryness of the mouth and skin, bone pain, nausea, vomiting, rash, sores in the mouth, hair loss, and changes in vision. Report any of these to your doctor or nurse right away. Tell your doctor if you are taking any vitamin A products.

Tell all the doctors, dentists, and pharmacists you visit that you are taking this drug.

- Most of the following side effects probably will not occur.
- Your doctor or nurse will want to discuss specific care instructions with you.
- They can help you understand these side effects and help you deal with them.

Side Effects:

More Common Side Effects

Headache
Fever
Dryness of skin and mucous
    membranes
Bone pain
Nausea

Vomiting
Rash
Itching
Sweating
Changes in vision

Less Common Side Effects

Difficulty breathing, fever, joint pain
    (retinoic acid-APL syndrome)
Dizziness
Difficulty sleeping
Confusion

Depression
Leg weakness
Slow speech
Facial numbness
Forgetfulness

Rare Side Effects

Irregular heartbeat
Flushing of face
Decreased or increased blood pressure
Inflammation of veins (phlebitis)
Heart failure
Bleeding in the gastrointestinal tract
Abdominal pain
Diarrhea
Constipation

Heartburn
Abdominal swelling
Inflammation of the liver (hepatitis)
Ulcer
Earache
Hearing loss
Changes in kidney function
Enlarged prostate

Side Effects / Symptoms of the Drug

Call your doctor or nurse right away if you have irregular heartbeats, difficulty breathing, blood in your stools, fever, or joint pain.

Other side effects not listed above can also occur in some patients.
Tell your doctor or nurse if you develop any problems.

FDA Approval: This drug is being studied for cancer treatment.

lomustine

Trade Names:
CCNU, CeeNU

Type of Drug:
Lomustine belongs to the general group of chemotherapy drugs known as alkylating agents. It is used to treat several types of cancer including brain cancer and Hodgkin's disease.

How Drug Works:
Lomustine stops the growth of cancer cells, which causes them to die.

How Drug Is Given:
Lomustine is a pill taken by mouth on an empty stomach at bedtime. Take an antinausea medicine 1 hour before. The pill is usually taken once every 6 weeks. The dose depends on your weight, whether you are taking other chemotherapy drugs with it, and how well your kidneys are working. Keep the medicine in a tightly closed container away from heat and moisture and out of the reach of children.

How Should I Take This Drug?
Take this drug exactly as directed by your doctor. If you do not understand these instructions, ask your doctor or nurse to explain them to you. This drug can be given at different strengths depending on the type of cancer being treated. Dosage may vary depending on your weight and your type of cancer.

 Read the following information. If you do not understand it or if any of it causes you special concern, check with your doctor.

Before taking this drug, tell your doctor:
- If you are trying to become pregnant, are pregnant, or breastfeeding. This drug may cause birth defects if either the male or female is taking it at the time of conception or during pregnancy. Men and women who are taking this drug need to use some kind of birth control. However, do not use oral contraceptives ("the pill") without checking with your doctor.
- If you think you may want to have children in the future. Many chemotherapy drugs can cause sterility.
- If you have any of the following medical problems: chickenpox or exposure to chickenpox, gout, heart disease, congestive heart failure, shingles, kidney stones, liver disease, or other forms of cancer.
- If you are taking any other prescription or over-the-counter drugs, including vitamins and herbals.

Should I avoid any other medicines, foods, alcohol, and/or activities?
Your prescription and nonprescription medicines may interact with other drugs, causing harm. Certain foods or alcohol can also interact with drug products. Never begin taking a new medicine—prescription or nonprescription—without asking your doctor or nurse if it will interact with alcohol, food, or other medicines. Some drug products can cause drowsiness and affect activities such as driving.

Precautions:
Lomustine can lower your blood counts (white blood cells, red blood cells, platelets). Your doctor will check your blood counts before and after each treatment to see its effect. Your doctor or nurse will give you specific instructions for low blood counts.

While you are being treated with lomustine, and after you stop treatment, do not have any immunizations (vaccinations) without your doctor's okay. Try to avoid contact with people who have recently taken the oral polio vaccine. Check with your doctor about this.

Lomustine can decrease your white blood cell count, especially 4 to 5 weeks after the drug is given. This can increase your risk of getting an infection. Report fever of 100.5°F or higher, or signs of infection such as pain in passing your urine, coughing, and bringing up sputum.

Lomustine can decrease your platelet count. This can increase your risk of bleeding. DO NOT take any aspirin or aspirin-containing medicines. Report unusual bruising, or bleeding such as nosebleeds, bleeding gums when you brush your teeth, or black, tarry stools.

Lomustine can cause nausea and vomiting. Ask your doctor or nurse to give you medicines to prevent or lessen this.

 Tell all the doctors, dentists, and pharmacists you visit that you are taking this drug.

- Most of the following side effects probably will not occur.
- Your doctor or nurse will want to discuss specific care instructions with you.
- They can help you understand these side effects and help you deal with them.

Side Effects:

More Common Side Effects
Nausea
Vomiting
Decreased white blood cell count with increased risk of infection
Decreased platelet count with increased risk of bleeding
Fetal changes if pregnancy occurs while taking lomustine

Less Common Side Effects
Loss of appetite
Weight loss
Weakness
Kidney changes with prolonged use of high doses

Rare Side Effects
Diarrhea
Confusion
Feeling sleepy or drowsy
Difficulty walking
Disorientation
Blurred vision

Other side effects not listed above can also occur in some patients.
Tell your doctor or nurse if you develop any problems.

FDA Approval: This drug is approved for cancer treatment.

mechlorethamine hydrochloride

Trade Names:
Mustargen, Nitrogen Mustard

Type of Drug:
Mechlorethamine hydrochloride belongs to the general group of chemotherapy drugs known as alkylating agents. It is used to treat Hodgkin's disease.

How Drug Works:
Mechlorethamine hydrochloride stops the growth of cancer cells, which causes the cells to die.

How Drug Is Given:
Mechlorethamine hydrochloride is given as an injection in a vein over 20 minutes. Tell the nurse if you feel pain, burning, or discomfort in the vein when it is given. You will get medicine to stop any nausea or vomiting before and after the mechlorethamine. The dose and how often you get mechlorethamine depends on your weight, your blood counts, how well your liver is working, and the type of cancer being treated. You will have your blood counts checked before each treatment; if they are too low, your treatment will be delayed. This medicine may be given in addition to other chemotherapy medicines. It can also be applied to the skin (topical) or given into a body cavity, like the lining around the lung. Keep the topical solution in a tightly closed container away from heat and moisture and out of the reach of children and pets.

 Read the following information. If you do not understand it or if any of it causes you special concern, check with your doctor.

Before taking this drug, tell your doctor:
• If you are trying to become pregnant, are pregnant, or breastfeeding. This drug may cause birth defects if either the male or female is taking it at the time of conception or during pregnancy. Men and women who are taking this drug need to use some kind of birth control. However, do not use oral contraceptives ("the pill") without checking with your doctor.
• If you think you may want to have children in the future. Many chemotherapy drugs can cause sterility.
• If you have any of the following medical problems: chickenpox or exposure to chickenpox, gout, heart disease, congestive heart failure, shingles, kidney stones, liver disease, or other forms of cancer.
• If you are taking any other prescription or over-the-counter drugs, including vitamins and herbals.

Should I avoid any other medicines, foods, alcohol, and/or activities?
Your prescription and nonprescription medicines may interact with other drugs, causing harm. Certain foods or alcohol can also interact with drug products. Never begin taking a new medicine—prescription or nonprescription—without asking your doctor or nurse if it will interact with alcohol, food, or other medicines. Some drug products can cause drowsiness and affect activities such as driving.

Precautions:
Mechlorethamine hydrochloride can lower your blood counts (white blood cells, red blood cells, platelets). Your doctor will check your blood counts before and after each treatment to see its effect. Your doctor or nurse will give you specific instructions if your blood counts are low.

Mechlorethamine hydrochloride can decrease your white blood cell count, especially 6 to 8 days after the drug is given. This can increase your risk of getting an infection. Report fever of 100.5°F or higher, or signs of infection such as pain in passing your urine, coughing, and bringing up sputum.

Mechlorethamine hydrochloride can decrease your platelet count. This can increase your risk of bleeding. DO NOT take any aspirin or aspirin-containing medicines. Report unusual bruising, or bleeding such as nosebleeds, bleeding gums when you brush your teeth, or black, tarry stools.

Mechlorethamine hydrochloride can cause nausea and vomiting. Ask your doctor or nurse to give you medicines to prevent or lessen this.

Mechlorethamine hydrochloride is given intravenously. If the drug accidentally leaks out of the vein where it is given, it may damage the tissue and cause scarring. Tell the nurse right away if you notice redness, pain, or swelling at the place of injection.

While you are being treated with mechlorethamine hydrochloride, and after you stop treatment, do not have any immunizations (vaccinations) without your doctor's okay. Try to avoid contact with people who have recently taken the oral polio vaccine. Check with your doctor about this.

Tell all the doctors, dentists, and pharmacists you visit that you are taking this drug.

- Most of the following side effects probably will not occur.
- Your doctor or nurse will want to discuss specific care instructions with you.
- They can help you understand these side effects and help you deal with them.

Side Effects:

More Common Side Effects

Decreased white blood cell count with increased risk of infection
Decreased platelet count with increased risk of bleeding
Nausea
Vomiting
Taste changes
Decreased appetite
Hair thinning
Fetal changes if pregnancy occurs while taking mechlorethamine hydrochloride

Less Common Side Effects

Hardening and darkening of vein used for injection
Chills
Fever
Diarrhea
Drowsiness
Headache

Rare Side Effects

Ringing in ears, hearing loss

Side Effects / Symptoms of the Drug

Because of the way this drug acts on the body, there is a chance that it can cause other side effects that may not occur until months or years after the drug is used. This drug can very rarely cause a second cancer such as leukemia. Discuss this with your doctor.

Other side effects not listed above can also occur in some patients.
Tell your doctor or nurse if you develop any problems.

FDA Approval: This drug is approved for cancer treatment.

megestrol acetate

Trade Name:
Megace

Type of Drug:
Megestrol acetate belongs to the general group of drugs known as hormones or hormone antagonists. It is used to treat several types of cancer, including advanced breast cancer and endometrial cancer. It is often used in higher doses to help increase appetite (see also page 426).

How Drug Works:
It is unclear how the drug, which is a progesterone (female hormone), stops cancer cells from growing, but the drug appears to compete for hormone receptor sites on the cell.

How Drug Is Given:
Megestrol acetate is a pill or liquid taken by mouth. The pill is usually taken 4 times a day. The dose is the same for all patients. Keep the medicine in a tightly closed container away from heat and moisture and out of the reach of children and pets.

How Should I Take This Drug?
Take this drug exactly as directed by your doctor. If you do not understand the instructions, ask your doctor or nurse to explain them to you. This drug can be given at different strengths depending on the type of cancer being treated. Dosage may vary depending on your weight and your type of cancer.

 Read the following information. If you do not understand it or if any of it causes you special concern, check with your doctor.

Before taking this drug, tell your doctor:
- If you are trying to become pregnant, are pregnant, or breastfeeding. This drug may cause birth defects if either the male or female is taking it at the time of conception or during pregnancy. Men and women who are taking this drug need to use some kind of birth control. However, do not use oral contraceptives ("the pill") without checking with your doctor.
- If you think you may want to have children in the future. Many chemotherapy drugs can cause sterility.
- If you have any of the following medical problems: chickenpox or exposure to chickenpox, gout, heart disease, congestive heart failure, shingles, kidney stones, liver disease, or other forms of cancer.
- If you are taking any other prescription or over-the-counter drugs, including vitamins and herbals.

Should I avoid any other medicines, foods, alcohol, and/or activities?
Your prescription and nonprescription medicines may interact with other drugs, causing harm. Certain foods or alcohol can also interact with drug products. Never begin taking a new medicine—prescription or nonprescription—without asking your doctor or nurse if it will interact with alcohol, food, or other medicines. Some drug products can cause drowsiness and may affect activities such as driving.

Precautions:
There are few side effects. If you develop side effects, talk to your doctor or nurse to find out how they can be lessened.

Tell all the doctors, dentists, and pharmacists you visit that you are taking this drug.

- Most of the following side effects probably will not occur.
- Your doctor or nurse will want to discuss specific care instructions with you.
- They can help you understand these side effects and help you deal with them.

Side Effects:

More Common Side Effects
Fluid retention

Less Common Side Effects
Weight gain

Rare Side Effects
Blood clot in leg or lungs
Nausea

Side Effects / Symptoms of the Drug
Tell your doctor or nurse right away if you develop any of the following: shortness of breath or difficulty breathing; coughing up blood; pain in your lower leg muscle (calf); crushing chest pain.

Other side effects not listed may also occur in some patients.
Tell your doctor or nurse if you develop any problems.

FDA Approval: This drug is approved for cancer treatment.

melphalan hydrochloride

Trade Names:
L-Phenylalanine Mustard, L-PAM, Alkeran, L-Sarcolysin

Type of Drug:
Melphalan hydrochloride belongs to the general group of chemotherapy drugs known as alkylating agents. It is used to treat multiple myeloma and ovarian cancer.

How Drug Works:
Melphalan hydrochloride stops the growth of cancer cells, causing them to die.

How Drug Is Given:
Melphalan hydrochloride is a pill taken by mouth. It can also be given in high doses as an injection in a vein (investigational). Take the pill on an empty stomach, usually once a day for 5 days, every 6 weeks. You will be given antinausea medicine before taking the high-dose melphalan. The dose depends on your size, why you are taking it, and what regimen is used. Keep the medicine in a tightly closed container away from heat and moisture and out of the reach of children and pets.

How Should I Take This Drug?
Take this drug exactly as directed by your doctor. If you do not understand the instructions, ask your doctor or nurse to explain them to you. This drug can be given at different strengths depending on the type of cancer being treated. Dosage may vary depending on your weight and your type of cancer.

 Read the following information. If you do not understand it or if any of it causes you special concern, check with your doctor.

Before taking this drug, tell your doctor:
- If you are trying to become pregnant, are pregnant, or breastfeeding. This drug may cause birth defects if either the male or female is taking it at the time of conception or during pregnancy. Men and women who are taking this drug need to use some kind of birth control. However, do not use oral contraceptives ("the pill") without checking with your doctor.
- If you think you may want to have children in the future. Many chemotherapy drugs can cause sterility.
- If you have any of the following medical problems: chickenpox or exposure to chickenpox, gout, heart disease, congestive heart failure, shingles, kidney stones, liver disease, or other forms of cancer.
- If you are taking any other prescription or over-the-counter drugs, including vitamins and herbals.

Should I avoid any other medicines, foods, alcohol, and/or activities?
Your prescription and nonprescription medicines may interact with other drugs, causing harm. Certain foods or alcohol can also interact with drug products. Never begin taking a new medicine—prescription or non-prescription—without asking your doctor or nurse if it will interact with alcohol, food, or other medicines. Some drug products can cause drowsiness and affect activities such as driving.

Precautions:
Melphalan hydrochloride can lower your blood counts (white blood cells, red blood cells, platelets). Your doctor will check your blood counts before and after each treatment to see its effect. Your doctor or nurse will give you specific instructions if your blood counts are low.

Melphalan hydrochloride can decrease your white blood cell count, especially 16 to 21 days after the drug is given. This can increase your risk of getting an infection. Report fever of 100.5°F or higher, or signs of infection such as pain in passing your urine, coughing, and bringing up sputum.

Melphalan hydrochloride can decrease your platelet count. This can increase your risk of bleeding. DO NOT take any aspirin or aspirin-containing medicines. Report unusual bruising, or bleeding such as nosebleeds, bleeding gums when you brush your teeth, or black, tarry stools.

While you are being treated with melphalan hydrochloride, and after you stop treatment, do not have any immunizations (vaccinations) without your doctor's okay. Try to avoid contact with people who have recently taken the oral polio vaccine. Check with your doctor about this.

Tell all the doctors, dentists, and pharmacists you visit that you are taking this drug.
- Most of the following side effects probably will not occur.
- Your doctor or nurse will want to discuss specific care instructions with you.
- They can help you understand these side effects and help you deal with them.

Side Effects:

More Common Side Effects
Nausea (at higher doses)
Vomiting (at higher doses)
Fetal changes if pregnancy occurs while taking this drug
Decreased white blood cell count with increased risk of infection
Decreased platelet count with increased risk of bleeding

Rare Side Effects
Severe allergic reaction (intravenous form)
Loss of appetite
Scarring of lung tissue with prolonged use
Hair loss
Rash
Itching

Side Effects / Symptoms of the Drug
Because of the way this drug acts on the body, there is a chance that it can cause other side effects that may not occur until months or years after the drug is used. This drug can very rarely cause a second cancer such as leukemia. Discuss this with your doctor.

Other side effects not listed above can also occur in some patients.
Tell your doctor or nurse if you develop any problems.

FDA Approval: This drug is approved for cancer treatment.

menogaril

Trade Name:
Menogarol

Type of Drug:
Menogaril belongs to the general group of chemotherapy drugs known as anthracycline antibiotics. It is being studied in several types of cancers.

How Drug Works:
Menogaril stops the growth of cancer cells, which are then destroyed.

How Drug Is Given:
Menogaril is given as an injection in a vein over 1 to 2 hours, or as directed in the investigational study. The dose depends on your size and the study protocol.

 Read the following information. If you do not understand it or if any of it causes you special concern, check with your doctor.

Before taking this drug, tell your doctor:
- If you are trying to become pregnant, are pregnant, or breastfeeding. This drug may cause birth defects if either the male or female is taking it at the time of conception or during pregnancy. Men and women who are taking this drug need to use some kind of birth control. However, do not use oral contraceptives ("the pill") without checking with your doctor.
- If you think you may want to have children in the future. Many chemotherapy drugs can cause sterility.
- If you have any of the following medical problems: chickenpox or exposure to chickenpox, gout, heart disease, congestive heart failure, shingles, kidney stones, liver disease, or other forms of cancer.
- If you are taking any other prescription or over-the-counter drugs, including vitamins and herbals.

Should I avoid any other medicines, foods, alcohol, and/or activities?
Your prescription and nonprescription medicines may interact with other drugs, causing harm. Certain foods or alcohol can also interact with drug products. Never begin taking a new medicine—prescription or non-prescription—without asking your doctor or nurse if it will interact with alcohol, food, or other medicines. Some drug products can cause drowsiness and affect activities such as driving.

Precautions:
While you are being treated with menogaril, and after you stop treatment, do not have any immunizations (vaccinations) without your doctor's okay. Try to avoid contact with people who have recently taken the oral polio vaccine. Check with your doctor about this.

Menogaril can lower your blood counts. Your doctor will check your blood counts before and after each treatment to see its effect. Your doctor or nurse will give you specific instructions if your blood counts are low.

Menogaril can decrease your white blood cell count, especially 2 to 3 weeks after the drug is given. This can increase your risk of getting an infection. Report fever of 100.5°F or higher, or signs of infection such as pain in passing your urine, coughing, and bringing up sputum.

Menogaril can decrease your platelet count. This can increase your risk of bleeding. DO NOT take any aspirin or aspirin-containing medicines. Report unusual bruising, or bleeding such as nosebleeds, bleeding gums when you brush your teeth, or black, tarry stools.

Getting a wig before starting treatment may make it easier to deal with hair loss. Talk to your nurse or doctor about this. If your insurance does not cover it, there may be other resources to help you. Hair loss is temporary, and your hair will grow back after treatment.

Menogaril can cause injury to the heart muscle when large total doses are given. Your doctor will do a heart function test before you receive your first treatment, and then during the treatments. This way, any damage can be found early. Talk to your doctor about this.

Tell all the doctors, dentists, and pharmacists you visit that you are taking this drug.

- Most of the following side effects probably will not occur.
- Your doctor or nurse will want to discuss specific care instructions with you.
- They can help you understand these side effects and help you deal with them.

Side Effects:

More Common Side Effects

Decreased white blood cell count with increased risk of infection
Loss of appetite
Sores in mouth or on lips
Irritation of vein used for giving the drug
Hair thinning

Less Common Side Effects

Decreased platelet count with increased risk of bleeding
Decrease in red blood cell count with increased risk of tiredness
Mild nausea
Mild vomiting
Redness and itching along vein during injection
Decreased strength of heart muscle

Side Effects / Symptoms of the Drug

Specific information is available from the drug investigational study.

Tell your doctor or nurse if you have nausea or vomiting. You will receive drugs to lessen this, and prevent it the next time you receive menogaril.

Tell your doctor or nurse if you get a sore mouth or lips. Ask your nurse about rinsing your mouth with warm salt water or dilute baking soda after meals and at bedtime.

Because of the way this drug acts on the body, there is a chance that it can cause side effects that may not occur until months or years after the drug is used. These side effects very rarely can include second cancers such as leukemia. Discuss this with your doctor.

Other side effects not listed above can also occur in some patients.
Tell your doctor or nurse if you develop any problems.

FDA Approval: This drug is being studied for cancer treatment.

mercaptopurine

Trade Names:
6-MP, Purinethol

Type of Drug:
Mercaptopurine belongs to a general group of chemotherapy drugs known as antimetabolites. It is used to treat several types of leukemia.

How Drug Works:
Mercaptopurine prevents cells from making DNA and RNA by interfering with the synthesis of nucleic acids, thus stopping the growth of cancer cells, and causing them to die.

How Drug Is Given:
Mercaptopurine is a pill given once a day, usually for 5 days, with or without food. The dose depends on your weight and the reason you are taking it. Keep the medicine in a tightly closed container away from heat and moisture and out of the reach of children and pets.

How Should I Take This Drug?
Take this drug exactly as directed by your doctor. If you do not understand the instructions, ask your doctor or nurse to explain them to you. This drug can be given at different strengths depending on the type of cancer being treated. Dosage may vary depending on your weight and your type of cancer.

 Read the following information. If you do not understand it or if any of it causes you special concern, check with your doctor.

Before taking this drug, tell your doctor:
- If you are trying to become pregnant, are pregnant, or breastfeeding. This drug may cause birth defects if either the male or female is taking it at the time of conception or during pregnancy. Men and women who are taking this drug need to use some kind of birth control. However, do not use oral contraceptives ("the pill") without checking with your doctor.
- If you think you may want to have children in the future. Many chemotherapy drugs can cause sterility.
- If you have any of the following medical problems: chickenpox or exposure to chickenpox, gout, heart disease, congestive heart failure, shingles, kidney stones, liver disease, or other forms of cancer.
- If you are taking any other prescription or over-the-counter drugs, including vitamins and herbals.

Should I avoid any other medicines, foods, alcohol, and/or activities?
Your prescription and nonprescription medicines may interact with other drugs, causing harm. Certain foods or alcohol can also interact with drug products. Never begin taking a new medicine—prescription or nonprescription—without asking your doctor or nurse if it will interact with alcohol, food, or other medicines. Some drug products can cause drowsiness and affect activities such as driving.

Precautions:
While you are being treated with mercaptopurine, and after you stop treatment, do not have any immunizations (vaccinations) without your doctor's okay. Try to avoid contact with people who have recently taken the oral polio vaccine. Check with your doctor about this.

Mercaptopurine can lower your blood counts (white blood cells, red blood cells, platelets). Your doctor will check your blood counts before and after each treatment to see its effect. Your doctor or nurse will give you specific instructions if your blood counts are low.

Mercaptopurine can decrease your white blood cell count, especially 5 days to 6 weeks after the drug is given. This can increase your risk of getting an infection. Report fever of 100.5°F or higher, or signs of infection such as pain in passing your urine, or coughing, and bringing up sputum.

Mercaptopurine can decrease your platelet count. This can increase your risk of bleeding. DO NOT take any aspirin or aspirin-containing medicines. Report unusual bruising, or bleeding such as nosebleeds, bleeding gums when you brush your teeth, or black, tarry stools.

The side effects of mercaptopurine can be increased in people who are taking allopurinol for gout. Tell your doctor if you are taking allopurinol.

 Tell all the doctors, dentists, and pharmacists you visit that you are taking this drug.
- -
- Most of the following side effects probably will not occur.
- Your doctor or nurse will want to discuss specific care instructions with you.
- They can help you understand these side effects and help you deal with them.

Side Effects:

More Common Side Effects
Decreased white blood cell count with increased risk of infection
Increased risk of infection
Decreased platelet count with increased risk of bleeding

Less Common Side Effects
Rash

Rare Side Effects
Nausea
Vomiting
Loss of appetite
Sores in mouth or on lips
Jaundice

Other side effects not listed above can also occur in some patients.
Tell your doctor or nurse if you develop any problems.

FDA Approval: This drug is approved for cancer treatment.

mesna

Trade Name:
Mesnex

Type of Drug:
Mesna belongs to a general group of drugs known as cytoprotective agents. It is used to decrease the risk of bleeding in the bladder due to ifosfamide or high-dose cyclophosphamide.

How Drug Works:
Mesna protects the bladder from damage by the chemotherapy drug ifosfamide. It must always be given with ifosfamide.

How Drug Is Given:
Mesna is a pill given by mouth or as an injection in a vein. It is usually given by vein over 15 minutes or a pill prior to the chemotherapy drug ifosfamide, then every 3 to 4 hours for 3 to 4 doses. It can also be given along with ifosfamide when given continuously for 24 hours for 3 or more days. Mesna is given for an additional 24 hours when given this way. The dose depends on the amount of ifosfamide, your size, and the type of cancer being treated. Keep the medicine in a tightly closed container away from heat and moisture and out of the reach of children and pets.

How Should I Take This Drug?
Take this drug exactly as directed by your doctor. If you do not understand the instructions, ask your doctor or nurse to explain them to you. This drug can be given at different strengths depending on the type of cancer being treated. Dosage may vary depending on your weight and your type of cancer.

 Read the following information. If you do not understand it or if any of it causes you special concern, check with your doctor.

Before taking this drug, tell your doctor:
- If you are trying to become pregnant, are pregnant, or breastfeeding. This drug may cause birth defects if either the male or female is taking it at the time of conception or during pregnancy. Men and women who are taking this drug need to use some kind of birth control. However, do not use oral contraceptives ("the pill") without checking with your doctor.
- If you think you may want to have children in the future. Many chemotherapy drugs can cause sterility.
- If you have any of the following medical problems: chickenpox or exposure to chickenpox, gout, heart disease, congestive heart failure, shingles, kidney stones, liver disease, or other forms of cancer.
- If you are taking any other prescription or over-the-counter drugs, including vitamins and herbals.

Should I avoid any other medicines, foods, alcohol, and/or activities?
Your prescription and nonprescription medicines may interact with other drugs, causing harm. Certain foods or alcohol can also interact with drug products. Never begin taking a new medicine—prescription or nonprescription—without asking your doctor or nurse if it will interact with alcohol, food, or other medicines. Some drug products can cause drowsiness and affect activities such as driving.

Precautions:
Mesna is given before and after, or during the infusion of ifosfamide. Tell your doctor or nurse right away if you see blood in your urine or if your urine is pink.

Tell all the doctors, dentists, and pharmacists you visit that you are taking this drug.

- Most of the following side effects probably will not occur.
- Your doctor or nurse will want to discuss specific care instructions with you.
- They can help you understand these side effects and help you deal with them.

Side Effects:

Rare Side Effects
Nausea
Vomiting
Diarrhea

Other side effects not listed above can also occur in some patients.
Tell your doctor or nurse if you develop any problems.

FDA Approval: This drug is approved for cancer treatment.

methotrexate

Trade Names:
Amethopterin, Folex, Mexate, MTX

Type of Drug:
Methotrexate belongs to a general group of chemotherapy drugs known as antimetabolites. It is used to treat choriocarcinoma, leukemia in the spinal fluid, osteogenic sarcoma, breast cancer, and head and neck cancers.

How Drug Works:
Methotrexate prevents cells from making DNA and RNA by interfering with the synthesis of nucleic acids, thus stopping the growth of cancer cells.

How Drug Is Given:
Methotrexate is given as a pill by mouth, as an injection in a vein for up to 20 minutes, or as an injection into a muscle. The pills are usually taken as a single dose at bedtime. If the pills cause stomach upset, take an antacid or antinausea pill 1 hour before taking the methotrexate. Methotrexate can also be injected into the spinal cord to kill any cancer cells there. If methotrexate is given in medium or high doses, leucovorin calcium is given 24 hours later, then every 6 hours for up to 8 doses to "rescue" normal cells. The dose depends on your size, the type of cancer being treated, and how well your kidneys are working. Keep the medicine in a tightly closed container away from heat and moisture and out of the reach of children and pets.

How Should I Take This Drug?
Take this drug exactly as directed by your doctor. If you do not understand the instructions, ask your doctor or nurse to explain them to you. This drug can be given at different strengths depending on the type of cancer being treated. Dosage may vary depending on your weight and your type of cancer.

 Read the following information. If you do not understand it or if any of it causes you special concern, check with your doctor.

Before taking this drug, tell your doctor:
• If you are trying to become pregnant, are pregnant, or breastfeeding. This drug may cause birth defects if either the male or female is taking it at the time of conception or during pregnancy. Men and women who are taking this drug need to use some kind of birth control. However, do not use oral contraceptives ("the pill") without checking with your doctor.
• If you think you may want to have children in the future. Many chemotherapy drugs can cause sterility.
• If you have any of the following medical problems: chickenpox or exposure to chickenpox, gout, heart disease, congestive heart failure, shingles, kidney stones, liver disease, or other forms of cancer.
• If you are taking any other prescription or over-the-counter drugs, including vitamins and herbals.

Should I avoid any other medicines, foods, alcohol, and/or activities?
Your prescription and nonprescription medicines may interact with other drugs, causing harm. Certain foods or alcohol can also interact with drug products. Never begin taking a new medicine—prescription or non-prescription—without asking your doctor or nurse if it will interact with alcohol, food, or other medicines. Some drug products can cause drowsiness and affect activities such as driving.

Precautions:
While you are being treated with methotrexate, and after you stop treatment, do not have any immunizations (vaccinations) without your doctor's okay. Try to avoid contact with people who have recently taken the oral polio vaccine. Check with your doctor about this.

It is important not to drink alcohol when receiving methotrexate. Otherwise, risk of liver damage is increased. Also, if you are taking folic acid, vitamin preparations that contain folic acid, or nonsteroidal anti-inflammatory drugs, make sure to tell your doctor before starting this drug.

Methotrexate can lower your blood counts (white blood cells, red blood cells, platelets). Your doctor will check your blood counts before and after each treatment to see its effect. Your doctor or nurse will give you specific instructions if your blood counts are low.

Methotrexate can decrease your white blood cell count, especially 7 to 9 days after the drug is given. This can increase your risk of getting an infection. Report fever of 100.5°F or higher, or signs of infection such as pain in passing your urine, or coughing, and bringing up sputum.

Methotrexate can decrease your platelet count. This can increase your risk of bleeding. DO NOT take any aspirin or aspirin-containing medicines. Report unusual bruising, or bleeding such as nosebleeds, bleeding gums when you brush your teeth, or black, tarry stools.

While receiving high-dose methotrexate, you will receive extra intravenous fluid with a medicine called sodium bicarbonate to flush the medicine through your kidneys. After the treatment, it is important to drink extra liquids and take the bicarbonate tablets as directed by your nurse or doctor.

Methotrexate can cause you to be very sensitive to sunlight or bright ultraviolet light. You can get a very bad sunburn. Wear sunglasses and protective clothing when out in strong sunlight. Always wear sunscreen when out in the sun.

Methotrexate is an effective drug for many cancers, and is given at doses that are low, medium, and high. At medium and high doses, severe side effects are prevented by giving it with leucovorin. Leucovorin MUST be taken exactly as directed. Leucovorin is also given when methotrexate is injected into the spinal canal to kill cancer cells in the spinal fluid.

 Tell all the doctors, dentists, and pharmacists you visit that you are taking this drug.

- Most of the following side effects probably will not occur.
- Your doctor or nurse will want to discuss specific care instructions with you.
- They can help you understand these side effects and help you deal with them.

Side Effects:

More Common Side Effects

Nausea (high dose)
Vomiting (high dose)
Sores in mouth or on lips
Diarrhea

Increased risk of sunburn
Skin changes in areas previously
    treated with radiation (radiation recall)
Loss of appetite

Less Common Side Effects

Decreased white blood cell count with increased risk of infection
Decreased platelet count with increased risk of bleeding
Kidney damage (high dose)

Rare Side Effects

Nausea (low and medium dose)
Vomiting (low and medium dose)
Liver toxicity
Lung collapse (high dose)
Allergic inflammation of the lung
    (high dose) with fever, cough, and
    shortness of breath

Hair loss
Rash, itching
Dizziness
Blurred vision

Other side effects not listed above can also occur in some patients.
Tell your doctor or nurse if you develop any problems.

FDA Approval: This drug is approved for cancer treatment.

methyl-CCNU

Trade Names:
MeCCNU, Semustine

Type of Drug:
Methyl-CCNU belongs to the general group of chemotherapy drugs known as alkylating agents. It is a nitrosourea and crosses the blood-brain barrier. It is used to treat several types of cancer, including some brain cancers.

How Drug Works:
Methyl-CCNU stops the growth of cancer cells, which causes the cells to die.

How Drug Is Given:
Methyl-CCNU is a capsule taken by mouth every 6 weeks as directed by the investigational study. Take the capsule at bedtime on an empty stomach, 3 to 4 hours after a meal. Take an antinausea medicine 1 hour before the dose. The dose depends on your size, the cancer being treated, and how well your liver is working. Keep the medicine in a tightly closed container away from heat and moisture and out of the reach of children and pets.

How Should I Take This Drug?
Take this drug exactly as directed by your doctor. If you do not understand the instructions, ask your doctor or nurse to explain them to you. This drug can be given at different strengths depending on the type of cancer being treated. Dosage may vary depending on your weight and your type of cancer.

 Read the following information. If you do not understand it or if any of it causes you special concern, check with your doctor.

Before taking this drug, tell your doctor:
- If you are trying to become pregnant, are pregnant, or breastfeeding. This drug may cause birth defects if either the male or female is taking it at the time of conception or during pregnancy. Men and women who are taking this drug need to use some kind of birth control. However, do not use oral contraceptives ("the pill") without checking with your doctor.
- If you think you may want to have children in the future. Many chemotherapy drugs can cause sterility.
- If you have any of the following medical problems: chickenpox or exposure to chickenpox, gout, heart disease, congestive heart failure, shingles, kidney stones, liver disease, or other forms of cancer.
- If you are taking any other prescription or over-the-counter drugs, including vitamins and herbals.

Should I avoid any other medicines, foods, alcohol, and/or activities?
Your prescription and nonprescription medicines may interact with other drugs, causing harm. Certain foods or alcohol can also interact with drug products. Never begin taking a new medicine—prescription or nonprescription—without asking your doctor or nurse if it will interact with alcohol, food, or other medicines. Some drug products can cause drowsiness and affect activities such as driving.

Precautions:
While you are being treated with Methyl-CCNU, and after you stop treatment, do not have any immunizations (vaccinations) without your doctor's okay. Try to avoid contact with people who have recently taken the oral polio vaccine. Check with your doctor about this.

Methyl-CCNU can lower your blood counts (white blood cells, red blood cells, platelets). Your doctor will check your blood counts before and after each treatment to see its effect. Your doctor or nurse will give you specific instructions if your blood counts are low.

Methyl-CCNU can decrease your white blood cell count, especially 4 to 8 weeks after the drug is given. This becomes cumulative, and may be more pronounced after the second or third drug dose. This can increase your risk of getting an infection. Report fever of 100.5°F or higher, or signs of infection such as pain in passing your urine or coughing, and bringing up sputum.

Methyl-CCNU can decrease your platelet count. This becomes cumulative and may be more pronounced after the second or third drug dose. This can increase your risk of bleeding. DO NOT take any aspirin or aspirin-containing medicines. Report unusual bruising, or bleeding such as nosebleeds, bleeding gums when you brush your teeth, or black, tarry stools.

Methyl-CCNU can cause nausea and vomiting. Ask your doctor or nurse to give you medicines to prevent or lessen this.

 Tell all the doctors, dentists, and pharmacists you visit that you are taking this drug.

- Most of the following side effects probably will not occur.
- Your doctor or nurse will want to discuss specific care instructions with you.
- They can help you understand these side effects and help you deal with them.

Side Effects:

More Common Side Effects
Decreased white blood cell count with increased risk of infection
Decreased platelet count with increased risk of bleeding
Nausea
Vomiting
Fetal abnormalities if pregnancy occurs while taking this drug

Less Common Side Effects
Tiredness (fatigue)

Rare Side Effects
Sores in mouth or on lips
Liver problems
Kidney problems
Feeling disoriented
Difficulty walking
Blurred vision
Change in vision
Scarring of lung tissue, with difficulty breathing

Side Effects / Symptoms of the Drug
Tell your doctor or nurse right away if your vision changes, or if you have wheezing or difficulty breathing.

Because of the way this drug acts on the body, there is a chance that it can cause other side effects that may not occur until months or years after the drug is used. These very rarely can include second cancers such as leukemia. Discuss this with your doctor.

Other side effects not listed above can also occur in some patients.
Tell your doctor or nurse if you develop any problems.

FDA Approval: This drug is being studied for cancer treatment.

mitomycin

Trade Names:
Mitomycin C, Mutamycin

Type of Drug:
Mitomycin belongs to a general group of chemotherapy drugs known as antibiotics but acts as an alkylating agent. It is used to treat gastric and anal cancers.

How Drug Works:
Mitomycin blocks DNA synthesis in the cell, which results in cell death.

How Drug Is Given:
Mitomycin is given by an injection in a vein over 20 minutes once every 6 to 8 weeks. Tell the nurse if you feel pain, burning, or discomfort in the vein when it is given. You will get medicine to stop any nausea or vomiting before the mitomycin, and to take afterward. The dose and how often you get the medicine depends on your weight, your blood counts, how well your kidneys are working, and the type of cancer being treated. You will have your blood counts checked before each treatment; if they are too low, your treatment will be delayed. This medicine may be given in addition to other chemotherapy medicines.

 Read the following information. If you do not understand it or if any of it causes you special concern, check with your doctor.

Before taking this drug, tell your doctor:
- If you are trying to become pregnant, are pregnant, or breastfeeding. This drug may cause birth defects if either the male or female is taking it at the time of conception or during pregnancy. Men and women who are taking this drug need to use some kind of birth control. However, do not use oral contraceptives ("the pill") without checking with your doctor.
- If you think you may want to have children in the future. Many chemotherapy drugs can cause sterility.
- If you have any of the following medical problems: chickenpox or exposure to chickenpox, gout, heart disease, congestive heart failure, shingles, kidney stones, liver disease, or other forms of cancer.
- If you are taking any other prescription or over-the-counter drugs, including vitamins and herbals.

Should I avoid any other medicines, foods, alcohol, and/or activities?
Your prescription and nonprescription medicines may interact with other drugs, causing harm. Certain foods or alcohol can also interact with drug products. Never begin taking a new medicine—prescription or non-prescription—without asking your doctor or nurse if it will interact with alcohol, food, or other medicines. Some drug products can cause drowsiness and affect activities such as driving.

Precautions:
While you are being treated with mitomycin, and after you stop treatment, do not have any immunizations (vaccinations) without your doctor's okay. Try to avoid contact with people who have recently taken the oral polio vaccine. Check with your doctor about this.

Mitomycin can lower your blood counts (white blood cells, red blood cells, platelets). Your doctor will check your blood counts before and after each treatment to see its effect. Your doctor or nurse will give you specific instructions if your blood counts are low.

Mitomycin can decrease your white blood cell count, especially 4 to 6 weeks after the drug is given. This can increase your risk of getting an infection. Report fever of 100.5°F or higher, or signs of infection such as pain in passing your urine, coughing, and bringing up sputum.

Mitomycin can cause a decrease in the platelet count. This can increase your risk of bleeding. DO NOT take any aspirin or aspirin-containing medicines. Report unusual bruising, or bleeding such as nosebleeds, bleeding gums when you brush your teeth, or black, tarry stools.

Mitomycin is given intravenously. If the drug accidentally leaks out of the vein where it is given, it may damage the tissue and cause scarring. Tell the nurse right away if you notice redness, pain, or swelling at the place of injection.

Getting a wig before starting treatment may make it easier to deal with hair loss. Talk to your nurse or doctor about this. If your insurance does not cover it, there may be other resources to help you. Hair loss is temporary, and your hair will grow back after treatment.

Mitomycin can cause severe nausea and vomiting. Ask your doctor or nurse to give you medicines to prevent or lessen this.

 Tell all the doctors, dentists, and pharmacists you visit that you are taking this drug.

- Most of the following side effects probably will not occur.
- Your doctor or nurse will want to discuss specific care instructions with you.
- They can help you understand these side effects and help you deal with them.

Side Effects:

More Common Side Effects
Decreased white blood cell count with increased risk of infection
Decreased platelet count with increased risk of bleeding
Nausea
Vomiting
Loss of appetite
Tiredness (fatigue)
Hair loss

Less Common Side Effects
Sores in mouth or on lips

Rare Side Effects
Inflammation of lungs with cough, difficulty breathing, pneumonia, blood in sputum
Kidney damage

Other side effects not listed above can also occur in some patients.
Tell your doctor or nurse if you develop any problems.

FDA Approval: This drug is approved for cancer treatment.

mitoxantrone

Trade Names:
Novantrone, DHAD, DHAQ

Type of Drug:
Mitoxantrone belongs to a general group of chemotherapy drugs known as antibiotics. It is used to treat leukemia, and prostate cancer together with steroids.

How Drug Works:
Mitoxantrone stops the growth of cancer cells, which are then destroyed.

How Drug Is Given:
Mitoxantrone is given by a shot in the vein over 5 to 20 minutes, daily for 3 days, or once every 3 weeks. You will get a mild antinausea medicine before the mitoxantrone. The dose and how often you get the medicine depends upon your size, your blood counts, how well your liver is working, and the type of cancer being treated. You will have your blood counts checked before each treatment; if they are too low, your treatment will be delayed. This medicine may be given in addition to other anticancer medicines.

 Read the following information. If you do not understand it or if any of it causes you special concern, check with your doctor.

Before taking this drug, tell your doctor:
- If you are trying to become pregnant, are pregnant, or breastfeeding. This drug may cause birth defects if either the male or female is taking it at the time of conception or during pregnancy. Men and women who are taking this drug need to use some kind of birth control. However, do not use oral contraceptives ("the pill") without checking with your doctor.
- If you think you may want to have children in the future. Many chemotherapy drugs can cause sterility.
- If you have any of the following medical problems: chickenpox or exposure to chickenpox, gout, heart disease, congestive heart failure, shingles, kidney stones, liver disease, or other forms of cancer.
- If you are taking any other prescription or over-the-counter drugs, including vitamins and herbals.

Should I avoid any other medicines, foods, alcohol, and/or activities?
Your prescription and nonprescription medicines may interact with other drugs, causing harm. Certain foods or alcohol can also interact with drug products. Never begin taking a new medicine—prescription or non-prescription—without asking your doctor or nurse if it will interact with alcohol, food, or other medicines. Some drug products can cause drowsiness and affect activities such as driving.

Precautions:
While you are being treated with mitoxantrone, and after you stop treatment, do not have any immunizations (vaccinations) without your doctor's okay. Try to avoid contact with people who have recently taken the oral polio vaccine. Check with your doctor about this.

Mitoxantrone can injure the heart muscle when large total doses are given. Your doctor will test your heart function before you receive your first treatment, and then during the treatment. This way, any damage can be found early.

Mitoxantrone can lower your blood counts (white blood cells, red blood cells, platelets). Your doctor will check your blood counts before and after each treatment to see its effect. Your doctor or nurse will give you specific instructions if your blood counts are low.

Mitoxantrone can decrease your white blood cell count, especially 9 to 10 days after the drug is given. This can increase your risk of getting an infection. Report fever of 100.5°F or higher, or signs of infection such as pain in passing your urine, or coughing, and bringing up sputum.

Mitoxantrone can decrease your platelet count. This can increase your risk of bleeding. DO NOT take any aspirin or aspirin-containing medicines. Report unusual bruising, or bleeding such as nosebleeds, bleeding gums when you brush your teeth, or black, tarry stools.

Mitoxantrone turns the urine blue/green for about 24 to 48 hours, and then the urine returns to a normal color. Rarely, the whites of the eyes may turn light blue for a brief time.

Mitoxantrone can cause an allergic reaction with itching, dizziness, flushed appearances, and rash. You will be watched closely by your doctor or nurse.

Tell all the doctors, dentists, and pharmacists you visit that you are taking this drug.

- Most of the following side effects probably will not occur.
- Your doctor or nurse will want to discuss specific care instructions with you.
- They can help you understand these side effects and help you deal with them.

Side Effects:

More Common Side Effects
Decreased white blood cell count with increased risk of infection
Mild nausea
Mild vomiting

Less Common Side Effects
Hair loss
Fetal damage if pregnancy occurs while receiving this drug

Rare Side Effects
Decreased platelet count with increased risk of bleeding
Allergic reaction with rash, difficulty breathing, itching, flushed appearance, and dizziness
Heart damage with congestive heart failure
Sores in your mouth or on lips

Other side effects not listed above can also occur in some patients.
Tell your doctor or nurse if you develop any problems.

FDA Approval: This drug is approved for cancer treatment.

nilutamide

Trade Name:
Nilandron

Type of Drug:
Nilutamide belongs to the general group of drugs called hormones or hormone antagonists. Antagonists block the effect of a hormone. Nilutamide is an androgen hormone antagonist. It is used to treat advanced prostate cancer.

How Drug Works:
Nilutamide stops the growth of cancer cells that depend on the male hormone testosterone to grow and divide.

How Drug Is Given:
Nilutamide is a pill given daily by mouth. Usually, for the first month you will receive twice the regular dose. Starting the second month, you will receive the regular dose. Take the pills once a day, with or without food. Keep the medicine in a tightly closed container away from heat and moisture and out of the reach of children and pets.

How Should I Take This Drug?
Take this drug exactly as directed by your doctor. If you do not understand the instructions, ask your doctor or nurse to explain them to you. This drug can be given at different strengths depending on the type of cancer being treated. Dosage may vary depending on your weight and your type of cancer.

 Read the following information. If you do not understand it or if any of it causes you special concern, check with your doctor.

Before taking this drug, tell your doctor:
- If you are trying to become pregnant, are pregnant, or breastfeeding. This drug may cause birth defects if either the male or female is taking it at the time of conception or during pregnancy. Men and women who are taking this drug need to use some kind of birth control. However, do not use oral contraceptives ("the pill") without checking with your doctor.
- If you think you may want to have children in the future. Many chemotherapy drugs can cause sterility.
- If you have any of the following medical problems: chickenpox or exposure to chickenpox, gout, heart disease, congestive heart failure, shingles, kidney stones, liver disease, or other forms of cancer.
- If you are taking any other prescription or over-the-counter drugs, including vitamins and herbals.

Should I avoid any other medicines, foods, alcohol, and/or activities?
Your prescription and nonprescription medicines may interact with other drugs, causing harm. Certain foods or alcohol can also interact with drug products. Never begin taking a new medicine—prescription or nonprescription—without asking your doctor or nurse if it will interact with alcohol, food, or other medicines. Some drug products can cause drowsiness and affect activities such as driving.

Precautions:
It is important to continue taking nilutamide, even if you feel well or if you have side effects. Talk to your doctor or nurse about ways to lessen the side effects.

Most people start taking this medicine the day of or the day after surgery.

Rarely, nilutamide can cause inflammation of the lungs. Tell your doctor immediately if you develop difficulty breathing. If you already have shortness of breath, report it if it becomes worse.

Rarely, nilutamide can cause inflammation of the liver. Tell your doctor if you develop nausea, vomiting, abdominal pain, or yellowing of the skin or whites of your eyes.

Rarely, men taking nilutamide who drink alcohol can get flushing of the face or feel bad or dizzy from low blood pressure. If this happens, you should stop drinking alcohol while taking the medicine.

Content:

oprelvekin

Trade Name:
Neumega

Type of Drug:
Oprelvekin belongs to a general class of substances called biologic response modifiers. It is used to increase the number of platelets in the body, especially in patients receiving chemotherapy.

How Drug Works:
Oprelvekin is a synthetic version of a substance made by the body called IL-II (interleukin II), which is a growth factor. It tells the body's bone marrow to make more platelet cells so that bleeding does not occur after chemotherapy.

How Drug Is Given:
Oprelvekin is given as a shot under the skin once a day. You or a family member may be taught to give the injection. Keep the syringes, needles, and supplies in a safe place, out of the reach of children and pets. The medicine should be kept in its original container in the refrigerator; you should take it out 1 hour before the shot is due. The dose depends on your weight, and the number of doses depends on your platelet count. Keep the used syringes and needles in a special container. Ask your nurse or doctor about this and when you should bring the filled container back to the office. Oprelvekin is usually started within 24 hours after you receive chemotherapy and continued until your platelet count has reached a certain level. It should not be given at least 2 days before your next treatment and should not be given for more than 2 days.

How Should I Take This Drug?
Take this drug exactly as directed by your doctor. If you do not understand the instructions, ask your doctor or nurse to explain them to you. This drug can be given at different strengths depending on the type of cancer being treated. Dosage may vary depending on your weight and your type of cancer.

 Read the following information. If you do not understand it or if any of it causes you special concern, check with your doctor.

Before taking this drug, tell your doctor:
• If you are trying to become pregnant, are pregnant, or breastfeeding. This drug may cause birth defects if either the male or female is taking it at the time of conception or during pregnancy. Men and women who are taking this drug need to use some kind of birth control. However, do not use oral contraceptives ("the pill") without checking with your doctor.
• If you think you may want to have children in the future. Many chemotherapy drugs can cause sterility.
• If you have any of the following medical problems: chickenpox or exposure to chickenpox, gout, heart disease, congestive heart failure, shingles, kidney stones, liver disease, or other forms of cancer.
• If you are taking any other prescription or over-the-counter drugs, including vitamins and herbals.

Should I avoid any other medicines, foods, alcohol, and/or activities?
Your prescription and nonprescription medicines may interact with other drugs, causing harm. Certain foods or alcohol can also interact with drug products. Never begin taking a new medicine—prescription or nonprescription—without asking your doctor or nurse if it will interact with alcohol, food, or other medicines. Some drug products can cause drowsiness and affect activities such as driving.

Precautions:
Tell your doctor or nurse if you get white patches or soreness in your mouth, or if you have difficulty swallowing. Your doctor will give you medicine to help lessen these side effects.

Tell your doctor if you are taking a water pill (diuretic). This drug can cause mild swelling of the ankles or fluid in the lungs.

Women who are pregnant or breastfeeding should not use this drug.

Tell all the doctors, dentists, and pharmacists you visit that you are taking this drug.
- -
- Most of the following side effects probably will not occur.
- Your doctor or nurse will want to discuss specific care instructions with you.
- They can help you understand these side effects and help you deal with them.

Side Effects:

More Common Side Effects
Mild swelling of ankles
Runny nose
Fluid in lungs
Difficulty breathing when exerting yourself

Less Common Side Effects
Shortness of breath
Dizziness
Sleep problems
Red eyes
Cough
Sore throat

Rare Side Effects
Irregular heartbeat
Blurred vision
Nausea
Vomiting
Sores in mouth
Diarrhea

Side Effects / Symptoms of the Drug
Tell your doctor or nurse right away if you develop shortness of breath or difficulty breathing or if you have swelling in your ankles.

Other side effects not listed above can also occur in some patients.
Tell your doctor or nurse if you develop any problems.

FDA Approval: This drug is approved for cancer treatment.

oxaliplatin

Trade Name:
Eloxatin

Type of Drug:
Oxaliplatin belongs to the general group of chemotherapy drugs known as alkylating agents. It is used together with 5-fluorouracil and leucovorin to treat metastatic colorectal cancer that has progressed or recurred within 6 months of being treated with 5-fluorouracil, leucovorin, and irinotecan.

How Drug Works:
Oxaliplatin stops the growth of cancer cells, which causes the cells to die.

How Drug Is Given:
Oxaliplatin is given as an injection in a vein over 2 hours. It can be mixed with a vitamin called leucovorin. It is usually followed by an injection of 5-fluorouracil, then a continuous infusion of 5-fluorouracil over 22 hours. This is repeated the next day without the oxaliplatin. It is important not to eat ice chips or drink anything cold before, during, or after getting the oxaliplatin. The dose depends on your weight, your blood counts, and the side effects of the medicine.

 Read the following information. If you do not understand it or if any of it causes you special concern, check with your doctor.

Before taking this drug, tell your doctor:
• If you are trying to become pregnant, are pregnant, or breastfeeding. This drug may cause birth defects if either the male or female is taking it at the time of conception or during pregnancy. Men and women who are taking this drug need to use some kind of birth control. However, do not use oral contraceptives ("the pill") without checking with your doctor.
• If you think you may want to have children in the future. Many chemotherapy drugs can cause sterility.
• If you have any of the following medical problems: chickenpox or exposure to chickenpox, gout, heart disease, congestive heart failure, shingles, kidney stones, liver disease, or other forms of cancer.
• If you are taking any other prescription or over-the-counter drugs, including vitamins and herbals.

Should I avoid any other medicines, foods, alcohol, and/or activities?
Your prescription and nonprescription medicines may interact with other drugs, causing harm. Certain foods or alcohol can also interact with drug products. Never begin taking a new medicine—prescription or non-prescription—without asking your doctor or nurse if it will interact with alcohol, food, or other medicines. Some drug products can cause drowsiness and affect activities such as driving.

Precautions:
While you are being treated with oxaliplatin, and after you stop treatment, do not have any immunizations (vaccinations) without your doctor's okay. Try to avoid contact with people who have recently taken the oral polio vaccine. Check with your doctor about this.

Oxaliplatin can cause nausea and vomiting. Your doctor or nurse will give you medicines to prevent the nausea and vomiting. If you do get this side effect, talk to your doctor or nurse right away about ways to lessen this.

Tell all the doctors, dentists, and pharmacists you visit that you are taking this drug.

- Most of the following side effects probably will not occur.
- Your doctor or nurse will want to discuss specific care instructions with you.
- They can help you understand these side effects and help you deal with them.

Side Effects:

More Common Side Effects
Nausea
Vomiting
Numbness and tingling in hands and/or feet due to nerve irritation
Numbness of lips
Diarrhea
Abdominal pain
Mouth sores
Difficulty breathing
Tiredness (fatigue)

Less Common Side Effects
Difficulty walking
Decreased white blood cell count with increased risk of infection
Decreased platelet count with increased risk of bleeding
Difficulty swallowing or breathing
Poor tolerance to cold temperatures
Allergic reaction with rash, itching, swelling lips or tongue, or sudden cough

Side Effects / Symptoms of the Drug
Tell your nurse or doctor if you have trouble breathing or your throat feels like it is closing in. This sensation is scary but it will go away.

Tell your nurse right away if you get a rash, hives, swelling of your lips or tongue, or a sudden cough. You may be having an allergic reaction that can be managed.

Also, make sure you dress warmly and avoid cold temperatures and cold objects.

Other side effects not listed above can also occur in some patients.
Tell your doctor or nurse if you develop any problems.

FDA Approval: This drug is approved for cancer treatment.

paclitaxel

Trade Name:
Taxol

Type of Drug:
Paclitaxel belongs to the general group of chemotherapy drugs known as taxanes. It is also called a mitotic inhibitor because of its effect on the cell during mitosis (cell division). It is used to treat breast, ovarian, and lung cancers, and Kaposi's sarcoma.

How Drug Works:
Paclitaxel stops cell division, resulting in cell death.

How Drug Is Given:
Paclitaxel is given by an injection in a vein over 1 hour, every 3 weeks, or in lower doses, weekly. You will probably get another medicine, dexamethasone, to take the night before and on the morning of treatment to lessen the chance you will have an allergic reaction. Also, you will probably get an antinausea medicine before the paclitaxel, especially if the medicine is given every 3 weeks. The dose depends on your weight, how well your liver is working, the side effects you are having, and how often the medicine is given.

 Read the following information. If you do not understand it or if any of it causes you special concern, check with your doctor.

Before taking this drug, tell your doctor:
- If you are trying to become pregnant, are pregnant, or breastfeeding. This drug may cause birth defects if either the male or female is taking it at the time of conception or during pregnancy. Men and women who are taking this drug need to use some kind of birth control. However, do not use oral contraceptives ("the pill") without checking with your doctor.
- If you think you may want to have children in the future. Many chemotherapy drugs can cause sterility.
- If you have any of the following medical problems: chickenpox or exposure to chickenpox, gout, heart disease, congestive heart failure, shingles, kidney stones, liver disease, or other forms of cancer.
- If you are taking any other prescription or over-the-counter drugs, including vitamins and herbals.

Should I avoid any other medicines, foods, alcohol, and/or activities?
Your prescription and nonprescription medicines may interact with other drugs, causing harm. Certain foods or alcohol can also interact with drug products. Never begin taking a new medicine—prescription or nonprescription—without asking your doctor or nurse if it will interact with alcohol, food, or other medicines. Some drug products can cause drowsiness and affect activities such as driving.

Precautions:
Paclitaxel can lower your blood counts (white blood cells, red blood cells, platelets). Your doctor will check your blood counts before and after each treatment to see how it affects your blood counts. Your doctor or nurse will give you specific instructions if your blood counts are low. When your blood counts are low, your treatment may be delayed or the dose could be reduced.

Paclitaxel can decrease your white blood cell count, especially 7 to 10 days after the drug is given. This can increase your risk of getting an infection. Report fever of 100.5°F or higher, or signs of infection such as pain in passing your urine, or coughing, and bringing up sputum.

Paclitaxel can decrease your platelet count. This can increase your risk of bleeding. DO NOT take any aspirin or aspirin-containing medicines. Report unusual bruising, or bleeding such as nosebleeds, bleeding gums when you brush your teeth, or black, tarry stools.

Getting a wig before starting treatment may make it easier to deal with hair loss. Talk to your nurse or doctor about this. If your insurance does not cover it, there may be other resources to help you. Hair loss is temporary, and your hair will grow back after treatment.

Rarely, you may have an allergic reaction when paclitaxel is given to you. You may receive medicines to prevent this.

While you are being treated with paclitaxel, and after you stop treatment, do not have any immunizations (vaccinations) without your doctor's okay. Try to avoid contact with people who have recently taken the oral polio vaccine. Check with your doctor about this.

 Tell all the doctors, dentists, and pharmacists you visit that you are taking this drug.

- Most of the following side effects probably will not occur.
- Your doctor or nurse will want to discuss specific care instructions with you.
- They can help you understand these side effects and help you deal with them.

Side Effects:

More Common Side Effects
Decreased white blood cell count with increased risk of infection
Tiredness (fatigue)
Numbness and tingling in hands and/or feet related to irritation of nerves in your extremities
Muscle and bone aches for 3 days
Hair loss
Nausea
Vomiting
Mild diarrhea
Mild stomatitis

Less Common Side Effects
Allergic reaction, which can include increased heart rate, wheezing, swelling of face

Rare Side Effects
Severe allergic reaction (anaphylaxis)
Decreased platelet count with increased risk of bleeding

Side Effects / Symptoms of the Drug
Tell your doctor or nurse right away if you develop burning or pain in your hands or feet.

Other side effects not listed above can also occur in some patients.
Tell your doctor or nurse if you develop any problems.

FDA Approval: This drug is approved for cancer treatment.

pegfilgrastim

Trade Name:
Neulasta

Type of Drug:
Pegfilgrastim is a protein cytokine that belongs to the general class of synthetic drugs called biologic response modifiers. It is used to increase the neutrophils (white blood cells) in the blood after chemotherapy.

How Drug Works:
Pegfilgrastim is similar to a cytokine, a substance made by the body's immune system. It stimulates the body's bone marrow to make more neutrophils, a type of white blood cell involved in fighting infections. It also makes them work better. Pegfilgrastim is a version of another drug, filgrastim, but has been changed so that it stays in the body longer.

How Drug Is Given:
Pegfilgrastim is given as a shot under the skin once in each chemotherapy cycle. You or a family member may be taught to give the injection. Keep the syringes, needles, and supplies in a safe place, out of the reach of children and pets. The medicine should be kept in its original container in the refrigerator; you should take it out 1 hour before the shot is due. The dose is the same for all patients based on weight, but your blood counts will be monitored to make sure you get the effect needed. Keep the used syringes and needles in a special container. Ask your doctor or nurse about this and when you should bring the filled container back to the office.

How Should I Take This Drug?
Take this drug exactly as directed by your doctor. If you do not understand the instructions, ask your doctor or nurse to explain them to you.

Read the following information. If you do not understand it or if any of it causes you special concern, check with your doctor.

Before taking this drug, tell your doctor:
- If you are trying to become pregnant, are pregnant, or breastfeeding. This drug may cause birth defects if either the male or female is taking it at the time of conception or during pregnancy. Men and women who are taking this drug need to use some kind of birth control. However, do not use oral contraceptives ("the pill") without checking with your doctor.
- If you think you may want to have children in the future. Many chemotherapy drugs can cause sterility.
- If you have any of the following medical problems: chickenpox or exposure to chickenpox, gout, heart disease, congestive heart failure, shingles, kidney stones, liver disease, or other forms of cancer.
- If you are taking any other prescription or over-the-counter drugs, including vitamins and herbals.

Should I avoid any other medicines, foods, alcohol, and/or activities?
Your prescription and nonprescription medicines may interact with other drugs, causing harm. Certain foods or alcohol can also interact with drug products. Never begin taking a new medicine—prescription or nonprescription—without asking your doctor or nurse if it will interact with alcohol, food, or other medicines. Some drug products can cause drowsiness and affect activities such as driving.

Precautions:
Pegfilgrastim should not be given 14 days before and up to 24 hours after the chemotherapy treatment.

You may feel pain in your bones, but it can be easily controlled. Talk to your nurse or doctor about ways to lessen this side effect.

Pegfilgrastim should not be used before high-dose chemotherapy is given.

Very rarely, patients receiving the parent drug filgrastim have an allergic reaction. Since pegfilgrastim contains the drug filgrastim, side effects in both drugs will be similar. Signs and symptoms to report right away are rash, itching, red blotches, difficulty breathing, or swollen face or lips.

Patients with sickle cell disease who receive Pegfilgrastim are at increased risk of having a sickle cell crisis. You should talk to your doctor about the risks and benefits and things you can do to reduce the chance of having a crisis.

Very rarely, patients receiving pegfilgrastim have had an increase in the size of their spleen. In some cases, the spleen has ruptured and a few people have died. If you get pain in your left upper abdomen or tip of the shoulder, tell your doctor right away.

Very rarely, patients receiving pegfilgrastim who have very low neutrophil counts (few infection-fighting cells) and blood infection (sepsis) also have severe breathing problems.

 Tell all the doctors, dentists, and pharmacists you visit that you are taking this drug.
- -
- Most of the following side effects probably will not occur.
- Your doctor or nurse will want to discuss specific care instructions with you.
- They can help you understand these side effects and help you deal with them.

Side Effects:

More Common Side Effects
Bone pain

Rare Side Effects
Allergic reaction with rash, itching, red blotches
Severe allergic reaction with swollen face or lips, difficulty breathing
Enlarged spleen
Ruptured spleen

Side Effects / Symptoms of the Drug
Go to the emergency room right away if you have any trouble breathing or have a swollen face or lips.

Call your doctor or nurse right away if you have pain and/or swelling in the left upper abdomen or tip of the shoulder.

Other side effects not listed above can also occur in some patients.
Tell your doctor or nurse if you develop any problems.

FDA Approval: This drug is approved for cancer treatment.

pentostatin

Trade Names:
Nipent, 2'-Deoxycoformycin, dCF

Type of Drug:
Pentostatin belongs to a general group of chemotherapy drugs known as antibiotics. It is used to treat hairy cell leukemia.

How Drug Works:
Pentostatin stops the growth of cancer cells, which causes cells to die.

How Drug Is Given:
Pentostatin is given by an injection in a vein over 5 to 30 minutes. The dose depends on your weight, how well your kidneys are functioning, and your blood counts.

 Read the following information. If you do not understand it or if any of it causes you special concern, check with your doctor.

Before taking this drug, tell your doctor:
• If you are trying to become pregnant, are pregnant, or breastfeeding. This drug may cause birth defects if either the male or female is taking it at the time of conception or during pregnancy. Men and women who are taking this drug need to use some kind of birth control. However, do not use oral contraceptives ("the pill") without checking with your doctor.
• If you think you may want to have children in the future. Many chemotherapy drugs can cause sterility.
• If you have any of the following medical problems: chickenpox or exposure to chickenpox, gout, heart disease, congestive heart failure, shingles, kidney stones, liver disease, or other forms of cancer.
• If you are taking any other prescription or over-the-counter drugs, including vitamins and herbals.

Should I avoid any other medicines, foods, alcohol, and/or activities?
Your prescription and nonprescription medicines may interact with other drugs, causing harm. Certain foods or alcohol can also interact with drug products. Never begin taking a new medicine—prescription or non-prescription—without asking your doctor or nurse if it will interact with alcohol, food, or other medicines. Some drug products can cause drowsiness and affect activities such as driving.

Precautions:
While you are being treated with pentostatin, and after you stop treatment, do not have any immunizations (vaccinations) without your doctor's okay. Try to avoid contact with people who have recently taken the oral polio vaccine. Check with your doctor about this.

Pentostatin can lower your blood counts (white blood cells, red blood cells, platelets). Your doctor will check your blood counts before and after each treatment to see how it affects your blood counts. Your doctor or nurse will give you specific instructions if your blood counts are low.

Pentostatin can decrease your white blood cell count, especially about 15 days after the drug is given. This can increase your risk of getting an infection. Report fever of 100.5°F or higher, or signs of infection such as pain in passing your urine, or coughing, and bringing up sputum.

Pentostatin can decrease your platelet count. This can increase your risk of bleeding. DO NOT take any aspirin or aspirin-containing medicines. Report unusual bruising, or bleeding such as nosebleeds, bleeding gums when you brush your teeth, or black, tarry stools.

Pentostatin is given intravenously. If the drug accidentally leaks out of the vein where it is given, it may damage the tissue and cause scarring. Tell the nurse right away if you notice redness, pain, or swelling at the place of injection.

Pentostatin can cause severe nausea and vomiting. Ask your doctor or nurse to give you medicines to prevent or lessen this.

Tell all the doctors, dentists, and pharmacists you visit that you are taking this drug.
- -
- Most of the following side effects probably will not occur.
- Your doctor or nurse will want to discuss specific care instructions with you.
- They can help you understand these side effects and help you deal with them.

Side Effects:

More Common Side Effects
Decreased white blood cell count with increased risk of infection
Decreased platelet count with increased risk of bleeding
Anemia
Nausea
Vomiting
Tiredness and sleepiness progressing to coma

Less Common Side Effects
Eye irritation

Rare Side Effects
Mild kidney damage (reversible)
Inflammation of the liver
Heart attack and anaphylactic reaction
Lung infiltrates and nodules in patients who have had bleomycin or radiation to the lungs

---

Other side effects not listed above can also occur in some patients.
Tell your doctor or nurse if you develop any problems.

FDA Approval: This drug is approved for cancer treatment.

plicamycin

Trade Names:
Mithracin, Mithramycin

Type of Drug:
Plicamycin belongs to the general group of chemotherapy drugs known as antibiotics. It is used to treat testicular cancer and rarely, to lower high blood calcium levels.

How Drug Works:
Plicamycin stops the growth of cancer cells, which causes cells to die.

How Drug Is Given:
Plicamycin is given by injection in a vein over 4 to 6 hours. The dose and how long the treatment is depends on your weight and the condition being treated (such as high calcium in the blood or cancer).

 Read the following information. If you do not understand it or if any of it causes you special concern, check with your doctor.

Before taking this drug, tell your doctor:
- If you are trying to become pregnant, are pregnant, or breastfeeding. This drug may cause birth defects if either the male or female is taking it at the time of conception or during pregnancy. Men and women who are taking this drug need to use some kind of birth control. However, do not use oral contraceptives ("the pill") without checking with your doctor.
- If you think you may want to have children in the future. Many chemotherapy drugs can cause sterility.
- If you have any of the following medical problems: chickenpox or exposure to chickenpox, gout, heart disease, congestive heart failure, shingles, kidney stones, liver disease, or other forms of cancer.
- If you are taking any other prescription or over-the-counter drugs, including vitamins and herbals.

Should I avoid any other medicines, foods, alcohol, and/or activities?
Your prescription and nonprescription medicines may interact with other drugs, causing harm. Certain foods or alcohol can also interact with drug products. Never begin taking a new medicine—prescription or nonprescription—without asking your doctor or nurse if it will interact with alcohol, food, or other medicines. Some drug products can cause drowsiness and affect activities such as driving.

Precautions:
While you are being treated with plicamycin, and after you stop treatment, do not have any immunizations (vaccinations) without your doctor's okay. Try to avoid contact with people who have recently taken the oral polio vaccine. Check with your doctor about this.

Plicamycin can lower your blood counts (white blood cells, red blood cells, platelets). Your doctor will check your blood counts before and after each treatment to see how it affects your blood counts. Your doctor or nurse will give you specific instructions if your blood counts are low.

Plicamycin can decrease your white blood cell count, especially 7 to 14 days after the drug is given. This may increase your risk of getting an infection. Report fever of 100.5°F or higher, or signs of infection such as pain in passing your urine, or coughing, and bringing up sputum.

Plicamycin can decrease your platelet count. This may increase your risk of bleeding. DO NOT take any aspirin or aspirin-containing medicines. Report unusual bruising, or bleeding, such as nosebleeds, bleeding gums when you brush your teeth, or black, tarry stools.

Plicamycin can cause nausea and vomiting. Ask your doctor or nurse to give you medicines to prevent or lessen this.

Getting a wig before starting treatment may make it easier to deal with hair loss. Talk to your nurse or doctor about this. If your insurance does not cover it, there may be other resources to help you. Hair loss is temporary, and your hair will grow back after treatment.

Plicamycin is given intravenously. If the drug accidentally leaks out of the vein where it is given, it can damage the tissue and cause scarring. Tell the nurse right away if you notice redness, pain, or swelling at the place of injection.

 Tell all the doctors, dentists, and pharmacists you visit that you are taking this drug.

- Most of the following side effects probably will not occur.
- Your doctor or nurse will want to discuss specific care instructions with you.
- They can help you understand these side effects and help you deal with them.

Side Effects:

More Common Side Effects
Nausea
Vomiting
Hair loss
Loss of appetite
Sores in mouth or on lips
Decreased platelet count with increased risk of bleeding
Decreased white blood cell count with increased risk of infection

Less Common Side Effects
Darkening of nail beds
Darkening of skin
Ridging of fingernails
Fetal abnormalities if given during pregnancy or if pregnancy occurs while taking this drug

Rare Side Effects
Decreased blood calcium level

Side Effects / Symptoms of the Drug
Report muscle stiffness, weakness, or twitching (signs of low calcium).

Report bleeding, fever, or infection right away.

Other side effects not listed above can also occur in some patients.
Tell your doctor or nurse if you develop any problems.

FDA Approval: This drug is approved for cancer treatment.

prednisone

Trade Names:
Apo-Prednisone, Orasone, Deltasone, Prednisone

Type of Drug:
Prednisone is a glucocorticoid steroid used to treat anorexia and cachexia and some cancers. It is similar to a steroid hormone made by the adrenal glands in the body.

How Drug Works:
Prednisone decreases inflammation by preventing white blood cells from completing an inflammatory reaction. This drug can cause lymphocytes, a type of white blood cell, to break apart and die. Thus it is an important drug used in combination with other chemotherapy agents to treat many different cancers.

How Drug Is Given:
Prednisone is given as a pill or liquid by mouth with food. If you are taking it once a day, take it with breakfast. If you are taking it 2 to 4 times a day, try to make sure it is evenly spaced out, and that you take it with milk or food at about the same time every day. Make sure to shake the liquid form before pouring the dose. If you have taken prednisone for a long time and your doctor has told you to stop now, make sure to taper it or stop it gradually. The dose depends on your weight and the reason you are taking it. Keep the medicine in a tightly closed container away from heat and moisture and out of the reach of children and pets.

How Should I Take This Drug?
Take this drug exactly as directed by your doctor. If you do not understand the instructions, ask your doctor or nurse to explain them to you. This drug can be given at different strengths depending on the type of cancer being treated. Dosage may vary depending on your weight and your type of cancer.

 Read the following information. If you do not understand it or if any of it causes you special concern, check with your doctor.

- If you are trying to become pregnant, are pregnant, or breastfeeding. This drug may cause birth defects if either the male or female is taking it at the time of conception or during pregnancy. Men and women who are taking this drug need to use some kind of birth control. However, do not use oral contraceptives ("the pill") without checking with your doctor.
- If you think you may want to have children in the future. Many chemotherapy drugs can cause sterility.
- If you have any of the following medical problems: chickenpox or exposure to chickenpox, gout, heart disease, congestive heart failure, shingles, kidney stones, liver disease, or other forms of cancer.
- If you are taking any other prescription or over-the-counter drugs, including vitamins and herbals.

Should I avoid any other medicines, foods, alcohol, and/or activities?
Your prescription and nonprescription medicines may interact with other drugs, causing harm. Certain foods or alcohol can also interact with drug products. Never begin taking a new medicine—prescription or nonprescription—without asking your doctor or nurse if it will interact with alcohol, food, or other medicines. Some drug products can cause drowsiness and affect activities such as driving.

Precautions:
While you are being treated with prednisone, and after you stop treatment, do not have any immunizations (vaccinations) without your doctor's okay. Try to avoid contact with people who have recently taken the oral polio vaccine. Check with your doctor about this.

If you have a stomach ulcer, you may not be able to take this drug, or may need extra medicines to protect your stomach. Check with your doctor about this. When you take this drug, if you develop stomach pain or vomit any blood, tell your doctor immediately.

This drug may suppress the immune system and increase your susceptibility to infections. In addition, the drug may mask the signs of infection such as fever.

The dose and number of days you should take the medicine will be prescribed by your doctor and depends upon whether you are being treated for anorexia or cancer.

If you take prednisone for a long time, do not stop the medicine abruptly, as this can cause a decrease in the adrenalin your body makes (adrenal insufficiency). Symptoms of this are nausea, loss of appetite, tiredness, dizziness, difficulty breathing, joint pain, depression, low blood sugar, and low blood pressure.

If you are a diabetic, this medicine will increase your blood sugar levels and you may need to take extra diabetes medicine. Talk to your doctor about this.

 Tell all the doctors, dentists, and pharmacists you visit that you are taking this drug.

- Most of the following side effects probably will not occur.
- Your doctor or nurse will want to discuss specific care instructions with you.
- They can help you understand these side effects and help you deal with them.

Side Effects:

More Common Side Effects
Delayed wound healing
Mood changes
Depression
Increased blood sugar
Increased appetite with weight gain
Bruising of the skin

Sleep disturbance
Increased risk of infection
Sodium and fluid retention with swelling
  in ankles, increased blood pressure,
  and congestive heart failure

Less Common Side Effects
Decrease in potassium blood level (symptoms are loss of appetite, muscle twitching, increased thirst, and increased urination)
Weakness
Fracture of weak bones
Fungal infections (white patches in the mouth, vagina)
Sweating
Diarrhea
Nausea
Headache
Increased heart rate
Loss of calcium from bones

Rare Side Effects
Cataracts
Personality changes
Blurred vision
Stomach ulcer that may bleed (hemorrhage)

Side Effects / Symptoms of the Drug
Tell your doctor or nurse right away if you develop any of the following: stomach pain or vomiting of blood; signs of infection such as fever, bad cough with sputum, burning when you pass your urine, or sore throat.

With prolonged use, the following changes may occur: round face, acne, abnormal hair growth on face, and purple spots on skin.

Report any changes or new problems to your doctor or nurse.

Other side effects not listed above can also occur in some patients.
Tell your doctor or nurse if you develop any problems.

FDA Approval: This drug is approved for cancer treatment.

procarbazine hydrochloride

Trade Name:
Matulane

Type of Drug:
Procarbazine hydrochloride is one of a group of miscellaneous chemotherapy drugs used to treat Hodgkin's disease and brain tumors.

How Drug Works:
Procarbazine hydrochloride stops the growth of cancer cells, which causes the cells to die.

How Drug Is Given:
Procarbazine hydrochloride is a pill taken by mouth usually daily for a specific number of days. Make sure you take an antinausea pill 1 hour before taking the medicine. Some people like to take the dose at bedtime. Your doctor or nurse will tell you what foods to avoid, like hard cheeses and Chianti wine that contain tyramine. The dose depends on your weight and the type of cancer being treated. Keep the medicine in a tightly closed container away from heat and moisture and out of the reach of children and pets.

How Should I Take This Drug?
Take this drug exactly as directed by your doctor. If you do not understand the instructions, ask your doctor or nurse to explain them to you. This drug can be given at different strengths depending on the type of cancer being treated. Dosage may vary depending on your weight and your type of cancer.

 Read the following information. If you do not understand it or if any of it causes you special concern, check with your doctor.

Before taking this drug, tell your doctor:
- If you are trying to become pregnant, are pregnant, or breastfeeding. This drug may cause birth defects if either the male or female is taking it at the time of conception or during pregnancy. Men and women who are taking this drug need to use some kind of birth control. However, do not use oral contraceptives ("the pill") without checking with your doctor.
- If you think you may want to have children in the future. Many chemotherapy drugs can cause sterility.
- If you have any of the following medical problems: chickenpox or exposure to chickenpox, gout, heart disease, congestive heart failure, shingles, kidney stones, liver disease, or other forms of cancer.
- If you are taking any other prescription or over-the-counter drugs, including vitamins and herbals.

Should I avoid any other medicines, foods, alcohol, and/or activities?
Your prescription and nonprescription medicines may interact with other drugs, causing harm. Certain foods or alcohol can also interact with drug products. Never begin taking a new medicine—prescription or nonprescription—without asking your doctor or nurse if it will interact with alcohol, food, or other medicines. Some drug products can cause drowsiness and affect activities such as driving.

Precautions:
While you are being treated with procarbazine hydrochloride, and after you stop treatment, do not have any immunizations (vaccinations) without your doctor's okay. Try to avoid contact with people who have recently taken the oral polio vaccine. Check with your doctor about this.

Procarbazine hydrochloride can lower your blood counts (white blood cells, red blood cells, platelets). Your doctor will check your blood counts before and after each treatment to see how it affects your blood counts. Your doctor or nurse will give you specific instructions if your blood counts are low.

Procarbazine hydrochloride can decrease your white blood cell count. This can increase your risk of getting an infection. Report fever of 100.5°F or higher, or signs of infection such as pain in passing your urine, or coughing, and bringing up sputum.

Procarbazine hydrochloride can decrease your platelet count, especially 28 days after the drug is given. This can increase your risk of bleeding. DO NOT take any aspirin or aspirin-containing medicines. Report unusual bruising, or bleeding such as nosebleeds, bleeding gums when you brush your teeth, or black, tarry stools.

Do not drink alcohol while taking procarbazine hydrochloride. It will cause a reaction, and you may develop a headache, difficulty breathing, nausea, vomiting, sweating, chest pain, low blood pressure, and changes in how you think and feel.

Procarbazine hydrochloride can cause nausea and vomiting. Ask your doctor or nurse to give you medicines to prevent or lessen this.

Procarbazine hydrochloride increases the effects of opioids, antihistamines, barbituates, and medicines to lower blood pressure. These medicines should be used with caution. If you are taking any of these, please discuss with your doctor.

 Tell all the doctors, dentists, and pharmacists you visit that you are taking this drug.

- Most of the following side effects probably will not occur.
- Your doctor or nurse will want to discuss specific care instructions with you.
- They can help you understand these side effects and help you deal with them.

Side Effects:

More Common Side Effects
Decreased white blood cell count with increased risk of infection
Decreased platelet count with increased risk of bleeding
Nausea
Vomiting
Feeling sleepy or drowsy
Depression
Difficulty sleeping
Nightmares
Nervousness
Flu-like symptoms (tiredness, headache, muscle aches, fever, stuffy nose)

Rare Side Effects
Diarrhea
Tremors, coma, convulsions
Numbness and tingling in hands and feet progressing to difficulty walking
Hair loss
Rash
Darkening of skin
Itching

Side Effects / Symptoms of the Drug
Call your doctor or nurse if you develop numbness or tingling in your hands and/or feet, confusion, mouth sores, diarrhea, or rash.

Other side effects not listed above can also occur in some patients.
Tell your doctor or nurse if you develop any problems.

FDA Approval: This drug is approved for cancer treatment.

raloxifene hydrochloride

Trade Name:
Evista

Type of Drug:
Raloxifene hydrochloride is a hormone or hormone blocker (antagonist) that belongs to a group of drugs called selective estrogen receptor modulators (SERMs). Raloxifene hydrochloride is being studied in women who are at high risk for development of breast cancer to see if it prevents cells from becoming cancerous. However, it is used to prevent osteoporosis because in cells like bone cells, it acts like estrogen to prevent bone loss (osteoporosis) in menopausal women. It also helps to lower the fat in the blood (low density lipids).

How Drug Works:
Raloxifene hydrochloride blocks estrogen from binding to certain cells, such as those in the breast. Some cancer cells depend on estrogen for their growth.

How Drug Is Given:
Raloxifene is a pill given once a day at about the same time each day, without regard to food. The dose is the same for all patients. Keep the medicine in a tightly closed container away from heat and moisture and out of the reach of children and pets.

How Should I Take This Drug?
Take this drug exactly as directed by your doctor. If you do not understand the instructions, ask your doctor or nurse to explain them to you.

 Read the following information. If you do not understand it or if any of it causes you special concern, check with your doctor.

Before taking this drug, tell your doctor:
- If you are trying to become pregnant, are pregnant, or breastfeeding. This drug may cause birth defects if either the male or female is taking it at the time of conception or during pregnancy. Men and women who are taking this drug need to use some kind of birth control. However, do not use oral contraceptives ("the pill") without checking with your doctor.
- If you think you may want to have children in the future. Many chemotherapy drugs can cause sterility.
- If you have any of the following medical problems: chickenpox or exposure to chickenpox, gout, heart disease, congestive heart failure, shingles, kidney stones, liver disease, or other forms of cancer.
- If you are taking any other prescription or over-the-counter drugs, including vitamins and herbals.

Should I avoid any other medicines, foods, alcohol, and/or activities?
Your prescription and nonprescription medicines may interact with other drugs, causing harm. Certain foods or alcohol can also interact with drug products. Never begin taking a new medicine—prescription or non-prescription—without asking your doctor or nurse if it will interact with alcohol, food, or other medicines. Some drug products can cause drowsiness and affect activities such as driving.

Precautions:
Drug or blood clotting levels may need to be checked more frequently if you are also taking Coumadin, a blood-thinning medicine.

Raloxifene hydrochloride can increase your risk for developing blood clots. If you travel or fly frequently, it is important to get up and walk around frequently so you are not in the same position for a long time. Call your nurse or doctor if you develop shortness of breath, chest pain, pain in your calf (leg) muscles, or redness or swelling of your legs; you may have a blood clot and should be seen by a doctor right away.

If you are pregnant or may be pregnant, you should not take this drug.

Tell all the doctors, dentists, and pharmacists you visit that you are taking this drug.

- Most of the following side effects probably will not occur.
- Your doctor or nurse will want to discuss specific care instructions with you.
- They can help you understand these side effects and help you deal with them.

Side Effects:

More Common Side Effects
Hot flashes
Trouble sleeping

Less Common Side Effects
Fluid weight gain
Headaches
Depression
Fever
Aches and pains in the joints
Leg cramps
Rash
Flu-like symptoms
Vaginal infections
Urinary tract infections

Rare Side Effects
Blood clots in the legs or lungs
Nausea
Vomiting
Heartburn
Passing gas

Side Effects / Symptoms of the Drug
Stop the drug and call your doctor or nurse right away if you develop sudden shortness of breath or pain, swelling, or redness in your legs.

Tell your doctor or nurse if you get a rash.

Other side effects not listed above can also occur in some patients.
Tell your doctor or nurse if you develop any problems.

FDA Approval: This drug is approved for cancer treatment.

raltitrexed

Trade Name:
Tomudex

Type of Drug:
Raltitrexed belongs to a general group of chemotherapy drugs known as antimetabolites. It is being studied in these cancers: colorectal, breast, ovary, pancreas, and nonsmall cell lung cancer.

How Drug Works:
The cancer cell is fooled into thinking that raltitrexed is a nutrient or building block; the cell takes in the drug, the DNA is damaged, and the cell cannot divide. This kills the cell.

How Drug Is Given:
Raltitrexed is given as an injection in a vein over 15 minutes, usually every 3 weeks. The dose depends on your weight, how well your kidneys are working, and the amount specified in the investigational study.

 Read the following information. If you do not understand it or if any of it causes you special concern, check with your doctor.

Before taking this drug, tell your doctor:
- If you are trying to become pregnant, are pregnant, or breastfeeding. This drug may cause birth defects if either the male or female is taking it at the time of conception or during pregnancy. Men and women who are taking this drug need to use some kind of birth control. However, do not use oral contraceptives ("the pill") without checking with your doctor.
- If you think you may want to have children in the future. Many chemotherapy drugs can cause sterility.
- If you have any of the following medical problems: chickenpox or exposure to chickenpox, gout, heart disease, congestive heart failure, shingles, kidney stones, liver disease, or other forms of cancer.
- If you are taking any other prescription or over-the-counter drugs, including vitamins and herbals.

Should I avoid any other medicines, foods, alcohol, and/or activities?
Your prescription and nonprescription medicines may interact with other drugs, causing harm. Certain foods or alcohol can also interact with drug products. Never begin taking a new medicine—prescription or nonprescription—without asking your doctor or nurse if it will interact with alcohol, food, or other medicines. Some drug products can cause drowsiness and affect activities such as driving.

Precautions:
Raltitrexed can cause lowering of your blood counts (white blood cells, red blood cells, platelets). Your doctor will check your blood counts before each treatment, and after to see how it affects your blood counts. Your doctor or nurse will give you specific instructions for lowered blood counts.

Do not take folate or folic acid vitamins, as this interferes with the drug's effect.

If you have received chemotherapy before, your dose might need to be decreased at first until your doctor knows how it will affect your blood counts.

Diarrhea may be severe. It is very important to call you doctor or nurse if your diarrhea does not go away in 24 hours. Your doctor or nurse will tell you more about this.

Tell all the doctors, dentists, and pharmacists you visit that you are taking this drug.

- Most of the following side effects probably will not occur.
- Your doctor or nurse will want to discuss specific care instructions with you.
- They can help you understand these side effects and help you deal with them.

Side Effects:

More Common Side Effects
Decreased white blood cells with increased risk of infection
Decreased platelets with increased risk of bleeding
Decreased red blood cells with increased risk of tiredness and anemia
Diarrhea
Sores in mouth
Nausea
Vomiting

Less Common Side Effects
Tiredness (fatigue)
Feeling sleepy or drowsy
Fever
Rash

Rare Side Effects
Hair loss
Skin infection
Pain
Loss of appetite

Side Effects / Symptoms of the Drug
Call your doctor or nurse right away if you get a fever of 100.5°F or higher and/or chills, if you are coughing up sputum, have burning when you pass your urine, or any signs or symptoms of an infection.

Call your doctor or nurse right away if you have any bleeding.

Other side effects not listed above can also occur in some patients.
Tell your doctor or nurse if you develop any problems.

FDA Approval: This drug is being studied for cancer treatment.

rituximab

Trade Name:
Rituxan

Type of Drug:
Rituximab is a monoclonal antibody that belongs to the general class of synthetic substances called biologic response modifiers. It is used to treat certain lymphomas that have lymphocytes with the CD20 receptor.

How Drug Works:
A monoclonal antibody is a protein that fits like a lock and key with a protein on the cancer cell. Rituximab (antibody) attaches to the CD20 protein (antigen) on certain cancerous lymphocytes (white blood cells). Once it attaches to the cells, it brings other immune cells to help kill the cancer cells.

How Drug Is Given:
Rituximab is given as an injection in a vein weekly for 4 weeks. The first infusion is given very slowly to see if you have a reaction. Later infusions are given a little faster if you tolerated the first one well. You will probably get other medicine to prevent a reaction if you have any trouble. The dose depends on your weight and the reason you are taking the drug. Tell your nurse if you begin to feel different at all during the treatment.

 Read the following information. If you do not understand it or if any of it causes you special concern, check with your doctor.

Before taking this drug, tell your doctor:
- If you are trying to become pregnant, are pregnant, or breastfeeding. This drug may cause birth defects if either the male or female is taking it at the time of conception or during pregnancy. Men and women who are taking this drug need to use some kind of birth control. However, do not use oral contraceptives ("the pill") without checking with your doctor.
- If you think you may want to have children in the future. Many chemotherapy drugs can cause sterility.
- If you have any of the following medical problems: chickenpox or exposure to chickenpox, gout, heart disease, congestive heart failure, shingles, kidney stones, liver disease, or other forms of cancer.
- If you are taking any other prescription or over-the-counter drugs, including vitamins and herbals.

Should I avoid any other medicines, foods, alcohol, and/or activities?
Your prescription and nonprescription medicines may interact with other drugs, causing harm. Certain foods or alcohol can also interact with drug products. Never begin taking a new medicine—prescription or nonprescription—without asking your doctor or nurse if it will interact with alcohol, food, or other medicines. Some drug products can cause drowsiness and affect activities such as driving.

Precautions:
While you are being treated with rituximab, and after you stop treatment, do not have any immunizations (vaccinations) without your doctor's okay. Try to avoid contact with people who have recently taken the oral polio vaccine. Check with your doctor about this.

Rituximab can often cause allergic reactions (fever and chills), especially the first treatment. Rarely, decreased blood pressure, swelling of face, and coughing can occur. Tell your nurse or doctor right away if you get a fever or chills, hives, nausea, itching, headache, shortness of breath, or swollen tongue or throat during your treatment. Your nurse will stop the infusion and evaluate you.

Tell all the doctors, dentists, and pharmacists you visit that you are taking this drug.
- -
- Most of the following side effects probably will not occur.
- Your doctor or nurse will want to discuss specific care instructions with you.
- They can help you understand these side effects and help you deal with them.

Side Effects:

More Common Side Effects
Allergic reaction with first infusion

Less Common Side Effects
Allergic reaction with second and later infusions
Nausea
Itching
Hives
Rash
Headache
Swelling of tongue or throat

Rare Side Effects
Tiredness (fatigue)
Cough with shortness of breath
Difficulty breathing
Decreased blood pressure
Flushing of face
Increased heart rate
Vomiting
Irregular heartbeat
Muscle aches
Dizziness
Decreased platelet count with increased risk of bleeding
Decreased white blood cell count with increased risk of infection

Side Effects / Symptoms of the Drug
Tell your doctor or nurse right away if you develop shortness of breath or difficulty breathing, have a fever over 100.5°F, have symptoms of infection such as coughing up sputum or burning when urinating, unusual bruising, or bleeding such as nosebleeds, bleeding of gums when you brush your teeth, or black, tarry stools.

Other side effects not listed above can also occur in some patients.
Tell your doctor or nurse if you develop any problems.

FDA Approval: This drug is approved for cancer treatment.

sargramostim

Trade Names:
Leukine, GM-CSF

Type of Drug:
Sargramostim is a protein cytokine that belongs to the general class of synthetic substances called biologic response modifiers. It is used to control and stimulate the growth of white blood cells and is used to help prevent infection due to low white blood cells following chemotherapy.

How Drug Works:
Sargramostim tells the body's bone marrow to make more special immune cells (monocytes and macrophages). It also stimulates the immune system to work better to fight infection.

How Drug Is Given:
Sargramostim is given as an injection under the skin or in a vein over 2 hours. You or a family member may be taught to give the injection under the skin. Keep the syringes, needles, and supplies in a safe place, out of the reach of children and pets. The medicine should be kept in its original container in the refrigerator; you should take it out 1 hour before the shot is due. The dose depends on your weight, and the number of doses depends on your white blood cell count. Keep the used syringes and needles in a special container. Ask your nurse or doctor about this, and when you should bring the filled container back to the office.

How Should I Take This Drug?
Take this drug exactly as directed by your doctor. If you do not understand the instructions, ask your doctor or nurse to explain them to you. This drug can be given at different strengths depending on the type of cancer being treated. Dosage may vary depending on your weight and your type of cancer.

 Read the following information. If you do not understand it or if any of it causes you special concern, check with your doctor.

Before taking this drug, tell your doctor:
- If you are trying to become pregnant, are pregnant, or breastfeeding. This drug may cause birth defects if either the male or female is taking it at the time of conception or during pregnancy. Men and women who are taking this drug need to use some kind of birth control. However, do not use oral contraceptives ("the pill") without checking with your doctor.
- If you think you may want to have children in the future. Many chemotherapy drugs can cause sterility.
- If you have any of the following medical problems: chickenpox or exposure to chickenpox, gout, heart disease, congestive heart failure, shingles, kidney stones, liver disease, or other forms of cancer.
- If you are taking any other prescription or over-the-counter drugs, including vitamins and herbals.

Should I avoid any other medicines, foods, alcohol, and/or activities?
Your prescription and nonprescription medicines may interact with other drugs, causing harm. Certain foods or alcohol can also interact with drug products. Never begin taking a new medicine—prescription or nonprescription—without asking your doctor or nurse if it will interact with alcohol, food, or other medicines. Some drug products can cause drowsiness and affect activities such as driving.

Precautions:
Sargramostim often causes a flu-like syndrome with fever, chills, tiredness, headache, and muscle aches. Talk to your nurse or doctor about ways to lessen these side effects.

Tell all the doctors, dentists, and pharmacists you visit that you are taking this drug.

- Most of the following side effects probably will not occur.
- Your doctor or nurse will want to discuss specific care instructions with you.
- They can help you understand these side effects and help you deal with them.

Side Effects:

More Common Side Effects
Flu-like symptoms such as fever, chills, tiredness, and muscle aches
Bone pain

Less Common Side Effects
Facial flushing
Rash
Redness and pain at the place of injection

Rare Side Effects
Difficulty breathing
Swelling of feet
Weight gain

Side Effects / Symptoms of the Drug
Talk to your doctor or nurse about ways to lessen the bone pain.

Other side effects not listed above can also occur in some patients.
Tell your doctor or nurse if you develop any problems.

FDA Approval: This drug is approved for cancer treatment.

streptozocin

Trade Name:
Zanosar

Type of Drug:
Streptozocin is a chemotherapy drug that belongs to a special group of alkylating agents called nitrosoureas. It is used to treat carcinoid tumors and pancreatic cancer.

How Drug Works:
Streptozocin stops the growth of cancer cells, which causes the cells to die.

How Drug Is Given:
Streptozocin is given as an injection in a vein over 1 to 2 hours. You will get antinausea medicine before the streptozocin. Tell your nurse right away if you feel any discomfort in the vein during the treatment. The dose depends on your weight and type of cancer being treated.

 Read the following information. If you do not understand it or if any of it causes you special concern, check with your doctor.

Before taking this drug, tell your doctor:
• If you are trying to become pregnant, are pregnant, or breastfeeding. This drug may cause birth defects if either the male or female is taking it at the time of conception or during pregnancy. Men and women who are taking this drug need to use some kind of birth control. However, do not use oral contraceptives ("the pill") without checking with your doctor.
• If you think you may want to have children in the future. Many chemotherapy drugs can cause sterility.
• If you have any of the following medical problems: chickenpox or exposure to chickenpox, gout, heart disease, congestive heart failure, shingles, kidney stones, liver disease, or other forms of cancer.
• If you are taking any other prescription or over-the-counter drugs, including vitamins and herbals.

Should I avoid any other medicines, foods, alcohol, and/or activities?
Your prescription and nonprescription medicines may interact with other drugs, causing harm. Certain foods or alcohol can also interact with drug products. Never begin taking a new medicine—prescription or non-prescription—without asking your doctor or nurse if it will interact with alcohol, food, or other medicines. Some drug products can cause drowsiness and affect activities such as driving.

Precautions:
While you are being treated with streptozocin, and after you stop treatment, do not have any immunizations (vaccinations) without your doctor's okay. Try to avoid contact with people who have recently taken the oral polio vaccine. Check with your doctor about this.

Streptozocin can change blood sugar levels. Take orange juice or a high-glucose food, and tell your nurse or doctor if you notice signs of low blood sugar, such as muscle weakness, sweating, flushing, restlessness, headache, confusion, or trembling. Tell your nurse or doctor if you notice signs of high blood sugar, such as increased thirst, increased urination, and increased hunger.

Streptozocin can cause nausea and vomiting. Ask your doctor or nurse to give you medicines to prevent or lessen this.

Tell all the doctors, dentists, and pharmacists you visit that you are taking this drug.

- Most of the following side effects probably will not occur.
- Your doctor or nurse will want to discuss specific care instructions with you.
- They can help you understand these side effects and help you deal with them.

Side Effects:

More Common Side Effects
Kidney damage (usually reversible)
Nausea
Vomiting
Liver damage with painless jaundice
Pain or burning in the vein where drug is given

Less Common Side Effects
Decreased blood sugar
Increased blood sugar

Rare Side Effects
Diarrhea
Abdominal cramping
Decreased white blood cell count with increased risk of infection
Decreased platelet count with increased risk of bleeding

Side Effects / Symptoms of the Drug
Streptozocin can increase your risk of getting an infection. Report fever of 100.5°F or higher, or signs of infection such as pain in passing your urine, or coughing, and bringing up sputum.

Streptozocin can increase your risk of bleeding. DO NOT take any aspirin or aspirin-containing medicines. Report unusual bruising, or bleeding such as nosebleeds, bleeding gums when you brush your teeth, or black, tarry stools.

Because of the way this drug acts on the body, there is a chance that it can cause other side effects that may not occur until months or years after the drug is used. These very rarely can include second cancers such as leukemia. Discuss this with your doctor.

Other side effects not listed above can also occur in some patients.
Tell your doctor or nurse if you develop any problems.

FDA Approval: This drug is approved for cancer treatment.

tamoxifen citrate

Trade Name:
Nolvadex

Type of Drug:
Tamoxifen citrate belongs to the general group of drugs known as hormones or hormone antagonists. It is used to prevent breast cancer in high-risk women; decrease the risk of getting invasive breast cancer in women with ductal cancer in situ (DCIS); prevent cancer from coming back after surgery, radiation, and chemotherapy; and to treat advanced breast cancer.

How Drug Works:
Tamoxifen citrate blocks estrogen by binding to estrogen receptors. When this occurs, the cancer cells that depend on estrogen to divide stop growing and die.

How Drug Is Given:
Tamoxifen citrate is a pill usually taken twice a day with an 8 oz glass of water, with or without food. The dose is the same for all patients and depends on the reason you are taking it. Keep the medicine in a tightly closed container away from heat and moisture and out of the reach of children and pets.

How Should I Take This Drug?
Take this drug exactly as directed by your doctor. If you do not understand the instructions, ask your doctor or nurse to explain them to you. This drug can be given at different strengths depending on the type of cancer being treated. Dosage may vary depending on your weight and your type of cancer.

 Read the following information. If you do not understand it or if any of it causes you special concern, check with your doctor.

Before taking this drug, tell your doctor:
- If you are trying to become pregnant, are pregnant, or breastfeeding. This drug may cause birth defects if either the male or female is taking it at the time of conception or during pregnancy. Men and women who are taking this drug need to use some kind of birth control. However, do not use oral contraceptives ("the pill") without checking with your doctor.
- If you think you may want to have children in the future. Many chemotherapy drugs can cause sterility.
- If you have any of the following medical problems: chickenpox or exposure to chickenpox, gout, heart disease, congestive heart failure, shingles, kidney stones, liver disease, or other forms of cancer.
- If you are taking any other prescription or over-the-counter drugs, including vitamins and herbals.

Should I avoid any other medicines, foods, alcohol, and/or activities?
Your prescription and nonprescription medicines may interact with other drugs, causing harm. Certain foods or alcohol can also interact with drug products. Never begin taking a new medicine—prescription or nonprescription—without asking your doctor or nurse if it will interact with alcohol, food, or other medicines. Some drug products can cause drowsiness and affect activities such as driving.

Precautions:
Tamoxifen may temporarily increase the calcium blood level when you start taking the medicine.

When you start taking tamoxifen, you may get a "flare" reaction. You will feel a temporary increase in bone and/or tumor pain. Tell your doctor if this does not go away in 1 to 2 weeks.

Tell all the doctors, dentists, and pharmacists you visit that you are taking this drug.

- Most of the following side effects probably will not occur.
- Your doctor or nurse will want to discuss specific care instructions with you.
- They can help you understand these side effects and help you deal with them.

Side Effects:

More Common Side Effects
Initial, temporary feeling of tiredness

Less Common Side Effects
Irregular menstrual bleeding
Vaginal discharge
Hot flashes
Milk production in the breast
Vaginal bleeding
"Flare" reaction when starting the drug

Rare Side Effects
Nausea
Vomiting
Visual changes
Rash
Swelling of hands or feet
Headache
Dizziness
Hair thinning
Mild decrease in white blood cell count with increased risk of infection
Mild decrease in platelet count with increased risk of bleeding
Increase in calcium blood level

Side Effects / Symptoms of the Drug
Tell your doctor or nurse right away if you have blurred vision, tumor or bone pain lasting more than 1 to 2 weeks, or if you have confusion or dizziness that does not go away.

Because of the way this drug acts on the body, there is a chance that it can cause other side effects that may not occur until months or years after the drug is used. Other side effects rarely can include second cancers, such as endometrial (uterine) cancer. Discuss this with your doctor.

Other side effects not listed above can also occur in some patients.
Tell your doctor or nurse if you develop any problems.

FDA Approval: This drug is approved for cancer treatment.

temozolomide

Trade Name:
Temodal

Type of Drug:
Temozolomide belongs to a general group of chemotherapy drugs called alkylating agents.

How Drug Works:
Temozolomide stops the growth of cancer cells, which causes them to die. The drug cannot tell the difference between normal cells and cancer cells, so some normal cells are injured, causing some of the side effects. This drug can cross into the brain, where it can kill hidden cancer cells. It is approved to treat a brain cancer called astrocytoma that does not shrink when other treatments have been tried.

How Drug Is Given:
Temozolomide is a capsule that comes in 4 sizes: 250 mg, 100 mg, 20 mg, and 5 mg. The capsules are taken once a day for 5 days every 4 weeks. The dose depends on your weight, whether you have received other chemotherapy before, and your blood counts. The capsules should be taken with an 8 oz glass of water on an empty stomach, either 1 hour before or 2 hours after eating. Try to take the capsules at the same time each day. Do not crush or dissolve the capsule. Keep the medicine in a tightly closed container away from heat and moisture and out of the reach of children and pets.

How Should I Take This Drug?
Take this drug exactly as directed by your doctor. If you do not understand the instructions, ask your doctor or nurse to explain them to you. This drug can be given at different strengths depending on the type of cancer being treated. Dosage may vary depending on your weight and your type of cancer.

 Read the following information. If you do not understand it or if any of it causes you special concern, check with your doctor.

Before taking this drug, tell your doctor:
- If you are trying to become pregnant, are pregnant, or breastfeeding. This drug may cause birth defects if either the male or female is taking it at the time of conception or during pregnancy. Men and women who are taking this drug need to use some kind of birth control. However, do not use oral contraceptives ("the pill") without checking with your doctor.
- If you think you may want to have children in the future. Many chemotherapy drugs can cause sterility.
- If you have any of the following medical problems: chickenpox or exposure to chickenpox, gout, heart disease, congestive heart failure, shingles, kidney stones, liver disease, or other forms of cancer.
- If you are taking any other prescription or over-the-counter drugs, including vitamins and herbals.

Should I avoid any other medicines, foods, alcohol, and/or activities?
Your prescription and nonprescription medicines may interact with other drugs, causing harm. Certain foods or alcohol can also interact with drug products. Never begin taking a new medicine—prescription or nonprescription—without asking your doctor or nurse if it will interact with alcohol, food, or other medicines. Some drug products can cause drowsiness and affect activities such as driving.

Precautions:
Temozolomide can lower your blood counts (white blood cells, red blood cells, platelets). Your doctor will check your blood counts before and after each treatment to see its effect. Your doctor or nurse will give you specific instructions if your blood counts are low.

Temozolomide can lower your white blood cell count, reaching the lowest point about 3 to 4 weeks after the treatment is given. This can increase your risk of getting an infection. Report fever of 100.5°F or higher, or signs of infection, such as pain in passing your urine or a productive cough (bringing up sputum).

Temozolomide can lower your platelet count and increase your risk of bleeding. DO NOT take any aspirin or aspirin-containing medicines. Report unusual bruising, bleeding such as nosebleeds, bleeding gums when you brush your teeth, or black, tarry stools.

Tell all the doctors, dentists, and pharmacists you visit that you are taking this drug.

- Most of the following side effects probably will not occur.
- Your doctor or nurse will want to discuss specific care instructions with you.
- They can help you understand these side effects and help you deal with them.

Side Effects:

More Common Side Effects
Decrease in white blood cell count with increased risk of infection
Decrease in platelet count with increased risk of bleeding
Nausea
Vomiting
Diarrhea
Constipation
Loss of appetite
Tiredness (fatigue)

Less Common Side Effects
Mouth sores
Rash
Itching
Slight hair loss
Tiredness
Headache

Rare Side Effects
Decreased red blood cell count with increased risk of tiredness and anemia
Difficulty walking
Dizziness

Other side effects not listed above can also occur in some patients.
Tell your doctor or nurse if you develop any problems.

FDA Approval: This drug is approved for cancer treatment.

teniposide

Trade Names:
VM-26, Vumon

Type of Drug:
Teniposide belongs to a general group of chemotherapy drugs called plant alkaloids. It is a topoisomerase inhibitor used to treat acute lymphoblastic leukemia.

How Drug Works:
Teniposide stops the growth of cancer cells, causing them to die.

How Drug Is Given:
Teniposide is given as an injection in a vein over 30 to 60 minutes. You will get antinausea medicine before the teniposide. The dose depends on your weight, your blood counts, and the type of cancer being treated.

 Read the following information. If you do not understand it or if any of it causes you special concern, check with your doctor.

Before taking this drug, tell your doctor:
- If you are trying to become pregnant, are pregnant, or breastfeeding. This drug may cause birth defects if either the male or female is taking it at the time of conception or during pregnancy. Men and women who are taking this drug need to use some kind of birth control. However, do not use oral contraceptives ("the pill") without checking with your doctor.
- If you think you may want to have children in the future. Many chemotherapy drugs can cause sterility.
- If you have any of the following medical problems: chickenpox or exposure to chickenpox, gout, heart disease, congestive heart failure, shingles, kidney stones, liver disease, or other forms of cancer.
- If you are taking any other prescription or over-the-counter drugs, including vitamins and herbals.

Should I avoid any other medicines, foods, alcohol, and/or activities?
Your prescription and nonprescription medicines may interact with other drugs, causing harm. Certain foods or alcohol can also interact with drug products. Never begin taking a new medicine—prescription or non-prescription—without asking your doctor or nurse if it will interact with alcohol, food, or other medicines. Some drug products can cause drowsiness and affect activities such as driving.

Precautions:
While you are being treated with teniposide, and after you stop treatment, do not have any immunizations (vaccinations) without your doctor's okay. Try to avoid contact with people who have recently taken the oral polio vaccine. Check with your doctor about this.

Teniposide can lower your blood counts (white blood cells, red blood cells, platelets). Your doctor will check your blood counts before and after each treatment to see its effect. Your doctor or nurse will give you specific instructions if your blood counts are low.

Teniposide can decrease your white blood cell count, especially 7 days after the drug is given. This can increase your risk of getting an infection. Report fever of 100.5°F or higher, or signs of infection such as pain in passing your urine, or coughing, and bringing up sputum.

Teniposide can decrease your platelet count. This can increase your risk of bleeding. DO NOT take any aspirin or aspirin-containing medicines. Report unusual bruising, or bleeding such as nosebleeds, bleeding gums when you brush your teeth, or black, tarry stools.

Tell all the doctors, dentists, and pharmacists you visit that you are taking this drug.
- Most of the following side effects probably will not occur.
- Your doctor or nurse will want to discuss specific care instructions with you.
- They can help you understand these side effects and help you deal with them.

Side Effects:

More Common Side Effects
Decreased white blood cell count with increased risk of infection
Decreased platelet count with increased risk of bleeding
Irritation of vein used for giving the drug

Less Common Side Effects
Nausea
Vomiting
Numbness and tingling in hands and/or feet due to peripheral nerve irritation
Decrease in blood pressure when drug is given
Fetal abnormalities if drug is taken during pregnancy or if pregnancy occurs while taking this drug

Rare Side Effects
Allergic reaction when drug is given with fever, chills, increased heart rate, difficulty breathing,
    flushing, back pain, or change in blood pressure
Hair loss
Sores in mouth or on lips
Abnormal values on liver function blood tests

Side Effects / Symptoms of the Drug
Tell your doctor or nurse right away if you have fever, chills, difficulty breathing, back pain, flushing, or rapid heartbeat when the drug is given.

Other side effects not listed above can also occur in some patients.
Tell your doctor or nurse if you develop any problems.

FDA Approval: This drug is approved for cancer treatment.

thalidomide

Trade Name:
Thalomid

Type of Drug:
Thalidomide is a very new cancer drug. While its exact mechanism in cancer treatment is not clearly understood yet, it appears to be an angiogenesis inhibitor.

How Drug Works:
Thalidomide appears to interfere with the growth of blood vessels. A group of cancer cells (tumor) must grow new blood vessels when it reaches the size of a pencil tip. Thalidomide interferes with the growth of these new blood vessels, and theoretically stops the cancer from growing larger than the size of a pencil tip. Thalidomide is being studied in combination with other agents, such as chemotherapy or biological therapy, to treat renal cell cancer and multiple myeloma.

How Drug Is Given:
Thalidomide is taken as a capsule with water, at least 1 hour after a meal. If you are only taking thalidomide once a day, take the capsule(s) 1 hour after your evening meal. The dose depends on the clinical study or protocol, as well as any side effects you may have from the drug. Patients must be enrolled in a clinical trial or in a government sponsored registry. Prescriptions can be written by precertified doctors. Only a 28-day supply will be given. You will be asked to sign a special consent and agree to birth control practices. Ask your doctor or nurse about this.

How Should I Take This Drug?
Take this drug exactly as directed by your doctor. If you do not understand the instructions, ask your doctor or nurse to explain them to you. This drug can be given at different strengths depending on the type of cancer being treated. Dosage may vary depending on your weight and your type of cancer.

 Read the following information. If you do not understand it or if any of it causes you special concern, check with your doctor.

Before taking this drug, tell your doctor:
- If you are trying to become pregnant, are pregnant, or breastfeeding. This drug may cause birth defects if either the male or female is taking it at the time of conception or during pregnancy. Men and women who are taking this drug need to use some kind of birth control. However, do not use oral contraceptives ("the pill") without checking with your doctor.
- If you think you may want to have children in the future. Many chemotherapy drugs can cause sterility.
- If you have any of the following medical problems: chickenpox or exposure to chickenpox, gout, heart disease, congestive heart failure, shingles, kidney stones, liver disease, or other forms of cancer.
- If you are taking any other prescription or over-the-counter drugs, including vitamins and herbals.

Should I avoid any other medicines, foods, alcohol, and/or activities?
Your prescription and nonprescription medicines may interact with other drugs, causing harm. Certain foods or alcohol can also interact with drug products. Never begin taking a new medicine—prescription or non-prescription—without asking your doctor or nurse if it will interact with alcohol, food, or other medicines. Some drug products can cause drowsiness and affect activities such as driving.

Precautions:
Thalidomide will cause damage to a developing fetus. Thus women of childbearing age must have a negative pregnancy test before starting the drug, and the test is repeated every 2 weeks for 2 months, then every month.

Women must use both barrier and hormonal contraception, and men must use barrier contraception. You should continue using the contraception for 1 month after the drug is discontinued.

Patients must be enrolled in a clinical trial or in a government monitored registry. Prescriptions can be written by precertified doctors. Only a 28-day supply will be given.

Thalidomide can make you very sleepy. You should not drive a car or operate heavy machinery until you know how this drug makes you feel.

Tell your doctor if you get the feeling of pins and needles in your fingers and toes and if it gets worse.

Thalidomide can make you feel dizzy when you change from a lying to sitting position, or from sitting to standing position. Try to change position very slowly, and make sure you have a secure surface to hold on to if needed.

 Tell all the doctors, dentists, and pharmacists you visit that you are taking this drug.
- -
- Most of the following side effects probably will not occur.
- Your doctor or nurse will want to discuss specific care instructions with you.
- They can help you understand these side effects and help you deal with them.

Side Effects:

More Common Side Effects
Birth defects in fetus
Numbness and tingling in hands and/or feet
Drowsiness
Dizziness
Mild constipation

Less Common Side Effects
Rash with itching
Feeling very tired

Rare Side Effects
Decreased white blood cell count with increased risk of infection
Allergic reaction
Slowed heartbeat

Side Effects / Symptoms of the Drug
If you are of childbearing age, it is very important to comply with contraception instructions. Talk to your doctor or nurse about this.

Stop the drug and call your doctor or nurse if you have numbness or tingling in your arms, hands, feet, or legs, or if you have trouble walking.

Other side effects not listed above can also occur in some patients.
Tell your doctor or nurse if you develop any problems.

FDA Approval: This drug is being studied for cancer treatment.

thioguanine

Trade Names:
6-TG, 6-Thioguanine, Tabloid

Type of Drug:
Thioguanine belongs to the general group of chemotherapy drugs known as antimetabolites. It is used to treat acute nonlymphocytic leukemia.

How Drug Works:
Thioguanine prevents cells from making DNA and RNA. This stops the growth of cancer cells and they eventually die.

How Drug Is Given:
Thioguanine is a pill taken by mouth once a day on an empty stomach, 1 hour before or 2 hours after a meal. If you get stomach upset, take an antinausea pill 1 hour before taking the thioguanine. The dose depends on your weight and the type of cancer being treated. Keep the medicine in a tightly closed container away from heat and moisture and out of the reach of children and pets.

How Should I Take This Drug?
Take this drug exactly as directed by your doctor. If you do not understand the instructions, ask your doctor or nurse to explain them to you. This drug can be given at different strengths depending on the type of cancer being treated. Dosage may vary depending on your weight and your type of cancer.

 Read the following information. If you do not understand it or if any of it causes you special concern, check with your doctor.

Before taking this drug, tell your doctor:
- If you are trying to become pregnant, are pregnant, or breastfeeding. This drug may cause birth defects if either the male or female is taking it at the time of conception or during pregnancy. Men and women who are taking this drug need to use some kind of birth control. However, do not use oral contraceptives ("the pill") without checking with your doctor.
- If you think you may want to have children in the future. Many chemotherapy drugs can cause sterility.
- If you have any of the following medical problems: chickenpox or exposure to chickenpox, gout, heart disease, congestive heart failure, shingles, kidney stones, liver disease, or other forms of cancer.
- If you are taking any other prescription or over-the-counter drugs, including vitamins and herbals.

Should I avoid any other medicines, foods, alcohol, and/or activities?
Your prescription and nonprescription medicines may interact with other drugs, causing harm. Certain foods or alcohol can also interact with drug products. Never begin taking a new medicine—prescription or nonprescription—without asking your doctor or nurse if it will interact with alcohol, food, or other medicines. Some drug products can cause drowsiness and affect activities such as driving.

Precautions:
While you are being treated with thioguanine, and after you stop treatment, do not have any immunizations (vaccinations) without your doctor's okay. Try to avoid contact with people who have recently taken the oral polio vaccine. Check with your doctor about this.

Thioguanine can lower your blood counts (white blood cells, red blood cells, platelets). Your doctor will check your blood counts periodically to see its effect. Your doctor or nurse will give you specific instructions if your blood counts are low.

Thioguanine can decrease your white blood cell count, especially 1 to 4 weeks after the drug is given. This can increase your risk of getting an infection. Report fever of 100.5°F or higher, or signs of infection such as pain in passing your urine, or coughing and bringing up sputum.

Thioguanine can decrease your platelet count. This can increase your risk of bleeding. DO NOT take any aspirin or aspirin-containing medicines. Report unusual bruising, or bleeding such as nosebleeds, bleeding gums when you brush your teeth, or black, tarry stools.

Thioguanine can cause nausea and vomiting. Ask your doctor or nurse to give you medicines to prevent or lessen this.

 Tell all the doctors, dentists, and pharmacists you visit that you are taking this drug.

- Most of the following side effects probably will not occur.
- Your doctor or nurse will want to discuss specific care instructions with you.
- They can help you understand these side effects and help you deal with them.

Side Effects:

More Common Side Effects
Nausea
Vomiting
Decreased platelet count with increased risk of bleeding
Decreased white blood cell count with increased risk of infection

Rare Side Effects
Loss of appetite
Sores in mouth or on lips
Unsteady gait
Liver toxicity

Other side effects not listed above can also occur in some patients.
Tell your doctor or nurse if you develop any problems.

FDA Approval: This drug is approved for cancer treatment.

thiotepa

Trade Names:
Thioplex, Triethylenethiophosphoramide

Type of Drug:
Thiotepa belongs to the general group of chemotherapy drugs known as alkylating agents. It is used to treat cancers of the breast, ovary, and bladder.

How Drug Works:
Thiotepa stops the growth of cancer cells, causing them to die.

How Drug Is Given:
Thiotepa is given by an injection in a vein, muscle, or under the skin. It can also be given directly into the bladder. The dose depends on your weight and the type of cancer being treated.

 Read the following information. If you do not understand it or if any of it causes you special concern, check with your doctor.

Before taking this drug, tell your doctor:
- If you are trying to become pregnant, are pregnant, or breastfeeding. This drug may cause birth defects if either the male or female is taking it at the time of conception or during pregnancy. Men and women who are taking this drug need to use some kind of birth control. However, do not use oral contraceptives ("the pill") without checking with your doctor.
- If you think you may want to have children in the future. Many chemotherapy drugs can cause sterility.
- If you have any of the following medical problems: chickenpox or exposure to chickenpox, gout, heart disease, congestive heart failure, shingles, kidney stones, liver disease, or other forms of cancer.
- If you are taking any other prescription or over-the-counter drugs, including vitamins and herbals.

Should I avoid any other medicines, foods, alcohol, and/or activities?
Your prescription and nonprescription medicines may interact with other drugs, causing harm. Certain foods or alcohol can also interact with drug products. Never begin taking a new medicine—prescription or non-prescription—without asking your doctor or nurse if it will interact with alcohol, food, or other medicines. Some drug products can cause drowsiness and affect activities such as driving.

Precautions:
While you are being treated with thiotepa, and after you stop treatment, do not have any immunizations (vaccinations) without your doctor's okay. Try to avoid contact with people who have recently taken the oral polio vaccine. Check with your doctor about this.

Thiotepa can lower your blood counts (white blood cells, red blood cells, platelets) when given intravenously. Your doctor will check your blood counts before and after each treatment to see its effect. Your doctor or nurse will give you specific instructions if your blood counts are low.

Thiotepa can decrease your white blood cell count, especially 5 to 30 days after the drug is given. This can increase your risk of getting an infection. Report fever of 100.5°F or higher, or signs of infection such as pain in passing your urine, or coughing and bringing up sputum.

Thiotepa can decrease your platelet count. This can increase your risk of bleeding. DO NOT take any aspirin or aspirin-containing medicines. Report unusual bruising, or bleeding such as nosebleeds, bleeding gums when you brush your teeth, or black, tarry stools.

Tell all the doctors, dentists, and pharmacists you visit that you are taking this drug.

- Most of the following side effects probably will not occur.
- Your doctor or nurse will want to discuss specific care instructions with you.
- They can help you understand these side effects and help you deal with them.

Side Effects:

More Common Side Effects
Decreased white blood cell count with increased risk of infection
Decreased platelet count with increased risk of bleeding
Nausea
Vomiting
Sterility (may be reversible)
Stopping of menstrual periods (usually resume in 6 to 8 months)

Less Common Side Effects
Tiredness (fatigue)
Dizziness
Headache
Fever
Pain at place of injection

Rare Side Effects
Loss of appetite
Allergic reaction

Side Effects / Symptoms of the Drug
Because of the way this drug acts on the body, there is a chance that it can cause other side effects that may not occur until months or years after the drug is used. These very rarely can include a second cancer such as leukemia. Discuss this with your doctor.

Other side effects not listed above can also occur in some patients.
Tell your doctor or nurse if you develop any problems.

FDA Approval: This drug is approved for cancer treatment.

topotecan hydrochloride

Trade Name:
Hycamtin

Type of Drug:
Topotecan hydrochloride belongs to the general group of chemotherapy drugs known as topoisomerase inhibitors. It is used to treat metastatic ovarian cancer and small cell lung cancer that has continued to grow after first-line therapy.

How Drug Works:
Topotecan hydrochloride stops the growth of cancer cells by preventing the development of elements necessary for cell division.

How Drug Is Given:
Topotecan hydrochloride is given by a shot in the vein over 30 minutes for 5 days, usually repeated every 3 to 4 weeks. You will get an antinausea medicine before the topotecan hydrochloride. The dose depends on your weight, your blood counts, how well your kidneys are working, and the type of cancer being treated. A pill form of the medicine is being tested.

 Read the following information. If you do not understand it or if any of it causes you special concern, check with your doctor.

Before taking this drug, tell your doctor:
- If you are trying to become pregnant, are pregnant, or breastfeeding. This drug may cause birth defects if either the male or female is taking it at the time of conception or during pregnancy. Men and women who are taking this drug need to use some kind of birth control. However, do not use oral contraceptives ("the pill") without checking with your doctor.
- If you think you may want to have children in the future. Many chemotherapy drugs can cause sterility.
- If you have any of the following medical problems: chickenpox or exposure to chickenpox, gout, heart disease, congestive heart failure, shingles, kidney stones, liver disease, or other forms of cancer.
- If you are taking any other prescription or over-the-counter drugs, including vitamins and herbals.

Should I avoid any other medicines, foods, alcohol, and/or activities?
Your prescription and nonprescription medicines may interact with other drugs, causing harm. Certain foods or alcohol can also interact with drug products. Never begin taking a new medicine—prescription or nonprescription—without asking your doctor or nurse if it will interact with alcohol, food, or other medicines. Some drug products can cause drowsiness and affect activities such as driving.

Precautions:
While you are being treated with topotecan hydrochloride, and after you stop treatment, do not have any immunizations (vaccinations) without your doctor's okay. Try to avoid contact with people who have recently taken the oral polio vaccine. Check with your doctor about this.

Topotecan hydrochloride can lower your blood counts (white blood cells, red blood cells, platelets). Your doctor will check your blood counts before and after each treatment to see its effect. Your doctor or nurse will give you specific instructions if your blood counts are low.

Topotecan hydrochloride can decrease your white blood cell count, especially about 11 days after the drug is given. This can increase your risk of getting an infection. Report fever of 100.5°F or higher, or signs of infection such as pain in passing your urine, coughing and bringing up sputum.

Topotecan hydrochloride can decrease your platelet count. This can increase your risk of bleeding. DO NOT take any aspirin or aspirin-containing medicines. Report unusual bruising, or bleeding such as nosebleeds, bleeding gums when you brush your teeth, or black, tarry stools.

Topotecan hydrochloride can cause severe nausea and vomiting. Your doctor or nurse will give you medicines to prevent the nausea and vomiting. If you do get this side effect, talk to your doctor or nurse right away about ways to lessen this.

Tell all the doctors, dentists, and pharmacists you visit that you are taking this drug.

- Most of the following side effects probably will not occur.
- Your doctor or nurse will want to discuss specific care instructions with you.
- They can help you understand these side effects and help you deal with them.

Side Effects:

More Common Side Effects
Decreased white blood cell count with increased risk of infection
Decreased platelet count with increased risk of bleeding
Decreased red blood cell count with increased risk for anemia and tiredness (fatigue)
Nausea
Vomiting
Diarrhea
Constipation
Abdominal pain

Rare Side Effects
Abnormal values of liver function blood tests

Other side effects not listed above can also occur in some patients.
Tell your doctor or nurse if you develop any problems.

FDA Approval: This drug is approved for cancer treatment.

toremifene citrate

Trade Name:
Fareston

Type of Drug:
Toremifene citrate belongs to the general group of drugs known as hormones or hormone antagonists. It is used to treat advanced breast cancer in postmenopausal women.

How Drug Works:
Toremifene citrate blocks estrogen. The cancer cells that depend on estrogen to divide, stop growing and die.

How Drug Is Given:
Toremifene citrate is a pill taken once a day with or without food. Try to take the pill at the same time every day. Keep the medicine in a tightly closed container away from heat and moisture and out of the reach of children and pets.

How Should I Take This Drug?
Take this drug exactly as directed by your doctor. If you do not understand the instructions, ask your doctor or nurse to explain them to you. This drug can be given at different strengths depending on the type of cancer being treated. Dosage may vary depending on your weight and your type of cancer.

 Read the following information. If you do not understand it or if any of it causes you special concern, check with your doctor.

Before taking this drug, tell your doctor:
- If you are trying to become pregnant, are pregnant, or breastfeeding. This drug may cause birth defects if either the male or female is taking it at the time of conception or during pregnancy. Men and women who are taking this drug need to use some kind of birth control. However, do not use oral contraceptives ("the pill") without checking with your doctor.
- If you think you may want to have children in the future. Many chemotherapy drugs can cause sterility.
- If you have any of the following medical problems: chickenpox or exposure to chickenpox, gout, heart disease, congestive heart failure, shingles, kidney stones, liver disease, or other forms of cancer.
- If you are taking any other prescription or over-the-counter drugs, including vitamins and herbals.

Should I avoid any other medicines, foods, alcohol, and/or activities?
Your prescription and nonprescription medicines may interact with other drugs, causing harm. Certain foods or alcohol can also interact with drug products. Never begin taking a new medicine—prescription or non-prescription—without asking your doctor or nurse if it will interact with alcohol, food, or other medicines. Some drug products can cause drowsiness and affect activities such as driving.

Precautions:
When you start taking toremifene citrate, you may get a "flare" reaction. You will feel a temporary increase in bone and/or tumor pain. Tell your doctor if this does not go away in 1 to 2 weeks.

Tell all the doctors, dentists, and pharmacists you visit that you are taking this drug.

  • Most of the following side effects probably will not occur.
  • Your doctor or nurse will want to discuss specific care instructions with you.
  • They can help you understand these side effects and help you deal with them.

Side Effects:

More Common Side Effects
Hot flashes

Less Common Side Effects
Irregular menstrual bleeding
Milk production in breasts
Vaginal discharge
Vaginal bleeding
"Flare" reaction when starting the drug

Rare Side Effects
Nausea
Vomiting
Loss of appetite
Tremors
Skin rash
Hair loss
Mild decrease in white blood cell and platelet count
Swelling of hands and feet

Other side effects not listed above can also occur in some patients.
Tell your doctor or nurse if you develop any problems.

FDA Approval: This drug is approved for cancer treatment.

tositumomab, I¹³¹ tositumomab

Trade Name:
Bexxar

Type of Drug:
Tositumomab is a monoclonal antibody that has a radioactive substance (iodine 131) attached to it. It belongs to the class called radioimmunotherapy agents.

How Drug Works:
The monoclonal antibody part of tositumomab is directed to the CD20 receptor located on B lymphocyte cells. This receptor is found on some normal lymphocytes and also lymphocytes that are cancerous, as in non-Hodgkin's lymphoma. The antibody attaches to the CD20 receptor and kills the cells by exposing the cell to radiation (iodine 131).

How Drug Is Given:
Tositumomab is given as an injection in a vein. Because it is radioactive, the dose depends on the time that it will stay in your body. To figure this out, a test taking 3 days is done before the treatment. About 1 week later, the treatment dose is given as 2 injections in a vein. The first shot (antibody) is given over 1 hour, then the second shot (antibody and radioactive iodine) is given 20 minutes later.

 Read the following information. If you do not understand it or if any of it causes you special concern, check with your doctor.

Before taking this drug, tell your doctor:
- If you are trying to become pregnant, are pregnant, or breastfeeding. This drug may cause birth defects if either the male or female is taking it at the time of conception or during pregnancy. Men and women who are taking this drug need to use some kind of birth control. However, do not use oral contraceptives ("the pill") without checking with your doctor.
- If you think you may want to have children in the future. Many chemotherapy drugs can cause sterility.
- If you have any of the following medical problems: chickenpox or exposure to chickenpox, gout, heart disease, congestive heart failure, shingles, kidney stones, liver disease, or other forms of cancer.
- If you are taking any other prescription or over-the-counter drugs, including vitamins and herbals.

Should I avoid any other medicines, foods, alcohol, and/or activities?
Your prescription and nonprescription medicines may interact with other drugs, causing harm. Certain foods or alcohol can also interact with drug products. Never begin taking a new medicine—prescription or non-prescription—without asking your doctor or nurse if it will interact with alcohol, food, or other medicines. Some drug products can cause drowsiness and affect activities such as driving.

Precautions:
You will receive a small amount of radiation and you will need to follow special instructions to prevent other people near you from being exposed to radiation. You should sleep alone for at least the first night after the treatment. Your doctor will tell you if this should continue for more nights, depending on the dose. You will need to keep at least 3 feet between you and other people for at least 2 days. Stay away from pregnant women and children if possible for this time or keep at least 9 feet between you and the woman or child if absolutely necessary for short periods. You should avoid commercial transportation and long car trips with others for at least the first 2 days as explained to you by your nurse or doctor.

It is important to drink at least one 12 oz glass of fluid every hour during the day for the first 2 days after the treatment. This means that you drink at least 3 quarts of fluid each day.

Many people receiving the treatment get mild flu-like symptoms after the treatment, including fever, nausea, and tiredness. Talk with your doctor or nurse about taking medicine to prevent fever and nausea.

While you are being treated with tositumomab, and after you stop treatment, do not have any immunizations (vaccinations) without your doctor's okay. Try to avoid contact with people who have recently taken the oral polio vaccine and people with infections.

Tositumomab can lower your blood counts (white blood cells, red blood cells, platelets). Your doctor will check your blood counts before and after each treatment. The blood counts reach their lowest point about 6 weeks after your treatment.

Tositumomab can lower your white blood cell count, reaching the lowest point about 6 weeks after the treatment is given. This can increase your risk of getting an infection. Report fever, of 100.5°F or higher, and signs of infection such as a productive cough or burning when you pass your urine.

Tositumomab can lower your platelet count. This can increase your risk of bleeding. DO NOT take any aspirin or aspirin-containing medicines. Report unusual bruising or bleeding, such as nosebleeds, bleeding when you brush your teeth, black, tarry stools, or heavy menstrual periods right away.

Rarely, you can have a severe allergic reaction to the monoclonal antibody. Your nurse or doctor will watch you very closely during the treatment.

You will also be given an iodine supplement by mouth during your treatments to block the I-131 effect on the thyroid gland.

 Tell all the doctors, dentists, and pharmacists you visit that you are taking this drug.
- Most of the following side effects probably will not occur.
- Your doctor or nurse will want to discuss specific care instructions with you.
- They can help you understand these side effects and help you deal with them.

Side Effects:

More Common Side Effects
Mild to moderate "flu-like" symptoms with fever, nausea, and weakness
Decreased white blood cell count with increased risk infection
Decreased platelet count with increased risk of bleeding
Decreased red blood cell count with increased risk of tiredness and anemia

Rare Side Effects
Severe allergic reaction with flushing, hives, difficulty breathing, decreased blood pressure, loss of skin color, and loss of consciousness

Side Effects / Symptoms of the Drug
Tell your doctor or nurse right away if you do not understand how to take care of yourself while receiving tositumomab.

Other side effects not listed above can also occur in some patients.
Tell your doctor or nurse if you develop any problems.

FDA Approval: This drug is being studied for cancer treatment.

trastuzumab

Trade Names:
rhuMAbHER2, Herceptin

Type of Drug:
Trastuzumab is a monoclonal antibody that belongs to the general class of synthetic substances called biologic response modifiers. It is used to treat breast cancer that over-expresses the HER-2 antigen.

How Drug Works:
Trastuzumab (monoclonal antibody) is a protein that fits like a lock and key with a protein (antigen) on certain breast cancer cells. This protein is called the epidermal growth factor receptor (HER-2). Once it attaches to the cells, it brings other immune cells to help kill the cancer cells. It is usually given with chemotherapy.

How Drug Is Given:
Trastuzumab is given by injection in a vein over 90 minutes the first time. If you don't have any problems, the next dose is given over 30 minutes. The dose depends on your weight. This medicine is often given with chemotherapy.

 Read the following information. If you do not understand it or if any of it causes you special concern, check with your doctor.

Before taking this drug, tell your doctor:
- If you are trying to become pregnant, are pregnant, or breastfeeding. This drug may cause birth defects if either the male or female is taking it at the time of conception or during pregnancy. Men and women who are taking this drug need to use some kind of birth control. However, do not use oral contraceptives ("the pill") without checking with your doctor.
- If you think you may want to have children in the future. Many chemotherapy drugs can cause sterility.
- If you have any of the following medical problems: chickenpox or exposure to chickenpox, gout, heart disease, congestive heart failure, shingles, kidney stones, liver disease, or other forms of cancer.
- If you are taking any other prescription or over-the-counter drugs, including vitamins and herbals.

Should I avoid any other medicines, foods, alcohol, and/or activities?
Your prescription and nonprescription medicines may interact with other drugs, causing harm. Certain foods or alcohol can also interact with drug products. Never begin taking a new medicine—prescription or nonprescription—without asking your doctor or nurse if it will interact with alcohol, food, or other medicines. Some drug products can cause drowsiness and affect activities such as driving.

Precautions:
Trastuzumab often can cause an allergic reaction with fever and chills. You will be watched closely during your first dose for any allergic symptoms.

Tell all the doctors, dentists, and pharmacists you visit that you are taking this drug.

- Most of the following side effects probably will not occur.
- Your doctor or nurse will want to discuss specific care instructions with you.
- They can help you understand these side effects and help you deal with them.

Side Effects:

More Common Side Effects
Fever
Chills

Less Common Side Effects
Severe heart problems when given with some chemotherapies (cyclophosphamides and the anthracyclines)
Congestive heart failure

Rare Side Effects
Severe allergic reaction
Generalized pain
Difficulty breathing
Abdominal pain
Tiredness (fatigue)
Nausea
Vomiting
Diarrhea
Liver failure with fluid buildup in the abdomen

Side Effects / Symptoms of the Drug
Tell your doctor or nurse right away if you have difficulty breathing, nausea and/or vomiting, or diarrhea.

Other side effects not listed above can also occur in some patients.
Tell your doctor or nurse if you develop any problems.

FDA Approval: This drug is approved for cancer treatment.

tretinoin

Trade Names:
Vesanoid, ATRA, All-Trans-Retinoic Acid

Type of Drug:
Tretinoin belongs to a general group called vitamins. It is derived from vitamin A and used to treat acute promyelocytic leukemia that has specific gene changes.

How Drug Works:
Tretinoin seems to stop the growth of leukemic cells, which are then destroyed. Since the growth of normal body cells may also be affected by tretinoin, other effects can occur. Some effects may not occur for months or years after the drug is used.

How Drug Is Given:
Tretinoin is a capsule taken by mouth with food in equal divided doses as directed by your doctor. The dose depends on your weight and side effects of the medicine. Keep the medicine in a tightly closed container away from heat and moisture and out of the reach of children and pets.

How Should I Take This Drug?
Take this drug exactly as directed by your doctor. If you do not understand the instructions, ask your doctor or nurse to explain them to you. This drug can be given at different strengths depending on the type of cancer being treated. Dosage may vary depending on your weight and your type of cancer.

 Read the following information. If you do not understand it or if any of it causes you special concern, check with your doctor.

Before taking this drug, tell your doctor:
• If you are trying to become pregnant, are pregnant, or breastfeeding. This drug may cause birth defects if either the male or female is taking it at the time of conception or during pregnancy. Men and women who are taking this drug need to use some kind of birth control. However, do not use oral contraceptives ("the pill") without checking with your doctor.
• If you think you may want to have children in the future. Many chemotherapy drugs can cause sterility.
• If you have any of the following medical problems: chickenpox or exposure to chickenpox, gout, heart disease, congestive heart failure, shingles, kidney stones, liver disease, or other forms of cancer.
• If you are taking any other prescription or over-the-counter drugs, including vitamins and herbals.

Should I avoid any other medicines, foods, alcohol, and/or activities?
Your prescription and nonprescription medicines may interact with other drugs, causing harm. Certain foods or alcohol can also interact with drug products. Never begin taking a new medicine—prescription or non-prescription—without asking your doctor or nurse if it will interact with alcohol, food, or other medicines. Some drug products can cause drowsiness and affect activities such as driving.

Precautions:
While you are being treated with tretinoin, and after you stop treatment, do not have any immunizations (vaccinations) without your doctor's okay. Try to avoid contact with people who have recently taken the oral polio vaccine. Check with your doctor about this.

Tell all the doctors, dentists, and pharmacists you visit that you are taking this drug.

- Most of the following side effects probably will not occur.
- Your doctor or nurse will want to discuss specific care instructions with you.
- They can help you understand these side effects and help you deal with them.

Side Effects:

More Common Side Effects
Headache
Fever
Dry mouth
Bone pain
Nausea
Vomiting
Rash

Less Common Side Effects
Dizziness
Sensation of pins and needles in hands and feet
Earache
Depression
Heartburn
Abdominal distention
Constipation or diarrhea
Syndrome of fever, difficulty breathing, weight gain, changes in chest x-ray, and fluid outside the lungs or heart
Sores in mouth or on lips
Itching
Sweating
Changes in vision
Skin changes
Irregular heartbeat
Changes in blood pressure
Flushing

Rare Side Effects
Heart damage
Ulcer
Inflammation of liver
Decreased hearing
Agitation
Hallucination
Sleepiness
Slow speech
Difficulty urinating
High triglyceride and cholesterol blood levels

Side Effects / Symptoms of the Drug
Tell your doctor or nurse right away if you develop fever, difficulty breathing, weight gain, or irregular heartbeat.

Other side effects not listed above can also occur in some patients.
Tell your doctor or nurse if you develop any problems.

FDA Approval: This drug is approved for cancer treatment.

trimetrexate

Trade Name:
Neutrexin

Type of Drug:
Trimetrexate belongs to the general group of chemtherapy drugs known as antimetabolites. It is used to treat several types of cancer including colon cancer. Trimetrexate is also used to treat a special bacterial infection in people with low immune function (pneumocystis carinii pneumonia).

How Drug Works:
Trimetrexate prevents cells from making DNA and RNA by interfering with the synthesis of nucleic acids. This stops the growth of cancer cells, causing them to die.

How Drug Is Given:
Trimetrexate is given as an injection in a vein over 60 minutes. The dose depends on your weight, how well your liver and kidneys are functioning, the level of protein in your blood, and the reason you are getting the medicine. The medicine will not be given if your liver function tests are too high, you have sores in your mouth, you have a high fever, or your blood counts are too low.

 Read the following information. If you do not understand it or if any of it causes you special concern, check with your doctor.

Before taking this drug, tell your doctor:
- If you are trying to become pregnant, are pregnant, or breastfeeding. This drug may cause birth defects if either the male or female is taking it at the time of conception or during pregnancy. Men and women who are taking this drug need to use some kind of birth control. However, do not use oral contraceptives ("the pill") without checking with your doctor.
- If you think you may want to have children in the future. Many chemotherapy drugs can cause sterility.
- If you have any of the following medical problems: chickenpox or exposure to chickenpox, gout, heart disease, congestive heart failure, shingles, kidney stones, liver disease, or other forms of cancer.
- If you are taking any other prescription or over-the-counter drugs, including vitamins and herbals.

Should I avoid any other medicines, foods, alcohol, and/or activities?
Your prescription and nonprescription medicines may interact with other drugs, causing harm. Certain foods or alcohol can also interact with drug products. Never begin taking a new medicine—prescription or non-prescription—without asking your doctor or nurse if it will interact with alcohol, food, or other medicines. Some drug products can cause drowsiness and affect activities such as driving.

Precautions:
While you are being treated with trimetrexate, and after you stop treatment, do not have any immunizations (vaccinations) without your doctor's okay. Try to avoid contact with people who have recently taken the oral polio vaccine. Check with your doctor about this.

Trimetrexate can lower your blood counts (white blood cells, red blood cells, platelets). Your doctor will check your blood counts before and after each treatment to see its effect. Your doctor or nurse will give you specific instructions if your blood counts are low.

Trimetrexate can decrease your white blood cell count. This can increase your risk of getting an infection. Report fever of 100.5°F or higher, or signs of infection such as pain in passing your urine, coughing, and bringing up sputum.

Trimetrexate can decrease your platelet count. This can increase your risk of bleeding. DO NOT take any aspirin or aspirin-containing medicines. Report unusual bruising, or bleeding such as nosebleeds, bleeding gums when you brush your teeth, or black, tarry stools.

Getting a wig before starting treatment may make it easier to deal with hair loss. Talk to your nurse or doctor about this. If your insurance does not cover it, there may be other resources to help you. Hair loss is temporary, and your hair will grow back after treatment.

Tell all the doctors, dentists, and pharmacists you visit that you are taking this drug.
- Most of the following side effects probably will not occur.
- Your doctor or nurse will want to discuss specific care instructions with you.
- They can help you understand these side effects and help you deal with them.

Side Effects:

More Common Side Effects
Decreased white blood cell count with increased risk of infection
Decreased platelet count with increased risk of bleeding
Hair loss

Less Common Side Effects
Nausea
Vomiting
Sores in mouth or on lips
Diarrhea
Difficulty breathing
Headache

Rare Side Effects
Severe difficulty in breathing

Side Effects / Symptoms of the Drug
Tell your doctor or nurse right away if you have difficulty breathing.

Other side effects not listed above can also occur in some patients.
Tell your doctor or nurse if you develop any problems.

FDA Approval: This drug is being studied for cancer treatment.

tumor necrosis factor

Trade Name:
(Investigational)

Type of Drug:
Tumor necrosis factor is a protein cytokine that is part of the immune system.

How Drug Works:
Tumor necrosis factor appears to stop some cancer cells from dividing. It causes damage to tumor blood vessels, killing the cancer cells. It activates and increases the effectiveness of a number of other immune cells.

How Drug Is Given:
Tumor necrosis factor is given as an injection in a vein, muscle, or under the skin. The dose depends on the investigational study.

 Read the following information. If you do not understand it or if any of it causes you special concern, check with your doctor.

Before taking this drug, tell your doctor:
- If you are trying to become pregnant, are pregnant, or breastfeeding. This drug may cause birth defects if either the male or female is taking it at the time of conception or during pregnancy. Men and women who are taking this drug need to use some kind of birth control. However, do not use oral contraceptives ("the pill") without checking with your doctor.
- If you think you may want to have children in the future. Many chemotherapy drugs can cause sterility.
- If you have any of the following medical problems: chickenpox or exposure to chickenpox, gout, heart disease, congestive heart failure, shingles, kidney stones, liver disease, or other forms of cancer.
- If you are taking any other prescription or over-the-counter drugs, including vitamins and herbals.

Should I avoid any other medicines, foods, alcohol, and/or activities?
Your prescription and nonprescription medicines may interact with other drugs, causing harm. Certain foods or alcohol can also interact with drug products. Never begin taking a new medicine—prescription or non-prescription—without asking your doctor or nurse if it will interact with alcohol, food, or other medicines. Some drug products can cause drowsiness and affect activities such as driving.

Precautions:
While you are being treated with tumor necrosis factor, and after you stop treatment, do not have any immunizations (vaccinations) without your doctor's okay. Try to avoid contact with people who have recently taken the oral polio vaccine. Check with your doctor about this.

Fever, shaking chills, and sweating can occur 1 to 6 hours after the drug is given. These symptoms will gradually disappear after repeated doses. Talk with your doctor or nurse about medication to prevent these side effects.

Tell all the doctors, dentists, and pharmacists you visit that you are taking this drug.
- -
- Most of the following side effects probably will not occur.
- Your doctor or nurse will want to discuss specific care instructions with you.
- They can help you understand these side effects and help you deal with them.

Side Effects:

More Common Side Effects
Fever
Chills
Rigors (rigid shaking chills)
Tiredness (fatigue)
Nausea
Vomiting
Weight loss

Less Common Side Effects
Muscle aches
Joint aches
Headache
Back pain
Decreased white blood cell count with increased risk of infection
Decreased platelet count with increased risk of bleeding

Rare Side Effects
Decreased blood pressure
Confusion
Difficulty speaking
Seizures
Difficulty breathing

Side Effects / Symptoms of the Drug
Tell your doctor or nurse right away if you have difficulty breathing, confusion, or any changes in your condition.

Other side effects not listed above can also occur in some patients.
Tell your doctor or nurse if you develop any problems.

FDA Approval: This drug is being studied for cancer treatment.

UFT (ftorafur and Uracil)

Trade Name:
Tegafur and Uracil

Type of Drug:
Ftorafur belongs to the general group of chemotherapy drugs known as antimetabolites. It is metabolized to 5-fluorouracil. Uracil is an amino acid that enhances the effect of 5-fluorouracil. UFT is a combination of Uracil and ftorafur. Together, they are used to treat several types of cancer including colon cancer.

How Drug Works:
UFT prevents cells from making DNA and RNA by interfering with the synthesis of nucleic acids. This stops the growth of cancer cells.

How Drug Is Given:
UFT (ftorafur and Uracil) is a capsule taken by mouth, in 3 divided doses. The dose depends on your weight and the investigational study. Keep the medicine in a tightly closed container away from heat and moisture and out of the reach of children and pets.

How Should I Take This Drug?
Take this drug exactly as directed by your doctor. If you do not understand the instructions, ask your doctor or nurse to explain them to you. This drug can be given at different strengths depending on the type of cancer being treated. Dosage may vary depending on your weight and your type of cancer.

 Read the following information. If you do not understand it or if any of it causes you special concern, check with your doctor.

Before taking this drug, tell your doctor:
- If you are trying to become pregnant, are pregnant, or breastfeeding. This drug may cause birth defects if either the male or female is taking it at the time of conception or during pregnancy. Men and women who are taking this drug need to use some kind of birth control. However, do not use oral contraceptives ("the pill") without checking with your doctor.
- If you think you may want to have children in the future. Many chemotherapy drugs can cause sterility.
- If you have any of the following medical problems: chickenpox or exposure to chickenpox, gout, heart disease, congestive heart failure, shingles, kidney stones, liver disease, or other forms of cancer.
- If you are taking any other prescription or over-the-counter drugs, including vitamins and herbals.

Should I avoid any other medicines, foods, alcohol, and/or activities?
Your prescription and nonprescription medicines may interact with other drugs, causing harm. Certain foods or alcohol can also interact with drug products. Never begin taking a new medicine—prescription or nonprescription—without asking your doctor or nurse if it will interact with alcohol, food, or other medicines. Some drug products can cause drowsiness and affect activities such as driving.

Precautions:
While you are being treated with UFT, and after you stop treatment, do not have any immunizations (vaccinations) without your doctor's okay. Try to avoid contact with people who have recently taken the oral polio vaccine. Check with your doctor about this.

UFT can lower your blood counts (white blood cells, red blood cells, platelets). Your doctor will check your blood counts before and after each treatment to see its effect. Your doctor or nurse will give you specific instructions if your blood counts are low.

UFT can decrease your white blood cell count, especially 14 days after the drug is given. This can increase your risk of getting an infection. Report fever of 100.5°F or higher, or signs of infection such as pain in passing your urine, or coughing and bringing up sputum.

UFT can decrease your platelet count. This can increase your risk of bleeding. DO NOT take any aspirin or aspirin-containing medicines. Report unusual bruising, or bleeding such as nosebleeds, bleeding gums when you brush your teeth, or black, tarry stools.

Tell all the doctors, dentists, and pharmacists you visit that you are taking this drug.
- Most of the following side effects probably will not occur.
- Your doctor or nurse will want to discuss specific care instructions with you.
- They can help you understand these side effects and help you deal with them.

Side Effects:

More Common Side Effects
Decreased white blood cell count with increased risk of infection
Decreased platelet count with increased risk of bleeding
Nausea
Vomiting
Loss of appetite
Diarrhea
Sores in mouth or on lips

Less Common Side Effects
Headaches
Numbness and tingling in the hands and feet
Skin pigmentation changes

Rare Side Effects
Dehydration if diarrhea is severe

Side Effects / Symptoms of the Drug
Tell your doctor or nurse immediately if you have diarrhea that does not go away, sores in mouth or on lips, fever, signs of infection, or bleeding.

Other side effects not listed above can also occur in some patients.
Tell your doctor or nurse if you develop any problems.

FDA Approval: This drug is being studied for cancer treatment.

valspodar

Trade Name:
Amdray

Type of Drug:
Valspodar is a chemotherapy sensitizer. Some cancer cells have a gene that allows them to get rid of the chemotherapy, which means that the cells are not damaged by the chemotherapy. A chemosensitizer stops the cells from getting rid of the chemotherapy so that the drug can remain in the cancer cells and kill them.

How Drug Works:
Valspodar binds to the surface of the cancer cell and blocks the gene. When the chemotherapy enters the cell, it is not removed. The chemotherapy stays in the cell, which causes the cell to die.

How Drug Is Given:
Valspodar is given by injection in a vein, then a continuous infusion. It is given 1 day before chemotherapy, and continued for 1 day after chemotherapy. The dose depends on the investigational study.

 Read the following information. If you do not understand it or if any of it causes you special concern, check with your doctor.

Before taking this drug, tell your doctor:
- If you are trying to become pregnant, are pregnant, or breastfeeding. This drug may cause birth defects if either the male or female is taking it at the time of conception or during pregnancy. Men and women who are taking this drug need to use some kind of birth control. However, do not use oral contraceptives ("the pill") without checking with your doctor.
- If you think you may want to have children in the future. Many chemotherapy drugs can cause sterility.
- If you have any of the following medical problems: chickenpox or exposure to chickenpox, gout, heart disease, congestive heart failure, shingles, kidney stones, liver disease, or other forms of cancer.
- If you are taking any other prescription or over-the-counter drugs, including vitamins and herbals.

Should I avoid any other medicines, foods, alcohol, and/or activities?
Your prescription and nonprescription medicines may interact with other drugs, causing harm. Certain foods or alcohol can also interact with drug products. Never begin taking a new medicine—prescription or non-prescription—without asking your doctor or nurse if it will interact with alcohol, food, or other medicines. Some drug products can cause drowsiness and affect activities such as driving.

Precautions:
Be sure to tell your doctor about all the medicines you are taking, because there may be some possible drug interactions.

Valspodar may cause a temporary increase in the amount of bilirubin in the blood (bilirubin is a pigment found in bile and blood and is related to how well the liver functions).

In clinical studies of high doses of this drug, valspodar caused neurological changes. You will be closely monitored for this. Report any changes in coordination, strength of leg muscles, gait, or walking ability right away to your doctor or nurse.

Other side effects include dizziness, lightheadedness, and numbness, beginning 1 hour after receiving valspodar and lasting 3 to 6 hours.

Tell all the doctors, dentists, and pharmacists you visit that you are taking this drug.

- Most of the following side effects probably will not occur.
- Your doctor or nurse will want to discuss specific care instructions with you.
- They can help you understand these side effects and help you deal with them.

Side Effects:

More Common Side Effects
Pain at injection site
Mild skin reactions at injection site

Less Common Side Effects
Nausea
Headache
Dizziness
Lightheadedness
Numbness around mouth
Sensation of pins and needles in the fingers or toes

Rare Side Effects
Loss of coordination
Difficulty walking
Severe allergic reaction with fever, chills, rash, hives, difficulty breathing, or swelling of face and lips

Side Effects / Symptoms of the Drug
Report any side effects right away.

Other side effects not listed above can also occur in some patients.
Tell your doctor or nurse if you develop any problems.

FDA Approval: This drug is being studied for cancer treatment.

vinblastine

Trade Name:
Velban

Type of Drug:
Vinblastine belongs to the general group of chemotherapy drugs known as plant (vinca) alkaloids. It is used to treat lymphomas, testicular cancer, and Kaposi's sarcoma.

How Drug Works:
Vinblastine stops cell division, resulting in cell death.

How Drug Is Given:
Vinblastine is given as an injection in a vein over 5 to 10 minutes. Tell the nurse if you feel pain, burning, or discomfort in the vein when it is given. The dose and how often you get the medicine depends on your weight, your blood counts, how well your liver is working, and the type of cancer being treated. You will have your blood counts checked before each treatment; if they are too low, your treatment will be delayed. This medicine may be given with other chemotherapy.

 Read the following information. If you do not understand it or if any of it causes you special concern, check with your doctor.

Before taking this drug, tell your doctor:
- If you are trying to become pregnant, are pregnant, or breastfeeding. This drug may cause birth defects if either the male or female is taking it at the time of conception or during pregnancy. Men and women who are taking this drug need to use some kind of birth control. However, do not use oral contraceptives ("the pill") without checking with your doctor.
- If you think you may want to have children in the future. Many chemotherapy drugs can cause sterility.
- If you have any of the following medical problems: chickenpox or exposure to chickenpox, gout, heart disease, congestive heart failure, shingles, kidney stones, liver disease, or other forms of cancer.
- If you are taking any other prescription or over-the-counter drugs, including vitamins and herbals.

Should I avoid any other medicines, foods, alcohol, and/or activities?
Your prescription and nonprescription medicines may interact with other drugs, causing harm. Certain foods or alcohol can also interact with drug products. Never begin taking a new medicine—prescription or nonprescription—without asking your doctor or nurse if it will interact with alcohol, food, or other medicines. Some drug products can cause drowsiness and affect activities such as driving.

Precautions:
Vinblastine can lower your blood counts (white blood cells, red blood cells, platelets). Your doctor will check your blood counts before and after each treatment to see its effect. Your doctor or nurse will give you specific instructions if your blood counts are low.

Vinblastine can decrease your white blood cell count 4 to 10 days after the drug is given. This can increase your risk of getting an infection. Report fever of 100.5°F or higher, or signs of infection such as pain in passing your urine, or coughing and bringing up sputum.

Vinblastine can cause a decrease in the platelet count. This can increase your risk of bleeding. DO NOT take any aspirin or aspirin-containing medicines. Report unusual bruising, or bleeding such as nosebleeds, bleeding gums when you brush your teeth, or black, tarry stools.

Vinblastine can cause constipation that may lead to a serious problem called paralytic ileus. Tell your doctor right away if you get constipation with severe abdominal pain or muscle cramping.

Getting a wig before starting treatment may make it easier to deal with hair loss. Talk to your nurse or doctor about this. If your insurance does not cover it, there may be other resources to help you. Hair loss is temporary, and your hair will grow back after treatment.

Vinblastine is given intravenously. If the drug accidentally leaks out of the vein where it is given, it may damage the tissue and cause scarring. Tell the nurse right away if you notice redness, pain, or swelling at the place of injection.

While you are being treated with vinblastine, and after you stop treatment, do not have any immunizations (vaccinations) without your doctor's okay. Try to avoid contact with people who have recently taken the oral polio vaccine. Check with your doctor about this.

 Tell all the doctors, dentists, and pharmacists you visit that you are taking this drug.

- Most of the following side effects probably will not occur.
- Your doctor or nurse will want to discuss specific care instructions with you.
- They can help you understand these side effects and help you deal with them.

Side Effects:

More Common Side Effects
Decreased white blood cell count with increased risk of infection
Decreased platelet count with increased risk of bleeding
Hair loss

Less Common Side Effects
Constipation
Numbness and tingling in the hands and/or feet related to peripheral nerve irritation

Rare Side Effects
Depression
Headache
Jaw pain
Difficulty emptying the bladder
Increased heart rate
Dizziness when changing position
Changes in vision
Nausea
Vomiting
Sores in mouth or on lips

Side Effects / Symptoms of the Drug
Call your doctor right away if you develop difficulty walking, cramping in your legs, or redness and pain of injection.

Other side effects not listed above can also occur in some patients.
Tell your doctor or nurse if you develop any problems.

FDA Approval: This drug is approved for cancer treatment.

vincristine

Trade Name:
Oncovin

Type of Drug:
Vincristine belongs to the general group of chemotherapy drugs known as plant (vinca) alkaloids. It is used to treat lymphoma and leukemia.

How Drug Works:
Vincristine stops cell division, resulting in cell death.

How Drug Is Given:
Vincristine is given by an injection in a vein over 2 to 5 minutes. Tell the nurse if you feel pain, burning, or discomfort in the vein when it is given. The dose and how often you get the medicine depends on your weight, how well your liver is working, and the type of cancer being treated. This medicine may be given with other chemotherapy.

 Read the following information. If you do not understand it or if any of it causes you special concern, check with your doctor.

Before taking this drug, tell your doctor:
- If you are trying to become pregnant, are pregnant, or breastfeeding. This drug may cause birth defects if either the male or female is taking it at the time of conception or during pregnancy. Men and women who are taking this drug need to use some kind of birth control. However, do not use oral contraceptives ("the pill") without checking with your doctor.
- If you think you may want to have children in the future. Many chemotherapy drugs can cause sterility.
- If you have any of the following medical problems: chickenpox or exposure to chickenpox, gout, heart disease, congestive heart failure, shingles, kidney stones, liver disease, or other forms of cancer.
- If you are taking any other prescription or over-the-counter drugs, including vitamins and herbals.

Should I avoid any other medicines, foods, alcohol, and/or activities?
Your prescription and nonprescription medicines may interact with other drugs, causing harm. Certain foods or alcohol can also interact with drug products. Never begin taking a new medicine—prescription or nonprescription—without asking your doctor or nurse if it will interact with alcohol, food, or other medicines. Some drug products can cause drowsiness and affect activities such as driving.

Precautions:
Vincristine can cause constipation that may lead to a serious problem called paralytic ileus. Tell your doctor right away if you get constipation with severe abdominal pain or muscle cramping. Before starting treatment, your doctor or nurse will likely discuss ways to reduce the occurrence of constipation.

Getting a wig before starting treatment may make it easier to deal with hair loss. Talk to your nurse or doctor about this. If your insurance does not cover it, there may be other resources to help you. Hair loss is temporary, and your hair will grow back after treatment.

Vincristine can cause numbness and tingling in the hands and/or feet. Tell your doctor if this side effect occurs, and if it makes it difficult to button your shirt or pick up a coin. Also tell your doctor right away if you get burning in your hands and/or feet or have difficulty walking.

Vincristine is given intravenously. If the drug accidentally leaks out of the vein where it is given, it may damage the tissue and cause scarring. Tell the nurse right away if you notice redness, pain, or swelling at the place of injection.

While you are being treated with vincristine, and after you stop treatment, do not have any immunizations (vaccinations) without your doctor's okay. Try to avoid contact with people who have recently taken the oral polio vaccine. Check with your doctor about this.

Tell all the doctors, dentists, and pharmacists you visit that you are taking this drug.

- Most of the following side effects probably will not occur.
- Your doctor or nurse will want to discuss specific care instructions with you.
- They can help you understand these side effects and help you deal with them.

Side Effects:

More Common Side Effects
Constipation
Hair loss
Numbness and tingling in hands and/or feet due to peripheral nerve irritation

Less Common Side Effects
Weakness
Muscle aches
Cramping
Stomach pain

Rare Side Effects
Double vision
Depression
Taste changes
Decreased white blood cell count with increased risk of infection
Decreased platelet count with increased risk of bleeding
Jaw pain
Headache
Impotence

Side Effects / Symptoms of the Drug
You will be asked if you are having any problem with the nerves in your hands and feet. Tell your doctor if you are having problems, like the sensation of "pins and needles" or if you have difficulty picking up a coin.

Other side effects not listed above can also occur in some patients.
Tell your doctor or nurse if you develop any problems.

FDA Approval: This drug is approved for cancer treatment.

vindesine

Trade Name:
Eldisine

Type of Drug:
Vindesine belongs to the general group of chemotherapy drugs known as plant (vinca) alkaloids. It is being studied in some types of cancer, including lung cancer.

How Drug Works:
Vindesine stops cell division, resulting in cell death.

How Drug Is Given:
Vindesine is given by injection in a vein. Tell the nurse if you feel pain, burning, or discomfort in the vein when it is given. The dose and how often you get the medicine depends on your weight, how well your liver is working, the type of cancer being treated, and the investigational study.

 Read the following information. If you do not understand it or if any of it causes you special concern, check with your doctor.

Before taking this drug, tell your doctor:
- If you are trying to become pregnant, are pregnant, or breastfeeding. This drug may cause birth defects if either the male or female is taking it at the time of conception or during pregnancy. Men and women who are taking this drug need to use some kind of birth control. However, do not use oral contraceptives ("the pill") without checking with your doctor.
- If you think you may want to have children in the future. Many chemotherapy drugs can cause sterility.
- If you have any of the following medical problems: chickenpox or exposure to chickenpox, gout, heart disease, congestive heart failure, shingles, kidney stones, liver disease, or other forms of cancer.
- If you are taking any other prescription or over-the-counter drugs, including vitamins and herbals.

Should I avoid any other medicines, foods, alcohol, and/or activities?
Your prescription and nonprescription medicines may interact with other drugs, causing harm. Certain foods or alcohol can also interact with drug products. Never begin taking a new medicine—prescription or nonprescription—without asking your doctor or nurse if it will interact with alcohol, food, or other medicines. Some drug products can cause drowsiness and affect activities such as driving.

Precautions:
Vindesine can lower your blood counts (white blood cells, red blood cells, platelets). Your doctor will check your blood counts before and after each treatment to see its effect. Your doctor or nurse will give you specific instructions if your blood counts are low.

Vindesine can decrease your white blood cell count, especially 5 to 10 days after the drug is given. This can increase your risk of getting an infection. Report fever of 100.5°F or higher, or signs of infection such as pain in passing your urine, or coughing and bringing up sputum.

Vindesine can decrease your platelet count. This can increase your risk of bleeding. DO NOT take any aspirin or aspirin-containing medicines. Report unusual bruising, or bleeding such as nosebleeds, bleeding gums when you brush your teeth, or black, tarry stools.

Vindesine can cause constipation that may lead to a serious problem called paralytic ileus. Tell your doctor right away if you get constipation with severe abdominal pain or muscle cramping. Before starting treatment, your doctor or nurse will likely discuss ways to reduce the occurrence of constipation.

Vindesine is given intravenously. If the drug accidentally leaks out of the vein where it is given, it may damage the tissue and cause scarring. Tell the nurse right away if you notice redness, pain, or swelling at the place of injection.

Getting a wig before starting treatment may make it easier to deal with hair loss. Talk to your nurse or doctor about this. If your insurance does not cover it, there may be other resources to help you. Hair loss is temporary, and your hair will grow back after treatment.

While you are being treated with vindesine, and after you stop treatment, do not have any immunizations (vaccinations) without your doctor's okay. Try to avoid contact with people who have recently taken the oral polio vaccine. Check with your doctor about this.

 Tell all the doctors, dentists, and pharmacists you visit that you are taking this drug.

- Most of the following side effects probably will not occur.
- Your doctor or nurse will want to discuss specific care instructions with you.
- They can help you understand these side effects and help you deal with them.

Side Effects:

More Common Side Effects
Decreased white blood cell count with increased risk of infection
Sensation of pins and needles in hands and/or feet as a result of peripheral nerve irritation
Constipation
Hair loss

Less Common Side Effects
Abdominal cramping
Muscle weakness
Nausea
Vomiting

Rare Side Effects
Decreased platelet count with increased risk of bleeding
Jaw pain
Hoarseness
Diarrhea

Side Effects / Symptoms of the Drug
Call your doctor or nurse right away if you develop difficulty walking, cramping in your legs, or redness and pain at the place of injection.

Other side effects not listed above can also occur in some patients.
Tell your doctor or nurse if you develop any problems.

FDA Approval: This drug is being studied for cancer treatment.

vinorelbine tartrate

Trade Name:
Navelbine

Type of Drug:
Vinorelbine tartrate belongs to the general group of chemotherapy drugs known as plant (vinca) alkaloids. It is used to treat lung cancer and breast cancers.

How Drug Works:
Vinorelbine tartrate stops cell division, resulting in cell death.

How Drug Is Given:
Vinorelbine tartrate is given by an injection in the vein over 5 to 10 minutes. Tell the nurse if you feel pain, burning, or discomfort in the vein when it is given. The dose depends on your weight, how well your liver is working, your blood counts, and the type of cancer being treated.

 Read the following information. If you do not understand it or if any of it causes you special concern, check with your doctor.

Before taking this drug, tell your doctor:
- If you are trying to become pregnant, are pregnant, or breastfeeding. This drug may cause birth defects if either the male or female is taking it at the time of conception or during pregnancy. Men and women who are taking this drug need to use some kind of birth control. However, do not use oral contraceptives ("the pill") without checking with your doctor.
- If you think you may want to have children in the future. Many chemotherapy drugs can cause sterility.
- If you have any of the following medical problems: chickenpox or exposure to chickenpox, gout, heart disease, congestive heart failure, shingles, kidney stones, liver disease, or other forms of cancer.
- If you are taking any other prescription or over-the-counter drugs, including vitamins and herbals.

Should I avoid any other medicines, foods, alcohol, and/or activities?
Your prescription and nonprescription medicines may interact with other drugs, causing harm. Certain foods or alcohol can also interact with drug products. Never begin taking a new medicine—prescription or nonprescription—without asking your doctor or nurse if it will interact with alcohol, food, or other medicines. Some drug products can cause drowsiness and affect activities such as driving.

Precautions:
Vinorelbine tartrate can lower your blood counts (white blood cells, red blood cells, platelets). Your doctor will check your blood counts before and after each treatment to see its effect. Your doctor or nurse will give you specific instructions if your blood counts are low.

Vinorelbine tartrate can decrease your white blood cell count, especially 7 days after the drug is given. This can increase your risk of getting an infection. Report fever of 100.5°F or higher, or signs of infection such as pain in passing your urine, or coughing and bringing up sputum.

Vinorelbine tartrate can decrease your platelet count. This can increase your risk of bleeding. DO NOT take any aspirin or aspirin-containing medicines. Report unusual bruising, or bleeding such as nosebleeds, bleeding gums when you brush your teeth, or black, tarry stools.

Vinorelbine tartrate is given intravenously. If the drug accidentally leaks out of the vein where it is given, it may damage the tissue and cause scarring. Tell the nurse right away if you notice redness, pain, or swelling at the place of injection.

While you are being treated with vinorelbine tartrate, and after you stop treatment, do not have any immunizations (vaccinations) without your doctor's okay. Try to avoid contact with people who have recently taken the oral polio vaccine. Check with your doctor about this.

Tell all the doctors, dentists, and pharmacists you visit that you are taking this drug.

- Most of the following side effects probably will not occur.
- Your doctor or nurse will want to discuss specific care instructions with you.
- They can help you understand these side effects and help you deal with them.

Side Effects:

More Common Side Effects
Decreased white blood cell count with increased risk of infection
Numbness and tingling in hands and/or feet due to peripheral nerve irritation
Increased blood values of liver function tests
Redness and tenderness at the place of injection
Darkening of vein used to give the drug

Less Common Side Effects
Nausea
Vomiting
Sores in mouth or on lips
Hair loss
Decreased platelet count with increased risk of bleeding

Rare Side Effects
Constipation

Side Effects / Symptoms of the Drug
Call your doctor or nurse right away if you develop difficulty walking, cramping in your legs, or redness and pain at the place of injection.

Other side effects not listed above can also occur in some patients.
Tell your doctor or nurse if you develop any problems.

FDA Approval: This drug is being studied for cancer treatment.

zolendronate

Trade Names:
Zometa, Zoledronic acid

Type of Drug:
Zolendronate is a chemotherapy drug that is a member of the bisphosphonate group used to lower calcium in the blood if it is too high. It is used to treat multiple myeloma or other solid tumors that have spread to the bones. This is usually in combination with other cancer treatments.

How Drug Works:
Zolendronate stops cancer cells from breaking down bone, thus stopping the calcium in the bone from going into the blood. It also seems to stop the cancer cells from growing in the bone, so it prevents new cancer spots in the bone. It may stop blood vessels from forming, so the cancer cells stop growing.

How Drug Is Given:
Zolendronate is given by injection in a vein over at least 15 minutes. You will probably also get fluid by vein to protect your kidneys. The dose is the same for all patients.

 Read the following information. If you do not understand it or if any of it causes you special concern, check with your doctor.

Before taking this drug, tell your doctor:
• If you are trying to become pregnant, are pregnant, or breastfeeding. This drug may cause birth defects if either the male or female is taking it at the time of conception or during pregnancy. Men and women who are taking this drug need to use some kind of birth control. However, do not use oral contraceptives ("the pill") without checking with your doctor.
• If you think you may want to have children in the future. Many chemotherapy drugs can cause sterility.
• If you have any of the following medical problems: chickenpox or exposure to chickenpox, gout, heart disease, congestive heart failure, shingles, kidney stones, liver disease, or other forms of cancer.
• If you are taking any other prescription or over-the-counter drugs, including vitamins and herbals.

Should I avoid any other medicines, foods, alcohol, and/or activities?
Your prescription and nonprescription medicines may interact with other drugs, causing harm. Certain foods or alcohol can also interact with drug products. Never begin taking a new medicine—prescription or non-prescription—without asking your doctor or nurse if it will interact with alcohol, food, or other medicines. Some drug products can cause drowsiness and affect activities such as driving.

Precautions:
You will have blood tests to check your kidney function before receiving this drug. Sometimes this drug can hurt the kidneys if given too fast.

Mild bone pain can be treated with over-the-counter drugs such as acetaminophen or ibuprofen.

Make sure you drink 2 to 3 quarts of fluid a day while receiving this drug.

Talk to your doctor or nurse about ways to prevent constipation.

If you develop nausea, talk to your doctor or nurse about taking antinausea medicine before the next treatment.

Tell all the doctors, dentists, and pharmacists you visit that you are taking this drug.
- Most of the following side effects probably will not occur.
- Your doctor or nurse will want to discuss specific care instructions with you.
- They can help you understand these side effects and help you deal with them.

Side Effects:

More Common Side Effects
Pain in the bone
Nausea and vomiting
Fever
Tiredness (fatigue)
Constipation

Less Common Side Effects
Decreased red blood cell count

Rare Side Effects
Loss of appetite
Injury to the kidneys
Increased kidney function blood tests

Other side effects not listed above can also occur in some patients.
Tell your doctor or nurse if you develop any problems.

FDA Approval: This drug is approved for cancer treatment.

Symptom Management Drugs

acetaminophen

Trade Names:
Acephen, Actamin, Anacin-3, Anesin, Apacet, Dapa, Datril, Genapap, Genebs, Gentabs, Halenol, Liquiprin, Meda Cap, Panadol, Panex, Suppap, Tempra, Tenol, Ty Caps, Tylenol

Type of Drug:
Acetaminophen belongs to a general group of drugs called nonopioid analgesics, or pain relieving medicines. It is also an antipyretic, which means it can lower body temperature when a fever is present.

How Drug Works:
Acetaminophen stops the body from making prostaglandins, which prevent pain receptors from passing the pain message to the brain. When this occurs, pain perception is decreased. This drug also reduces fever by helping the body to expand blood vessels so that heat is lost through sweating.

How Drug Is Given:
Acetaminophen is given by mouth as a pill or capsule or by suppository rectally. The dose depends upon why the drug is taken and by how well your liver is working. Take the pill or capsule with a glass of water or juice. Coat the suppository with Vaseline if necessary and insert in the rectum with a gloved finger. Keep the medicine in a tightly closed container away from heat and moisture and out of the reach of children and pets.

How Should I Take This Drug?
Take this drug exactly as directed by your doctor. If you do not understand the instructions, ask your doctor or nurse to explain them to you.

 Read the following information. If you do not understand it or if any of it causes you special concern, check with your doctor.

Before taking this drug, tell your doctor if you are taking any other prescription or over-the-counter drugs, including vitamins and herbals.

Should I avoid any other medicines, foods, alcohol, and/or activities?
Your prescription and nonprescription medicines may interact with other drugs, causing harm. Certain foods or alcohol can also interact with drug products. Never begin taking a new medicine—prescription or nonprescription—without asking your doctor or nurse if it will interact with alcohol, food, or other medicines. Some drugs can cause drowsiness and affect activities such as driving.

Precautions:
Acetaminophen can cause liver damage. Your doctor may suggest decreasing the dose or how often you take the medicine if you have liver or kidney damage.

It is important not to drink alcohol if you are taking acetaminophen as this may increase the chance of liver damage. Ask your doctor or nurse to tell you more about this.

Acetaminophen may be given with opioid pain relievers (analgesics) to provide more effective pain relief. Acetaminophen is also given to bring a fever down or to prevent a fever from occurring.

Since fever can be a sign of an infection, and taking acetaminophen on a regular basis could cover up an important sign of infection, ask your doctor if you should take acetaminophen when you have a fever. Your doctor may wish to learn about the fever first, then instruct you to take acetaminophen.

Tell all the doctors, dentists, and pharmacists you visit that you are taking this drug.

- Most of the following side effects probably will not occur.
- Your doctor or nurse will want to discuss specific care instructions with you.
- They can help you understand these side effects and help you deal with them.

Side Effects:

Rare Side Effects
Liver damage

Other side effects not listed above can also occur in some patients.
Tell your doctor or nurse if you develop any problems.

FDA Approval: Yes

acyclovir

Trade Name:
Zovirax

Type of Drug:
Acyclovir belongs to the general class of drugs called antiviral agents.

How Drug Works:
Acyclovir interferes with the virus making DNA, so the virus cannot reproduce. Acyclovir is used to treat herpes simplex, herpes zoster, and cytomegalovirus.

How Drug Is Given:
Acyclovir is given by mouth, by vein, or by applying ointment to the skin. The dose depends on your size, how it is given, and the reason you are taking the drug. If you are taking the oral form, keep the medicine in a tightly closed container away from heat and moisture and out of the reach of children and pets.

How Should I Take This Drug?
Take this drug exactly as directed by your doctor. If you do not understand the instructions, ask your doctor or nurse to explain them to you.

 Read the following information. If you do not understand it or if any of it causes you special concern, check with your doctor.

Before taking this drug, tell your doctor if you are taking any other prescription or over-the-counter drugs, including vitamins and herbals.

Should I avoid any other medicines, foods, alcohol, and/or activities?
Your prescription and nonprescription medicines may interact with other drugs, causing harm. Certain foods or alcohol can also interact with drug products. Never begin taking a new medicine—prescription or nonprescription—without asking your doctor or nurse if it will interact with alcohol, food, or other medicines. Some drugs can cause drowsiness and affect activities such as driving.

Precautions:
All drugs used to fight microorganisms can cause allergic reactions. Stop the drug and tell your nurse or doctor right away if you develop a rash, hives, red blotches on your skin, difficulty breathing, or chest pain.

The dose of acyclovir will be reduced if you have any kidney problems. Your doctor will monitor your kidney function through blood tests while you are receiving acyclovir, especially when you receive it in the vein.

Tell all the doctors, dentists, and pharmacists you visit that you are taking this drug.
- -
- Most of the following side effects probably will not occur.
- Your doctor or nurse will want to discuss specific care instructions with you.
- They can help you understand these side effects and help you deal with them.

Side Effects:

Less Common Side Effects
Increase in kidney function blood and urine tests
Nausea
Vomiting
Diarrhea
Pain and irritation at place of injection

Rare Side Effects
Skin rash
Tremors
Hives
Itching
Dizziness
Confusion
Seizures
Tiredness (fatigue)

Side Effects / Symptoms of the Drug
Call your doctor or nurse right away if you develop rash, fever, or chills.

Other side effects not listed above can also occur in some patients.
Tell your doctor or nurse if you develop any problems.

FDA Approval: Yes

allopurinol

Trade Names:
Aloprim, Zurinol, Zyloprim

Type of Drug:
Allopurinol is a cytoprotective agent that belongs to the class of drugs called enzyme inhibitors.

How Drug Works:
Allopurinol blocks an enzyme necessary for making uric acid. When a large number of cancer cells are killed, they release substances that increase the production of uric acid. This is called tumor lysis syndrome. This large amount of uric acid can damage the kidneys. Allopurinol decreases the amount of uric acid made and thus protects the kidneys from the high levels of uric acid in the blood and urine. Allopurinol is used in the initial treatment of patients with leukemia, lymphoma, and small cell lung cancer.

How Drug Is Given:
Allopurinol is given by mouth and by vein injection if you are unable to take the pill. When taken to treat gout, the dose is fixed. When taken to decrease uric acid levels due to chemotherapy, the dose depends upon your size and laboratory values such as uric acid and kidney function.

How Should I Take This Drug?
Take this drug exactly as directed by your doctor. If you do not understand the instructions, ask your doctor or nurse to explain them to you.

 Read the following information. If you do not understand it or if any of it causes you special concern, check with your doctor.

Before taking this drug, tell your doctor if you are taking any other prescription or over-the-counter drugs, including vitamins and herbals.

Should I avoid any other medicines, foods, alcohol, and/or activities?
Your prescription and nonprescription medicines may interact with other drugs, causing harm. Certain foods or alcohol can also interact with drug products. Never begin taking a new medicine—prescription or nonprescription—without asking your doctor or nurse if it will interact with alcohol, food, or other medicines. Some drugs can cause drowsiness and affect activities such as driving.

Precautions:
Allopurinol can interact with many other drugs. Make sure that you tell your doctor about all the medicines you are taking.

Allopurinol may increase blood levels of liver function tests.

The dose of allopurinol will be reduced if you have kidney problems.

STOP the drug immediately if you develop a rash. Call your doctor or nurse right away.

When given to decrease uric acid, allopurinol is given with intravenous fluids so that the kidneys are protected.

Rarely, allopurinol can cause an allergic reaction with fever, chills, joint ache, rash, itching, nausea, vomiting, and changes in blood counts. If any of these occur, stop taking the drug and tell your doctor right away.

Overall, allopurinol is usually well tolerated.

Tell all the doctors, dentists, and pharmacists you visit that you are taking this drug.

- Most of the following side effects probably will not occur.
- Your doctor or nurse will want to discuss specific care instructions with you.
- They can help you understand these side effects and help you deal with them.

Side Effects:

Less Common Side Effects
Drowsiness
Headache
Sleepiness

Rare Side Effects
Seizures
Agitation
Changes in mental status
Tremor
Allergic reaction (rash, fever, chills, nausea, vomiting, joint pain)
Hair thinning
Severe skin rash with peeling of the skin

Side Effects / Symptoms of the Drug
If a severe skin rash with peeling should occur, stop taking the drug right away and call your doctor.

Other side effects not listed above can also occur in some patients.
Tell your doctor or nurse if you develop any problems.

FDA Approval: Yes

alprazolam

Trade Name:
Xanax

Type of Drug:
Alprazolam is used to reduce anxiety and belongs to a general class of drugs called benzodiazepines.

How Drug Works:
Alprazolam binds to receptors in the central nervous system resulting in decreased anxiety, muscle relaxation, and decrease in seizures.

How Drug Is Given:
Alprazolam is taken in pill form, with food or milk if the drug upsets your stomach. At first the dose is lower and gradually increased if needed over 3 to 4 days, as directed by your doctor. Once the right dose is found, the drug can be continued for up to 4 months. When stopping the drug, it is important to decrease the dose gradually, instead of just stopping it. Elderly patients may receive lower doses. Keep the medicine in a tightly closed container and out of the reach of children and pets.

How Should I Take This Drug?
Take this drug exactly as directed by your doctor. If you do not understand the instructions, ask your doctor or nurse to explain them to you.

 Read the following information. If any of it causes you special concern, check with your doctor.

Before taking this drug, tell your doctor if you are taking any other prescription or over-the-counter drugs, including vitamins and herbals.

Should I avoid any other medicines, foods, alcohol, and/or activities?
Your prescription and nonprescription medicines may interact with other drugs, causing harm. Certain foods or alcohol can also interact with drug products. Never begin taking a new medicine—prescription or nonprescription—without asking your doctor or nurse if it will interact with alcohol, food, or other medicines. Some drugs can cause drowsiness and affect activities such as driving.

Precautions:
Alprazolam should be used cautiously if you have liver or kidney problems. Talk with your doctor or nurse about this.

After starting alprazolam, if you feel "manic" or very excited and are overly active (hyperactive), stop the drug and call your doctor or nurse. You should not take the drug.

At first, you may feel drowsy, tired, lethargic, or weak, or be slightly confused and/or have a headache. This will go away with continued use. If such symptoms continue, tell your doctor. The dose of the drug might need to be reduced.

Alprazolam is used for the short-term (less than 4 months) relief of anxiety associated with depression and panic disorder. It can cause psychological dependence (addiction) as well as physical dependence (body goes into withdrawal if the drug is suddenly stopped). It should not be taken to manage everyday stress. When taken as directed by your doctor or nurse, this will not be a problem.

Alprazolam should not be used if you are pregnant or breastfeeding.

Tell all the doctors, dentists, and pharmacists you visit that you are taking this drug.

- Most of the following side effects probably will not occur.
- Your doctor or nurse will want to discuss specific care instructions with you.
- They can help you understand these side effects and help you deal with them.

Side Effects:

More Common Side Effects
Drowsiness (when first starting the drug)
Tiredness (fatigue) (when first starting the drug)
Weakness (when first starting the drug)
Confusion (when first starting the drug)
Headache (when first starting the drug)
Dry mouth
Decreased mental alertness

Less Common Side Effects
Nausea
Vomiting
Change in body weight

Rare Side Effects
Vivid dreams
Bizarre behavior
Change in heart rate
Change in blood pressure
Palpitations
Swelling of feet
Rash
Itching
Hives

Side Effects / Symptoms of the Drug
Take care in walking around or changing position if you are drowsy. Stop the drug and call your doctor or nurse if the drowsiness does not go away, or if you have trouble walking or moving because of it.

Other side effects not listed above can also occur in some patients.
Tell your doctor or nurse if you develop any problems.

FDA Approval: Yes

amikacin sulfate

Trade Name:
Amikin

Type of Drug:
Amikacin sulfate is an antibiotic that belongs to a group of drugs called aminoglycosides.

How Drug Works:
Amikacin sulfate blocks protein synthesis in bacteria, resulting in death of the organism. Amikacin sulfate is effective against many gram-negative bacteria and some gram–positive bacteria.

How Drug Is Given:
Amikacin sulfate is given as a shot into the muscle (intramuscular) or an injection into a vein over 20 to 30 minutes, 2 to 3 times a day. The dose depends upon your size, and the number of days of treatment depend upon the type of infection.

 Read the following information. If you do not understand it or if any of it causes you special concern, check with your doctor.

Before taking this drug, tell your doctor if you are taking any other prescription or over-the-counter drugs, including vitamins and herbals.

Should I avoid any other medicines, foods, alcohol, and/or activities?
Your prescription and nonprescription medicines may interact with other drugs, causing harm. Certain foods or alcohol can also interact with drug products. Never begin taking a new medicine—prescription or non-prescription—without asking your doctor or nurse if it will interact with alcohol, food, or other medicines. Some drugs can cause drowsiness and affect activities such as driving.

Precautions:
Tell your doctor if you have any drug allergies, especially to antibiotic drugs.

Amikacin sulfate can cause injury to the nerve for hearing (eighth cranial nerve, auditory). Tell your doctor or nurse right away if you feel dizzy, have difficulty walking, ringing in your ears (tinnitus), a roaring sound in your ears, or any decrease in hearing. The drug should be stopped and changed to another effective drug.

Amikacin sulfate can damage your kidneys. Your doctor will monitor blood tests to find this early, if it occurs. Tell your doctor if you have ever had any kidney problems.

All antibiotics can cause allergic reactions. Stop the drug and tell your doctor or nurse right away if you develop a rash, hives, red blotches on your skin, difficulty breathing, or chest pain.

Tell all the doctors, dentists, and pharmacists you visit that you are taking this drug.

- Most of the following side effects probably will not occur.
- Your doctor or nurse will want to discuss specific care instructions with you.
- They can help you understand these side effects and help you deal with them.

Side Effects:

More Common Side Effects
Nausea
Headache
Feeling sleepy or drowsy

Less Common Side Effects
Dizziness
Ringing in ears (tinnitus)
Roaring sound in ears
Difficulty walking
Tremors

Rare Side Effects
Decreased hearing
Kidney damage
Numbness and tingling of hands and feet related to nerve irritation
Vomiting
Decreased white blood cell count with increased risk of infection
Decreased platelet count with increased risk of bleeding
Decreased red blood cell count with increased risk of tiredness (fatigue)
Diarrhea related to infection of the intestinal lining (pseudomembranous colitis)

Side Effects / Symptoms of the Drug
Stop the drug and call your doctor or nurse right away if you get diarrhea that does not stop, abdominal cramping, and blood and/or pus in the stool. This needs to be treated right away.

Stop the drug and call your doctor or nurse right away if you get ringing in your ears (tinnitus), a roaring sound in your ears, or hearing loss.

Other side effects not listed above can also occur in some patients.
Tell your doctor or nurse if you develop any problems.

FDA Approval: Yes

amitriptyline hydrochloride

Trade Name:
Elavil

Type of Drug:
Amitriptyline hydrochloride is used to reduce anxiety or depression. It belongs to a general class of drugs called tricyclic antidepressants.

How Drug Works:
Amitriptyline hydrochloride increases the amount of serotonin and norepinephrine in the brain, so that the feeling of depression is prevented or relieved. By a separate mechanism, amitriptyline hydrochloride also may reduce peripheral nerve pain.

How Drug Is Given:
Amitriptyline hydrochloride is a pill taken by mouth, with food if the medicine upsets your stomach. The dose is low when the drug is started and gradually increased, as directed by your doctor. Amitriptyline hydrochloride can also be given by a shot into a muscle if needed. Keep the medicine in a tightly closed container and out of the reach of children and pets.

How Should I Take This Drug?
Take this drug exactly as directed by your doctor. If you do not understand the instructions, ask your doctor or nurse to explain them to you.

 Read the following information. If you do not understand it or if any of it causes you special concern, check with your doctor.

Before taking this drug, tell your doctor if you are taking any other prescription or over-the-counter drugs, including vitamins and herbals.

Should I avoid any other medicines, foods, alcohol, and/or activities?
Your prescription and nonprescription medicines may interact with other drugs, causing harm. Certain foods or alcohol can also interact with drug products. Never begin taking a new medicine—prescription or nonprescription—without asking your doctor or nurse if it will interact with alcohol, food, or other medicines. Some drugs can cause drowsiness and affect activities such as driving.

Precautions:
Tell your doctor if you are taking any of the following drugs as they may have serious interactions with amitriptyline hydrochloride: Coumadin, monamine oxidase inhibitors or other antidepressant drugs, or amphetamines.

Tell your doctor if you have had a heart attack (myocardial infarction), have a seizure disorder, or have benign prostatic hypertrophy (BPH) as you should not take amitriptyline hydrochloride.

Tell your doctor if you have urine retention, narrow-angle glaucoma, hyperthyroidism, liver problems, or thoughts of suicide. This drug should be used very cautiously if you have any of these conditions.

Once you start taking amitriptyline hydrochloride, it may take 2 weeks or longer for the antidepressant effect to work. This medicine can be used to help you get to sleep at night, and this effect starts right away. Pain relief usually starts right away as well.

Try to take your dose of the medicine at bedtime so it will help you sleep better. Abruptly stopping the drug can cause anxiety, dizziness, nausea and vomiting, and tiredness. The drug should be gradually discontinued.

Since amitriptyline hydrochloride affects the central nervous system (CNS), do not take other drugs or substances that are known CNS depressants, such as alcohol, sedatives, and hypnotics.

Tell all the doctors, dentists, and pharmacists you visit that you are taking this drug.
- Most of the following side effects probably will not occur.
- Your doctor or nurse will want to discuss specific care instructions with you.
- They can help you understand these side effects and help you deal with them.

Side Effects:

More Common Side Effects
Drowsiness
Dizziness
Weakness
Feeling sleepy or drowsy
Tiredness (fatigue)
Dry mouth

Less Common Side Effects
Confusion (especially in the elderly)
Hallucinations
Increased heart rate
Loss of appetite
Vomiting
Urinary retention
Disorientation
Decreased blood pressure when changing positions
Increased blood pressure
Nausea
Diarrhea

Rare Side Effects
Fine tremors
Rigidity
Difficulty speaking
Difficulty swallowing
Numbness and tingling in the hands and/or feet related to nerve irritation
Blurred vision
Electrical changes in the heart
Abdominal cramping
Increase in liver function blood levels
Rash
Hives
Redness of the skin
Increased sensitivity to sunlight

Side Effects / Symptoms of the Drug
The drowsiness and/or dizziness usually goes away within 1 to 2 weeks. Do not drive or operate heavy machinery if you feel drowsy or dizzy.

Take care in walking around or changing position if you are drowsy. Stop the drug and call your doctor or nurse if the drowsiness does not go away, or if you have trouble walking or moving because of it.

Tell your doctor or nurse if you get fine tremors, feel like your body is rigid, or have difficulty speaking or swallowing. You can be given another medicine to take away these problems.

Other side effects not listed above can also occur in some patients.
Tell your doctor or nurse if you develop any problems.

FDA Approval: Yes

amoxicillin

Trade Names:
Amoxil, Polymox, Trimox, Wymox

Type of Drug:
Amoxicillin is an antibiotic that belongs to the class of drugs called penicillins. Amoxicillin is used to treat gram-negative and some gram-positive bacteria. It is used to treat infections in the lungs, throat, sinuses, kidneys, bladder, and skin.

How Drug Works:
Amoxicillin stops bacteria from making their protein cell wall, so the bacteria die. Penicillins can do this because they contain a special beta-lactam ring.

How Drug Is Given:
Amoxicillin is a capsule taken by mouth 1 to 4 times a day. Take on an empty stomach, either 1 hour before or 2 hours after eating. The dose and frequency depend on the infection being treated. Keep the medicine in a tightly closed container and out of the reach of children and pets.

How Should I Take This Drug?
Take this drug exactly as directed by your doctor. If you do not understand the instructions, ask your doctor or nurse to explain them to you.

 Read the following information. If you do not understand it or if any of it causes you special concern, check with your doctor.

Before taking this drug, tell your doctor if you are taking any other prescription or over-the-counter drugs, including vitamins and herbals.

Should I avoid any other medicines, foods, alcohol, and/or activities?
Your prescription and nonprescription medicines may interact with other drugs, causing harm. Certain foods or alcohol can also interact with drug products. Never begin taking a new medicine—prescription or nonprescription—without asking your doctor or nurse if it will interact with alcohol, food, or other medicines. Some drugs can cause drowsiness and affect activities such as driving.

Precautions:
Tell your doctor if you have any drug allergies, especially to antibiotics.

All antibiotics can cause allergic reactions. Stop the drug and tell your doctor or nurse right away if you develop a rash, hives, fever and chills, red blotches on your skin, or difficulty breathing.

Use of antibiotics can change the normal organisms in your body. Women are at risk for fungal infections. Tell your nurse or doctor if you have vaginal itching or discharge.

Tell all the doctors, dentists, and pharmacists you visit that you are taking this drug.
- Most of the following side effects probably will not occur.
- Your doctor or nurse will want to discuss specific care instructions with you.
- They can help you understand these side effects and help you deal with them.

Side Effects:

More Common Side Effects
Nausea
Diarrhea

Less Common Side Effects
Vomiting
Vaginal itching
Vaginal candidiasis (fungal infection)

Rare Side Effects
Diarrhea related to infection of the intestinal lining (pseudomembranous colitis)
Decreased white blood cell count with increased risk of infection
Decreased red blood cell count with increased risk of anemia and tiredness (fatigue)
Decreased clotting of the blood with risk of bleeding
Allergic reaction with rash, hives, fever, chills, swelling of face and lips, and difficulty breathing

Side Effects / Symptoms of the Drug
Stop the drug and tell your doctor or nurse right away if you get diarrhea that does not stop, stomach cramping, or blood in your stool.

Stop the drug and call your doctor or nurse right away if you develop a rash, fever, chills, swelling of lips or face, or difficulty breathing. This can be serious.

Other side effects not listed above can also occur in some patients.
Tell your doctor or nurse if you develop any problems.

FDA Approval: Yes

amoxicillin with clavulanate

Trade Name:
Augmentin

Type of Drug:
Amoxicillin with clavulanate is an antibiotic that belongs to the class of drugs called penicillins. Amoxicillin with clavulanate is used to treat gram-negative and some gram-positive bacteria. It is used to treat infections in the lungs, throat, sinuses, kidneys, bladder, and skin.

How Drug Works:
Amoxicillin stops bacteria from making their protein cell wall, so the bacteria die. Penicillins can do this because they contain a special beta-lactam ring. Some bacteria contain an enzyme that breaks down the beta-lactam ring so that it does not work anymore, and the antibiotic no longer kills the bacteria. Clavulanate stops this enzyme, so that the bacteria can still be killed by the amoxicillin.

How Drug Is Given:
Amoxicillin is combined with clavulanate in a pill taken twice a day by mouth. Take it on an empty stomach, 1 hour before or 2 hours after eating. The dose and frequency depend on the infection being treated and kidney function. Keep the medicine in a tightly closed container and out of the reach of children and pets.

How Should I Take This Drug?
Take this drug exactly as directed by your doctor. If you do not understand the instructions, ask your doctor or nurse to explain them to you.

 Read the following information. If you do not understand it or if any of it causes you special concern, check with your doctor.

Before taking this drug, tell your doctor if you are taking any other prescription or over-the-counter drugs, including vitamins and herbals.

Should I avoid any other medicines, foods, alcohol, and/or activities?
Your prescription and nonprescription medicines may interact with other drugs, causing harm. Certain foods or alcohol can also interact with drug products. Never begin taking a new medicine—prescription or nonprescription—without asking your doctor or nurse if it will interact with alcohol, food, or other medicines. Some drugs can cause drowsiness and affect activities such as driving.

Precautions:
Tell your doctor if you are allergic to any drugs, especially to antibiotics.

All antibiotics can cause allergic reactions. Stop taking the drug and tell your doctor or nurse right away if you develop a rash, hives, fever and chills, red blotches on your skin, or difficulty breathing.

Amoxicillin with clavulanate can interact with other drugs. These include aminoglycosides, rifampin, probenecid, and allopurinol. Be sure to tell your doctor or nurse if you are taking these drugs.

Use of antibiotics can change the normal organisms in your body. Women are at risk for fungal infections. Tell your nurse or doctor if you have vaginal itching or discharge.

Tell all the doctors, dentists, and pharmacists you visit that you are taking this drug.

- Most of the following side effects probably will not occur.
- Your doctor or nurse will want to discuss specific care instructions with you.
- They can help you understand these side effects and help you deal with them.

Side Effects:

More Common Side Effects
Nausea
Diarrhea

Less Common Side Effects
Vomiting
Vaginal itching
Vaginal candidiasis (fungal infection)

Rare Side Effects
Diarrhea related to infection of the intestinal lining (pseudomembranous colitis)
Decreased white blood cell count with increased risk of infection
Decreased clotting of the blood with risk of bleeding
Allergic reaction with rash, hives, fever, chills, swelling of face or lips, and difficulty breathing

Side Effects / Symptoms of the Drug
Stop the drug and tell your doctor or nurse if you develop a rash, fever, chills or swelling of your face or throat.

Other side effects not listed above can also occur in some patients.
Tell your doctor or nurse if you develop any problems.

FDA Approval: Yes

amphotericin B, amphotericin B cholesteryl, amphotericin B lipid complex, sulfate complex, liposomal amphotericin B

Trade Names:
Abelcet, Ambisome, Amphotec, Fungizone

Type of Drug:
Amphotericin B is used to treat fungal and protozoal infections.

How Drug Works:
Amphotericin B damages fungal membranes, prevents reproduction, and kills fungi at high doses. It is used to treat fungal infections in the blood and spinal cord. The liposomal form of the drug decreases the side effects of the drug, including those involving the kidneys.

How Drug Is Given:
Amphotericin B can be given in different ways. It is usually given every other day by a shot into a vein. The first dose is very small and given over 6 hours. The dose is gradually increased, and the infusion time decreased. When given into the spinal column (intrathecally), it is given 2 to 3 times a week. The dose and type of amphotericin B given depend on your weight and how well your kidneys are working.

 Read the following information. If you do not understand it or if any of it causes you special concern, check with your doctor.

Before taking this drug, tell your doctor if you are taking any other prescription or over-the-counter drugs, including vitamins and herbals.

Should I avoid any other medicines, foods, alcohol, and/or activities?
Your prescription and nonprescription medicines may interact with other drugs, causing harm. Certain foods or alcohol can also interact with drug products. Never begin taking a new medicine—prescription or non-prescription—without asking your doctor or nurse if it will interact with alcohol, food, or other medicines. Some drugs can cause drowsiness and affect activities such as driving.

Precautions:
Amphotericin B can damage your kidneys, so your doctor will check your kidney function before your first treatment and periodically throughout the treatment. Most people have some changes in their kidney function. This returns to normal after treatment is finished or stopped.

All drugs used to fight infections can cause allergic reactions. Tell your nurse or doctor right away if you develop a rash, hives, red blotches on your skin, difficulty breathing, or tightness in your chest.

Amphotericin B can cause you to feel poorly during the first infusion. The side effects will go away, and with future doses will stop completely. You will be given a test dose first to see how you react. The side effects include fever, chills starting 1 to 3 hours after the drug is given, nausea, vomiting, increased breathing rate, headache, and feeling "blah." Your nurse or doctor will give you medicine to take away the chills and tight feeling and to stop the nausea.

Women who are pregnant and patients with kidney problems should use this drug with caution.

Amphotericin B can be used for a long period to treat serious fungal or protozoal infections. Often, you will receive the drug in the hospital. Sometimes, you will go home and receive your treatments there. The infusion usually runs for several hours, daily, or every other day.

Tell all the doctors, dentists, and pharmacists you visit that you are taking this drug.
- -
- Most of the following side effects probably will not occur.
- Your doctor or nurse will want to discuss specific care instructions with you.
- They can help you understand these side effects and help you deal with them.

Side Effects:

More Common Side Effects
Changes in kidney function
Decreased red blood cell count with increased risk of anemia and tiredness (fatigue)
Pain at place of injection
Decrease in blood potassium level
Nausea
Vomiting
Cramping
Fever
Rigors

Less Common Side Effects
Kidney damage
Vomiting
Loss of appetite
Heartburn
Abdominal pain
Diarrhea

Rare Side Effects
Increased blood pressure
Irregular heart beat
Wheezing
Inflammation of lung
Hearing loss
Ringing in ears (tinnitus)
Blurred or double vision
Numbness in hands and/or feet
Seizures
Decreased white blood cell count with increased risk of infection
Decreased platelet count with increased risk of bleeding
Blood in stool

Side Effects / Symptoms of the Drug
Call your doctor or nurse if you develop rash, fever, or chills. Your nurse or doctor will give you medicine to make you feel better. You will probably receive medicines before the next treatment to prevent these problems.

Other side effects not listed above can also occur in some patients.
Tell your doctor or nurse if you develop any problems.

FDA Approval: Yes

ampicillin sodium combined with sulbactam sodium

Trade Name:
Unasyn

Type of Drug:
Ampicillin sodium combined with sulbactam sodium is an antibiotic that belongs to the class of drugs called penicillins. It is used to treat infections caused by gram-negative and some gram-positive bacteria. It is used to treat infections of the lungs, throat, sinuses, kidneys, bladder, and skin.

How Drug Works:
Ampicillin and forms of ampicillin stops bacteria from making their protein cell wall, so the bacteria die. Penicillins are able to do this because they contain a special beta-lactam ring. Some bacteria contain an enzyme that breaks down the beta-lactam ring so that it doesn't work anymore, and the antibiotic no longer kills the bacteria. Sulbactam sodium stops this enzyme, so that the bacteria can still be killed by the ampicillin sodium.

How Drug Is Given:
Ampicillin sodium combined with sulbactam sodium is given as a shot into a vein over 10 to 15 minutes, or by shot into the muscle, 4 times a day. The dose and length of treatment depend on the type of infection being treated.

 Read the following information. If you do not understand it or if any of it causes you special concern, check with your doctor.

Before taking this drug, tell your doctor if you are taking any other prescription or over-the-counter drugs, including vitamins and herbals.

Should I avoid any other medicines, foods, alcohol, and/or activities?
Your prescription and nonprescription medicines may interact with other drugs, causing harm. Certain foods or alcohol can also interact with drug products. Never begin taking a new medicine—prescription or non-prescription—without asking your doctor or nurse if it will interact with alcohol, food, or other medicines. Some drugs can cause drowsiness and affect activities such as driving.

Precautions:
Tell your doctor if you have any drug allergies, especially to antibiotic drugs.

All antibiotics can cause allergic reactions. Stop taking the drug and tell your doctor or nurse right away if you develop a rash, hives, fever and chills, red blotches on your skin, or difficulty breathing.

Use of antibiotics can change the normal organisms in your body. Women are at risk for getting fungal infections. Tell your nurse or doctor if you have vaginal itching or discharge.

Ampicillin and forms of ampicillin may decrease the effectiveness of oral contraceptives (birth control pills). Women should add barrier contraception while taking the antibiotics.

Ampicillin sodium combined with sulbactam sodium can interact with many other medicines. Some of these are aminoglycosids, rifampin, probenicid, and oral contraceptives. Make sure you tell your doctor about all the medicines you are taking.

Ampicillin sodium combined with sulbactam sodium should be used with caution if you are pregnant or breastfeeding.

The dose of ampicillin sodium combined with sulbactam sodium will be reduced if kidney disease is present.

Tell all the doctors, dentists, and pharmacists you visit that you are taking this drug.
- Most of the following side effects probably will not occur.
- Your doctor or nurse will want to discuss specific care instructions with you.
- They can help you understand these side effects and help you deal with them.

Side Effects:

More Common Side Effects
Nausea
Diarrhea

Less Common Side Effects
Vomiting
Vaginal itching
Vaginal candidiasis (fungal infection)

Rare Side Effects
Diarrhea related to infection of the intestinal lining (pseudomembranous colitis)
Decreased white blood cell count with increased risk of infection
Decreased red blood cell count with increased risk of anemia and tiredness (fatigue)
Decreased clotting of the blood with risk of bleeding
Allergic reaction with rash, hives, fever, chills, swelling of face or lips, and difficulty breathing

Other side effects not listed above can also occur in some patients.
Tell your doctor or nurse if you develop any problems.

FDA Approval: Yes

aspirin, acetylsalicylic acid

Trade Names:
ASA, Aspergum, Bayer Aspirin, Easprin, Ecotrin, Empirin

Type of Drug:
Aspirin belongs to a general class of nonopioid analgesics (pain-relieving medicines) called salicylates, which belong to a larger category called nonsteroidal anti-inflammatory drugs (NSAIDs).

How Drug Works:
Aspirin blocks the synthesis of prostaglandins. This prevents pain receptors from passing the pain message to the brain so that pain perception is decreased. This drug is also an anti-inflammatory drug that relieves pain and reduces fever.

How Drug Is Given:
Aspirin is given as a pill or capsule, or as a rectal suppository. Because aspirin can irritate the stomach, it may be given with milk, food, or at least 8 oz of water. Keep the medicine in a tightly closed container and out of the reach of children and pets. Keep the suppositories in a safe place out of the reach of children and pets.

How Should I Take This Drug?
Take this drug exactly as directed by your doctor. If you do not understand the instructions, ask your doctor or nurse to explain them to you.

 Read the following information. If you do not understand it or if any of it causes you special concern, check with your doctor.

Before taking this drug, tell your doctor if you are taking any other prescription or over-the-counter drugs, including vitamins and herbals.

Should I avoid any other medicines, foods, alcohol, and/or activities?
Your prescription and nonprescription medicines may interact with other drugs, causing harm. Certain foods or alcohol can also interact with drug products. Never begin taking a new medicine—prescription or nonprescription—without asking your doctor or nurse if it will interact with alcohol, food, or other medicines. Some drugs can cause drowsiness and affect activities such as driving.

Precautions:
It you have asthma, inflammation of the nose (rhinitis), or nasal polyps, take aspirin cautiously. Talk to your doctor or nurse about this as aspirin can cause bronchospasms, or tightening of your breathing tubes.

DO NOT take aspirin if you are also taking Coumadin or other medicines to prevent blood clots, methotrexate, other nonsteroidal anti-inflammatory drugs, or have liver damage. Talk with your doctor or nurse about this.

If you take too much aspirin, you can have ringing in the ears (tinnitus), decreased hearing, nausea, vomiting, diarrhea, mental confusion, headache, sweating, fast breathing, lethargy, and dizziness. Be careful not to exceed recommended dosages.

Aspirin may increase the risk of bleeding. You should not take aspirin if you are receiving chemotherapy that decreases your platelet count, or have stomach or intestinal ulcers, bleeding problems, or bleeding in your gastrointestinal tract. Talk to your doctor or nurse if you have questions.

Aspirin must be stopped 3 or more days before a surgical procedure. Make sure you tell your doctor if you are taking aspirin.

Tell all the doctors, dentists, and pharmacists you visit that you are taking this drug.
- -
   • Most of the following side effects probably will not occur.
   • Your doctor or nurse will want to discuss specific care instructions with you.
   • They can help you understand these side effects and help you deal with them.

Side Effects:

More Common Side Effects
Increased bleeding time
Heartburn
Increased bruising
Sweating

Less Common Side Effects
Bleeding in the gastrointestinal tract
Flushing
Ringing in the ears (tinnitis)
Hearing loss
Dizziness

Rare Side Effects
Decreased platelet count with increased risk of bleeding
Decreased white blood cell count with increased risk of infection
Decreased red blood cell count with increased risk of anemia and tiredness (fatigue)
Drowsiness
Confusion
Headache
Nausea
Vomiting
Diarrhea
Loss of appetite
Inflammation of the liver
Rash
Hives
Wheezing
Increased heart rate
Changes in blood levels of sugar, potassium, and/or sodium

Other side effects not listed above can also occur in some patients.
Tell your doctor or nurse if you develop any problems.

FDA Approval: Yes

azithromycin

Trade Name:
Zithromax

Type of Drug:
Azithromycin is an antibiotic. It is used to treat infections caused by gram-negative bacteria as well as staphylococcal ("staph") infections.

How Drug Works:
Azithromycin prevents bacteria from making the proteins needed for continued growth. This makes the bacteria die.

How Drug Is Given:
Azithromycin is given as a pill by mouth on an empty stomach, either 1 hour before or 2 hours after eating. The dose is the same for all adults, starting with 2 tablets on the first day, then 1 tablet each day for the next 4 days. Keep the medicine in a tightly closed container and out of the reach of children and pets. Azithromycin can also be given as a shot into a vein, over 1 to 3 hours.

How Should I Take This Drug?
Take this drug exactly as directed by your doctor. If you do not understand the instructions, ask your doctor or nurse to explain them to you.

 Read the following information. If you do not understand it or if any of it causes you special concern, check with your doctor.

Before taking this drug, tell your doctor if you are taking any other prescription or over-the-counter drugs, including vitamins and herbals.

Should I avoid any other medicines, foods, alcohol, and/or activities?
Your prescription and nonprescription medicines may interact with other drugs, causing harm. Certain foods or alcohol can also interact with drug products. Never begin taking a new medicine—prescription or nonprescription—without asking your doctor or nurse if it will interact with alcohol, food, or other medicines. Some drugs can cause drowsiness and affect activities such as driving.

Precautions:
Tell your doctor if you are allergic to any drugs, especially to antibiotics such as erythromycin.

Taking antibiotics can change the normal organisms in your body. Women are at risk for fungal infections. Tell your nurse or doctor if you develop vaginal itching or discharge.

Antacids can decrease the effectiveness of the antibiotic. If you take antacids, take the antibiotic pill at least 1 hour before or 2 hours after an antacid.

Tell all the doctors, dentists, and pharmacists you visit that you are taking this drug.
- Most of the following side effects probably will not occur.
- Your doctor or nurse will want to discuss specific care instructions with you.
- They can help you understand these side effects and help you deal with them.

Side Effects:

Less Common Side Effects
Abdominal pain
Diarrhea
Nausea
Vomiting

Rare Side Effects
Diarrhea related to infection of the intestinal lining (pseudomembranous colitis)
Inflammation of the kidneys
Joint pain
Serious allergic reaction including fever, chills, rash, hives, difficulty breathing, swelling of face or lips
Dizziness
Headache
Itching

Side Effects / Symptoms of the Drug
Stop the drug and tell your doctor or nurse right away if you get diarrhea that does not stop, stomach cramping, and blood in your stool.

Stop the drug and tell your doctor or nurse right away if you develop a rash, fever, chills, hives, and swelling in your lips or face. This can be serious.

Other side effects not listed above can also occur in some patients.
Tell your doctor or nurse if you develop any problems.

FDA Approval: Yes

aztreonam

Trade Name:
Azactam

Type of Drug:
Aztreonam is an antibiotic.

How Drug Works:
Aztreonam stops bacteria from making their protein cell wall, so the bacteria die. Aztreonam is used to treat gram-negative infections of the urinary and lower respiratory tract, infections involving the female reproductive organs, abdomen, and infections throughout the body (septicemia).

How Drug Is Given:
Aztreonam is given by an injection in the vein over 20 to 60 minutes, or as an injection into a muscle 2 to 4 times a day. The dose and length of treatment depend on the type of infection.

 Read the following information. If you do not understand it or if any of it causes you special concern, check with your doctor.

Before taking this drug, tell your doctor if you are taking any other prescription or over-the-counter drugs, including vitamins and herbals.

Should I avoid any other medicines, foods, alcohol, and/or activities?
Your prescription and nonprescription medicines may interact with other drugs, causing harm. Certain foods or alcohol can also interact with drug products. Never begin taking a new medicine—prescription or non-prescription—without asking your doctor or nurse if it will interact with alcohol, food, or other medicines. Some drugs can cause drowsiness and affect activities such as driving.

Precautions:
Tell your doctor if you have any drug allergies, especially to antibiotic drugs.

All antibiotics can cause allergic reactions. Stop the drug and tell your doctor or nurse right away if you develop a rash, hives, red blotches on your skin, difficulty breathing, or chest tightness.

Use of antibiotics can change the normal organisms your body. Women are at risk of getting fungal infections. Tell your nurse or doctor if you get vaginal itching or discharge.

DO NOT drink alcohol until 3 days after you stop taking this drug. It can cause a dangerous drug interaction (flushing, throbbing headache, shortness of breath, nausea, vomiting, sweating, chest pain, increased blood pressure, increased heart rate, "black out," weakness, and blurred vision).

Patients with kidney or liver problems should use this drug with caution.

___Tell all the doctors, dentists, and pharmacists you visit that you are taking this drug.___
- -
- Most of the following side effects probably will not occur.
- Your doctor or nurse will want to discuss specific care instructions with you.
- They can help you understand these side effects and help you deal with them.

Side Effects:

More Common Side Effects
Nausea
Vomiting
Diarrhea
Loss of appetite

Less Common Side Effects
Vaginal itching
Vaginal candidiasis (fungal infection)

Rare Side Effects
Diarrhea related to infection of the intestinal lining (pseudomembranous colitis)
Rash
Hives
Itching
Decreased white blood cell count with increased risk of infection
Decreased platelet count with increased risk of bleeding
Decreased platelet count with increased risk of anemia and tiredness (fatigue)
Dizziness
Headache
Sleepiness
Irritation of the vein used for giving the drug
Pain and swelling at place of injection
Change in blood pressure and heart rate

Side Effects / Symptoms of the Drug
Stop the drug and call your doctor or nurse right away if you get diarrhea that does not stop, abdominal cramping, and blood and/or pus in the stool. This needs to be treated right away.

Other side effects not listed above can also occur in some patients.
Tell your doctor or nurse if you develop any problems.

FDA Approval: Yes

bisacodyl

Trade Name:
Dulcolax

Type of Drug:
Bisacodyl belongs to the class of drugs called stimulant laxatives.

How Drug Works:
Bisacodyl stimulates (irritates) the smooth muscle of the intestines. This causes the normal forward movement of the intestines (peristalsis). It increases water in the intestines, resulting in a bowel movement.

How Drug Is Given:
Bisacodyl is given as a pill or as a rectal suppository. The dose of the pill may depend on how often you take laxatives. The suppository is available in one dose. Take the pill on an empty stomach, more than 1 hour after taking antacids or drinking milk. Do not crush the pill. Keep the medicine in a tightly closed container and out of the reach of children and pets.

How Should I Take This Drug?
Take this drug exactly as directed by your doctor. If you do not understand the instructions, ask your doctor or nurse to explain them to you.

 Read the following information. If you do not understand it or if any of it causes you special concern, check with your doctor.

Before taking this drug, tell your doctor if you are taking any other prescription or over-the-counter drugs, including vitamins and herbals.

Should I avoid any other medicines, foods, alcohol, and/or activities?
Your prescription and nonprescription medicines may interact with other drugs, causing harm. Certain foods or alcohol can also interact with drug products. Never begin taking a new medicine—prescription or nonprescription—without asking your doctor or nurse if it will interact with alcohol, food, or other medicines. Some drugs can cause drowsiness and affect activities such as driving.

Precautions:
You will probably have an urge to move your bowels 6 to 10 hours after taking the pills, and 15 minutes to 1 hour after taking the suppository.

Talk to your doctor before taking bisacodyl if you have nausea, vomiting, abdominal pain, or blood in the stool, or if you have not had a bowel movement in several days. There may be something else wrong besides constipation.

If you use laxatives all the time, your body may forget the normal process of moving your bowels. You then become dependent on the laxative. If you are taking opioid pain relievers, you will need to take a laxative regularly.

To prevent constipation, try to drink 2 to 3 quarts of fluid a day, increase the amount of bran, fruits, and vegetables in your diet (try to eat 5 fruits and vegetables daily), eat vegetable fiber or cereal, and do gentle exercise as tolerated.

Some laxatives can cause diarrhea. It is important to replace the fluid that you lose through diarrhea. Try to drink 2 to 3 quarts of fluid a day. Fluids with electrolytes, such as chicken broth or sports drinks, are helpful in replacing potassium and salt that are lost in diarrhea.

Tell all the doctors, dentists, and pharmacists you visit that you are taking this drug.
- -
  • Most of the following side effects probably will not occur.
  • Your doctor or nurse will want to discuss specific care instructions with you.
  • They can help you understand these side effects and help you deal with them.

Side Effects:

More Common Side Effects
Mild rectal burning as suppository is absorbed
Loss of normal reflexes to move bowels when used on a long-term basis

Less Common Side Effects
Dehydration due to fluid loss in diarrhea
Diarrhea
Loss of electrolytes

Other side effects not listed above can also occur in some patients.
Tell your doctor or nurse if you develop any problems.

FDA Approval: Yes

bupropion hydrochloride

Trade Name:
Wellbutrin

Type of Drug:
Bupropion hydrochloride is an aminoketone antidepressant used to relieve anxiety or depression.

How Drug Works:
The action of bupropion hydrochloride is not known. It increases the amount of serotonin and norepinephrine in the brain, thus relieving or preventing the feeling of depression.

How Drug Is Given:
Bupropion hydrochloride pills can be either short-acting (immediate release) or long-lasting (sustained release). The short-acting pills are usually taken twice a day, morning and night, for 3 days to start and then 3 times a day as directed by your doctor. The long-lasting pills are usually taken once a day in the morning for a few days to start. If you are doing okay with this dose, your doctor will usually increase the dose so you take 1 pill in the morning and 1 in the evening. The dose depends on your size and other factors. Keep the medicine in a tightly closed container and out of the reach of children or pets. If you are also taking Zyban tablets to stop smoking, do not take bupropion hydrochloride until you talk to your doctor; they are the same medicine.

How Should I Take This Drug?
Take this drug exactly as directed by your doctor. If you do not understand the instructions, ask your doctor or nurse to explain them to you.

 Read the following information. If you do not understand it or if any of it causes you special concern, check with your doctor.

Before taking this drug, tell your doctor if you are taking any other prescription or over-the-counter drugs, including vitamins and herbals.

Should I avoid any other medicines, foods, alcohol, and/or activities?
Your prescription and nonprescription medicines may interact with other drugs, causing harm. Certain foods or alcohol can also interact with drug products. Never begin taking a new medicine—prescription or nonprescription—without asking your doctor or nurse if it will interact with alcohol, food, or other medicines. Some drugs can cause drowsiness and affect activities such as driving.

Precautions:
Tell your doctor if you are taking any of the following drugs as they may have serious interactions with bupropion hydrochloride: Tegretol, cimetidine, phenobarbital, Dilantin, monoamine oxidase inhibitors (or other antidepressant medicines), and/or L-dopa (or other seizure medicines).

Tell your doctor if you have recently had a heart attack (myocardial infarction), have frequent bouts of chest pain, or have urinary retention.

This drug contains the same medicine as the drug Zyban, which is used to help people stop smoking. DO NOT take both these drugs. Talk with your doctor or nurse about this.

If you have a history of seizures, you should not take this drug.

DO NOT drink alcohol while taking this drug.

When starting this drug, some people may feel more restless, agitated, or anxious, or they may have more trouble sleeping. This should go away after a few days. If not, call your doctor or nurse to see what can be done, or if the drug should be stopped.

Tell all the doctors, dentists, and pharmacists you visit that you are taking this drug.
- -
- Most of the following side effects probably will not occur.
- Your doctor or nurse will want to discuss specific care instructions with you.
- They can help you understand these side effects and help you deal with them.

Side Effects:

More Common Side Effects
Increased restlessness (when first starting the drug)
Agitation (when first starting the drug)
Anxiety (when first starting the drug)
Difficulty sleeping (when first starting the drug)

Less Common Side Effects
Hostility
Decreased concentration
Lack of coordination
Confusion
Dizziness
Increased heart rate
Change in blood pressure
Urinary retention

Rare Side Effects
Euphoria
Paranoia
Anxiety
Palpitations
Swelling of feet
Irregular heartbeats
Dry mouth
Change in appetite
Nausea
Diarrhea
Constipation
Changes in weight
Changes in taste
Increased urination
Rash
Itching of skin
Hives
Impotence
Irregular menstrual periods

Other side effects not listed above can also occur in some patients.
Tell your doctor or nurse if you develop any problems.

FDA Approval: Yes

buspirone hydrochloride

Trade Name:
BuSpar

Type of Drug:
Buspirone hydrochloride belongs to a general class of drugs called antianxiety agents.

How Drug Works:
The action of buspirone hydrochloride is not known, but it affects the many neurotransmitters in the brain that bring about the feeling of anxiety.

How Drug Is Given:
Buspirone hydrochloride tablets are taken by mouth the same time each day. Food increases absorption, so if you take it with food, make sure you always take it with food. If you do not take it with food, then make sure you always take it on an empty stomach. Do not take the pill with grapefruit juice. The dose depends upon how much of the medicine you need to make you feel better. Your doctor will start you on a low-dosage pill twice a day and will increase the dose as needed every 2 to 3 days until you feel better. Keep pills in a tightly closed container and out of the reach of children and pets.

How Should I Take This Drug?
Take this drug exactly as directed by your doctor. If you do not understand the instructions, ask your doctor or nurse to explain them to you. This drug can be given at different strengths depending on the type of cancer being treated. Dosage may vary depending on your body weight and the type of cancer being treated.

 Read the following information. If you do not understand it or if any of it causes you special concern, check with your doctor.

Before taking this drug, tell your doctor if you are taking any other prescription or over-the-counter drugs, including vitamins and herbals.

Should I avoid any other medicines, foods, alcohol, and/or activities?
Your prescription and nonprescription medicines may interact with other drugs, causing harm. Certain foods or alcohol can also interact with drug products. Never begin taking a new medicine—prescription or non-prescription—without asking your doctor or nurse if it will interact with alcohol, food, or other medicines. Some drugs can cause drowsiness and affect activities such as driving.

Precautions:
Tell your doctor if you are taking any of the following drugs as they may have serious interactions with buspirone hydrochloride: haloperidol, antidepressants (monamine oxidase inhibitors), or sedatives.

Once you start taking buspirone hydrochloride, you may not see the full effect of this drug for 3 to 4 weeks.

DO NOT drink alcohol while you are taking this drug.

Tell all the doctors, dentists, and pharmacists you visit that you are taking this drug.

- Most of the following side effects probably will not occur.
- Your doctor or nurse will want to discuss specific care instructions with you.
- They can help you understand these side effects and help you deal with them.

Side Effects:

Less Common Side Effects
Dizziness
Drowsiness
Headache

Rare Side Effects
Tiredness (fatigue)
Nightmares
Weakness
Numbness and tingling in hands and/or feet
Nausea
Dry mouth
Vomiting
Diarrhea
Constipation

Other side effects not listed above can also occur in some patients.
Tell your doctor or nurse if you develop any problems.

FDA Approval: Yes

calcitonin-salmon

Trade Names:
Calcimar, Miacalcin

Type of Drug:
Calcitonin-salmon is a thyroid hormone that helps decrease blood calcium levels. It is used in patients whose cancer causes an increase in calcium in the blood.

How Drug Works:
Calcitonin-salmon blocks bone breakdown (absorption), thus preventing the bone from releasing more calcium into the blood. It helps the kidneys rid the body of the excess calcium in the blood. It also makes changes in the gastrointestinal system that help decrease calcium entering the body through food.

How Drug Is Given:
Calcitonin-salmon is given as an injection in the muscle or under the skin, or it can be inhaled through the nose. If your doctor orders the injection, you or a family member will learn how to give it, usually once or twice a day. Many people who get just 1 injection a day like to have it at night. Keep the medicine in its original container in the refrigerator. The dose depends upon your size, but your doctor may start with a smaller dose and gradually increase the dose. The nasal spray is usually given once a day, about the same time every day. Keep the equipment in a safe, dry place and out of the reach of children and pets.

How Should I Take This Drug?
Take this drug exactly as directed by your doctor. If you do not understand the instructions, ask your doctor or nurse to explain them to you.

 Read the following information. If you do not understand it or if any of it causes you special concern, check with your doctor.

Before taking this drug, tell your doctor if you are taking any other prescription or over-the-counter drugs, including vitamins and herbals.

Should I avoid any other medicines, foods, alcohol, and/or activities?
Your prescription and nonprescription medicines may interact with other drugs, causing harm. Certain foods or alcohol can also interact with drug products. Never begin taking a new medicine—prescription or nonprescription—without asking your doctor or nurse if it will interact with alcohol, food, or other medicines. Some drugs can cause drowsiness and affect activities such as driving.

Precautions:
Calcitonin-salmon is made of protein, so it can cause allergic reactions. Your doctor may ask you to have a skin test first to see if you have allergies.

You may also receive intravenous fluids, since it is important for your kidneys to make a lot of urine.

Tell all the doctors, dentists, and pharmacists you visit that you are taking this drug.
- -
• Most of the following side effects probably will not occur.
• Your doctor or nurse will want to discuss specific care instructions with you.
• They can help you understand these side effects and help you deal with them.

Side Effects:

More Common Side Effects
Flushing of face, hands, and/or feet after injection
Tingling in hands and/or feet after injection

Less Common Side Effects
Nausea that lasts a short time
Vomiting that lasts a short time
Decreased appetite
Diarrhea
Abdominal pain

Rare Side Effects
Rash
Hives
Headache
Chills
Low calcium blood levels (if drug is very effective)

Other side effects not listed above can also occur in some patients.
Tell your doctor or nurse if you develop any problems.

FDA Approval: Yes

camphorated opium tincture

Trade Name:
Paregoric

Type of Drug:
Camphorated opium tincture is an opium agent used to control diarrhea.

How Drug Works:
Camphorated opium tincture stops the forward movement of the intestines (peristalsis), so that the stool moves slowly. This allows the water to be absorbed from the stool so the stool becomes more firm. Camphorated opium tincture also decreases the release of digestive secretions.

How Drug Is Given:
Camphorated opium tincture is taken by mouth, mixed in water. It will look cloudy white. Your doctor will tell you how often to take it, usually 1 to 4 times a day, or after each loose stool (bowel movement), but not more than 6 times a day. It is important not to take more than your doctor tells you. The drug should be stored in a closed container and protected from light. Keep it out of the reach of children and pets.

How Should I Take This Drug?
Take this drug exactly as directed by your doctor. If you do not understand the instructions, ask your doctor or nurse to explain them to you.

 Read the following information. If you do not understand it or if any of it causes you special concern, check with your doctor.

Before taking this drug, tell your doctor if you are taking any other prescription or over-the-counter drugs, including vitamins and herbals.

Should I avoid any other medicines, foods, alcohol, and/or activities?
Your prescription and nonprescription medicines may interact with other drugs, causing harm. Certain foods or alcohol can also interact with drug products. Never begin taking a new medicine—prescription or non-prescription—without asking your doctor or nurse if it will interact with alcohol, food, or other medicines. Some drug products can cause drowsiness and affect activities such as driving.

Precautions:
Camphorated opium tincture should not be used to treat diarrhea caused by poisoning or by infection of the intestinal lining (pseudomembranous colitis) caused by antibiotics.

To decrease the diarrhea, change your diet. Try to eat small, frequent meals that are warm or at room temperature. Avoid foods that cause gas (such as broccoli or beans), fatty foods (such as bacon or cheeses), citrus fruits and juices, and high lactose-foods (such as milk or ice cream). Eat foods high in sodium and potassium (such as soups or sports drinks). Eat foods high in soluble fiber (such as rice or bananas). Avoid foods high in insoluble fiber (such as cereal or nuts). Try to drink at least eight oz glasses of water a day. To add calories, dilute with fruit juice.

If camphorated opium tincture is used for a long time, physical dependence may develop and the body will go into withdrawal if the drug is stopped abruptly. It is a controlled substance.

Do not confuse camphorated opium tincture with tincture of opium, which is 25 times more potent.

Tell all the doctors, dentists, and pharmacists you visit that you are taking this drug.
- Most of the following side effects probably will not occur.
- Your doctor or nurse will want to discuss specific care instructions with you.
- They can help you understand these side effects and help you deal with them.

Side Effects:

More Common Side Effects
Nausea

Less Common Side Effects
Vomiting

Rare Side Effects
Constipation

Side Effects / Symptoms of the Drug
Tell your doctor or nurse if the diarrhea does not go away after 48 hours.

Other side effects not listed above can also occur in some patients.
Tell your doctor or nurse if you develop any problems.

FDA Approval: Yes

carbenicillin indanyl sodium

Trade Names:
Geocillin, Geopen

Type of Drug:
Carbenicillin indanyl sodium is an antibiotic. It belongs to the class of extended-spectrum penicillins.

How Drug Works:
Carbenicillin indanyl sodium stops bacteria from making their protein cell wall, so the bacteria die. Carbenicillin indanyl sodium is used to treat both gram-positive and gram-negative bacterial infections.

How Drug Is Given:
Carbenicillin indanyl sodium is usually given as a pill but can also be given as an injection. The dose of the pills depends upon the type of infection. The usual dose is 1 or 2 pills every 6 hours by mouth with a full glass of water on an empty stomach. You should take the pill(s) at least 1 hour before or 2 hours after meals, at about the same time every day. If you have high blood pressure, you may need to restrict your salt intake even more because carbenicillin pills have a lot of salt in the tablets. The dose of the injection depends upon your weight. Keep the medicine in a tightly closed container and out of the reach of children and pets.

How Should I Take This Drug?
Take this drug exactly as directed by your doctor. If you do not understand the instructions, ask your doctor or nurse to explain them to you.

 Read the following information. If you do not understand it or if any of it causes you special concern, check with your doctor.

Before taking this drug, tell your doctor if you are taking any other prescription or over-the-counter drugs, including vitamins and herbals.

Should I avoid any other medicines, foods, alcohol, and/or activities?
Your prescription and nonprescription medicines may interact with other drugs, causing harm. Certain foods or alcohol can also interact with drug products. Never begin taking a new medicine—prescription or nonprescription—without asking your doctor or nurse if it will interact with alcohol, food, or other medicines. Some drugs can cause drowsiness and affect activities such as driving.

Precautions:
Tell your doctor if you have any drug allergies, especially to antibiotic drugs.

All antibiotics can cause allergic reactions. Stop the drug and tell your doctor or nurse right away if you develop a rash, hives, red blotches on your skin, difficulty breathing, or chest tightness.

Tell all the doctors, dentists, and pharmacists you visit that you are taking this drug.
- -
- Most of the following side effects probably will not occur.
- Your doctor or nurse will want to discuss specific care instructions with you.
- They can help you understand these side effects and help you deal with them.

Side Effects:

More Common Side Effects
Nausea
Vomiting
Diarrhea
Loss of appetite

Less Common Side Effects
Vaginal itching
Vaginal candidiasis (fungal infection)

Rare Side Effects
Diarrhea related to infection of the intestinal lining (pseudomembranous colitis)
Rash
Hives
Itching
Decreased white blood cell count with increased risk of infection
Decreased red blood cell count with increased risk of anemia and tiredness (fatigue)

Side Effects / Symptoms of the Drug
Stop the drug and call your doctor or nurse right away if you develop a rash, fever, muscle aches, or blood in your urine. This can be a serious reaction and needs to be treated right away.

Stop the drug and call your doctor or nurse right away if you get diarrhea that does not stop, abdominal cramping, and blood and/or pus in the stool. This needs to be treated right away.

Other side effects not listed above can also occur in some patients.
Tell your doctor or nurse if you develop any problems.

FDA Approval: Yes

caspofungin

Trade Name:
Cancidas

Type of Drug:
Caspofungin is an antifungal antibiotic.

How Drug Works:
Caspofungin prevents fungus from making its cell wall, blocking the formation of a sugar needed for the fungus to grow. This results in death of the fungus.

How Drug Is Given:
Caspofungin is given as an injection in the vein over 1 hour. The dose is the same for all adults; if you have liver problems, the dose may be lowered. Caspofungin is given once a day for about 1 month. The first dose will be larger than the rest of the daily doses.

 Read the following information. If you do not understand it or if any of it causes you special concern, check with your doctor.

Before taking this drug, tell your doctor if you are taking any other prescription or over-the-counter drugs, including vitamins and herbals.

Should I avoid any other medicines, foods, alcohol, and/or activities?
Your prescription and nonprescription medicines may interact with other drugs, causing harm. Certain foods or alcohol can also interact with drug products. Never begin taking a new medicine—prescription or non-prescription—without asking your doctor or nurse if it will interact with alcohol, food, or other medicines. Some drugs can cause drowsiness and affect activities such as driving.

Precautions:
If you have had an allergic reaction to an antibiotic before, be sure to tell your doctor or nurse.

All antibiotics can cause allergic reactions. Tell your doctor or nurse right away if you develop a rash, hives, fever and chills, red blotches on your skin, difficulty breathing, or swelling in your face and lips.

Tell all the doctors, dentists, and pharmacists you visit that you are taking this drug.

- Most of the following side effects probably will not occur.
- Your doctor or nurse will want to discuss specific care instructions with you.
- They can help you understand these side effects and help you deal with them.

Side Effects:

More Common Side Effects
Redness and irritation of the injection site

Less Common Side Effects
Nausea
Vomiting
Headache

Rare Side Effects
Itching
Allergic reaction with fever and chills, rash, hives, difficulty breathing, or swelling of face and lips

Other side effects not listed above can also occur in some patients.
Tell your doctor or nurse if you develop any problems.

FDA Approval: Yes

cefaclor

Trade Name:
Ceclor

Type of Drug:
Cefaclor is an antibiotic that belongs to a group of drugs called cephalosporins.

How Drug Works:
Cefaclor stops bacteria from making their protein cell wall, so the bacteria die. Cefaclor is used to treat infections of the lungs, urinary tract, skin and soft tissue, and gall bladder, as well as infection in the blood (septicemia).

How Drug Is Given:
Cefaclor is taken by mouth 3 times a day with a full glass of water on an empty stomach. If you have stomach problems with the dose, then your doctor may tell you to take the pill(s) with food. Try to take the medicine at the same time each day for 7 to 10 days as directed. Cefaclor also comes as a slow-release pill that is given every 12 hours. The dose of cefaclor depends on the infection being treated. Keep the medicine in a tightly closed container and out of the reach of children and pets.

How Should I Take This Drug?
Take this drug exactly as directed by your doctor. If you do not understand the instructions, ask your doctor or nurse to explain them to you.

 Read the following information. If you do not understand it or if any of it causes you special concern, check with your doctor.

Before taking this drug, tell your doctor if you are taking any other prescription or over-the-counter drugs, including vitamins and herbals.

Should I avoid any other medicines, foods, alcohol, and/or activities?
Your prescription and nonprescription medicines may interact with other drugs, causing harm. Certain foods or alcohol can also interact with drug products. Never begin taking a new medicine—prescription or nonprescription—without asking your doctor or nurse if it will interact with alcohol, food, or other medicines. Some drugs can cause drowsiness and affect activities such as driving.

Precautions:
Tell your doctor if you have any allergies to antibiotics. All antibiotics can cause allergic reactions. Stop the drug and tell your doctor or nurse right away if you develop a rash, hives, red blotches on your skin, difficulty breathing, or chest tightness.

Use of antibiotics can change the normal organisms in your body. Women are at risk of getting fungal infections. Tell your nurse or doctor if you get vaginal itching or discharge.

Patients with kidney problems should use this drug with caution.

Tell all the doctors, dentists, and pharmacists you visit that you are taking this drug.

• Most of the following side effects probably will not occur.
• Your doctor or nurse will want to discuss specific care instructions with you.
• They can help you understand these side effects and help you deal with them.

Side Effects:

More Common Side Effects
Nausea
Vomiting
Diarrhea
Loss of appetite

Less Common Side Effects
Vaginal itching
Vaginal candidiasis (fungal infection)

Rare Side Effects
Diarrhea related to infection of the intestinal lining (pseudomembranous colitis)
Rash
Hives
Itching
Decreased white blood cell count with increased risk of infection
Decreased red blood cell count with increased risk of anemia and tiredness (fatigue)
Dizziness
Headache
Sleepiness

Side Effects / Symptoms of the Drug
Stop the drug and call your doctor or nurse right away if you develop a rash, fever, muscle aches, or blood in your urine. This can be a serious reaction and needs to be treated right away.

Stop the drug and call your doctor or nurse right away if you get diarrhea that does not stop, abdominal cramping, and blood and/or pus in the stool. This needs to be treated right away.

Other side effects not listed above can also occur in some patients.
Tell your doctor or nurse if you develop any problems.

FDA Approval: Yes

cefamandole nafate

Trade Name:
Mandol

Type of Drug:
Cefamandole nafate is an antibiotic that belongs to a group of drugs called cephalosporins.

How Drug Works:
Cefamandole nafate stops bacteria from making their protein cell wall, so the bacteria die. Cefamandole nafate is used to treat infections of the lungs, urinary tract, skin and soft tissue, and gall bladder, as well as infections of the blood (septicemia).

How Drug Is Given:
Cefamandole nafate is given as an injection in a vein over 15 to 30 minutes, or as an injection into the muscle. The dose depends upon the type of infection and whether you have any problems with your kidneys. The dose is given every 6 to 8 hours.

 Read the following information. If you do not understand it or if any of it causes you special concern, check with your doctor.

Before taking this drug, tell your doctor if you are taking any other prescription or over-the-counter drugs, including vitamins and herbals.

Should I avoid any other medicines, foods, alcohol, and/or activities?
Your prescription and nonprescription medicines may interact with other drugs, causing harm. Certain foods or alcohol can also interact with drug products. Never begin taking a new medicine—prescription or nonprescription—without asking your doctor or nurse if it will interact with alcohol, food, or other medicines. Some drugs can cause drowsiness and affect activities such as driving.

Precautions:
Tell your doctor if you have any drug allergies, especially to antibiotic drugs. All antibiotics can cause allergic reactions. Stop the drug and tell your doctor or nurse right away if you develop a rash, hives, red blotches on your skin, difficulty breathing, or chest tightness.

Use of antibiotics can change the normal organisms in your body. Women are at risk of getting fungal infections. Tell your nurse or doctor if you get vaginal itching or discharge.

Patients with kidney problems and patients with a history of colitis (bowel irritation and inflammation) should use this drug with caution.

Do not drink alcohol until 3 days after this drug is stopped. It can cause a dangerous drug interaction (flushing, throbbing headache, shortness of breath, nausea, vomiting, sweating, chest pain, increased blood pressure, increased heart rate, "black out," weakness, and blurred vision).

Tell all the doctors, dentists, and pharmacists you visit that you are taking this drug.
- Most of the following side effects probably will not occur.
- Your doctor or nurse will want to discuss specific care instructions with you.
- They can help you understand these side effects and help you deal with them.

Side Effects:

More Common Side Effects
Nausea
Vomiting
Diarrhea
Loss of appetite

Less Common Side Effects
Vaginal itching
Pain at place of injection
Hardening of vein used for giving drug
Vaginal candidiasis (fungal infection)

Rare Side Effects
Diarrhea related to infection of the intestinal membrane (psuedomembranous colitis)
Rash
Hives
Itching
Decreased white blood cell count with increased risk of infection
Decreased red blood cell count with increased risk of anemia and tiredness (fatigue)
Dizziness
Headache
Sleepiness

Side Effects / Symptoms of the Drug
Stop the drug and call your doctor or nurse right away if you develop a rash, fever, muscle aches, or blood in your urine. This can be a serious reaction and needs to be treated right away.

Stop the drug and call your doctor or nurse right away if you get diarrhea that does not stop, abdominal cramping, and blood and/or pus in the stool. This needs to be treated right away.

Other side effects not listed above can also occur in some patients.
Tell your doctor or nurse if you develop any problems.

FDA Approval: Yes

cefazolin sodium

Trade Names:
Ancel, Kefzol

Type of Drug:
Cefazolin sodium is an antibiotic that belongs to a group of drugs called cephalosporins.

How Drug Works:
Cefazolin sodium stops bacteria from making their protein cell wall, so the bacteria die. Cefazolin sodium is used to treat infections of the lungs, urinary tract, skin and soft tissue, gall bladder, and abdomen.

How Drug Is Given:
Cefazolin sodium is given as an injection in the vein over 30 minutes or as an injection in the muscle 2 to 4 times a day. The dose depends on the type of infection and how well your kidneys are working.

 Read the following information. If you do not understand it or if any of it causes you special concern, check with your doctor.

Before taking this drug, tell your doctor if you are taking any other prescription or over-the-counter drugs, including vitamins and herbals.

Should I avoid any other medicines, foods, alcohol, and/or activities?
Your prescription and nonprescription medicines may interact with other drugs, causing harm. Certain foods or alcohol can also interact with drug products. Never begin taking a new medicine—prescription or nonprescription—without asking your doctor or nurse if it will interact with alcohol, food, or other medicines. Some drugs can cause drowsiness and affect activities such as driving.

Precautions:
Tell your doctor if you have any allergies to antibiotics. All antibiotics can cause allergic reactions. Stop the drug and tell your doctor or nurse right away if you develop a rash, hives, red blotches on your skin, difficulty breathing, or chest pain.

Use of antibiotics can change the normal organisms in your body. Women are at risk of getting fungal infections. Tell your nurse or doctor if you get vaginal itching or discharge.

Patients with kidney problems or with history of colitis (colon inflammation) should use this drug with caution.

Tell all the doctors, dentists, and pharmacists you visit that you are taking this drug.
- Most of the following side effects probably will not occur.
- Your doctor or nurse will want to discuss specific care instructions with you.
- They can help you understand these side effects and help you deal with them.

Side Effects:

More Common Side Effects
Nausea
Vomiting
Diarrhea
Loss of appetite

Less Common Side Effects
Vaginal itching
Pain at place of injection
Hardening of vein used for giving the drug
Vaginal candidiasis (fungal infections)

Rare Side Effects
Diarrhea related to infection of the intestinal lining (pseudomembranous colitis)
Rash
Hives
Itching
Decreased white blood cell count with increased risk of infection
Decreased red blood cell count with increased risk of anemia and tiredness (fatigue)
Dizziness
Headache
Sleepiness
Fever, chills

Side Effects / Symptoms of the Drug
Stop the drug and call your doctor or nurse right away if you develop a rash, fever, muscle aches, or blood in your urine. This can be a serious reaction and needs to be treated right away.

Stop the drug and call your doctor or nurse right away if you get diarrhea that does not stop, abdominal cramping, and blood and/or pus in the stool. This needs to be treated right away.

Other side effects not listed above can also occur in some patients.
Tell your doctor or nurse if you develop any problems.

FDA Approval: Yes

cefdinir

Trade Name:
Omnicef

Type of Drug:
Cefdinir belongs to the general class of drugs called cephalosporin broad-spectrum antibiotics.

How Drug Works:
Cefdinir prevents bacteria from making their cell wall, causing the cell to die. Cefdinir is active against some bacteria that are resistant to penicillin medicines. Cefdinir is used to treat mild or moderate infections: community-acquired pneumonia, worsening bronchitis, sinusitis, pharyngitis, or tonsillitis.

How Drug Is Given:
Cefdinir is given by mouth with or without food in the morning and night for 10 days. Take the pill with a large glass of water, and preferably at the same time each day. The dose depends upon the type of infection and whether you have any problems with your kidneys. Keep the medicine in a tightly closed container and out of the reach of children and pets.

How Should I Take This Drug?
Take this drug exactly as directed by your doctor. If you do not understand the instructions, ask your doctor or nurse to explain them to you.

 Read the following information. If you do not understand it or if any of it causes you special concern, check with your doctor.

Before taking this drug, tell your doctor if you are taking any other prescription or over-the-counter drugs, including vitamins and herbals.

Should I avoid any other medicines, foods, alcohol, and/or activities?
Your prescription and nonprescription medicines may interact with other drugs, causing harm. Certain foods or alcohol can also interact with drug products. Never begin taking a new medicine—prescription or nonprescription—without asking your doctor or nurse if it will interact with alcohol, food, or other medicines. Some drugs can cause drowsiness and affect activities such as driving.

Precautions:
Tell your doctor if you have an allergy to penicillin or other antibiotics called cephalosporins. You should not take cefdinir if you have these allergies.

If you have any kidney problems, your doctor will reduce the amount of drug you receive.

If you are taking antacids that contain magnesium or aluminum, take cefdinir at least 2 hours before or after the antacid.

If you are taking iron or iron supplements, take cefdinir at least 2 hours before or after the iron.

Tell your doctor if you are taking probenecid, as the dose of cefdinir will need to be reduced.

If you use a clinitest to test your urine for sugar, cefdinir may cause a false positive. You should use Clinistix or Tes-tape.

Taking antibiotics can change the normal organisms in your body. Women are at risk for fungal infections. Tell your nurse or doctor if you get vaginal itching or discharge.

Tell all the doctors, dentists, and pharmacists you visit that you are taking this drug.

- Most of the following side effects probably will not occur.
- Your doctor or nurse will want to discuss specific care instructions with you.
- They can help you understand these side effects and help you deal with them.

Side Effects:

More Common Side Effects
Diarrhea

Less Common Side Effects
Nausea
Headache

Rare Side Effects
Abdominal discomfort
Decreased appetite
Heartburn
Constipation
Red colored stool if taking iron
Dizziness
Tiredness (fatigue)
Difficulty sleeping
Sleepiness
Rash
Vaginal itching
Diarrhea related to infection of the intestinal lining (pseudomembraneous colitis)

Side Effects / Symptoms of the Drug
If you develop diarrhea with stomach cramping or blood in your stool, call your doctor.

Stop the drug and call your doctor or nurse right away if you get a rash, hives, fever, flushing, chills, and swelling in the face.

Call your doctor or nurse if you develop vaginal itching or a white discharge. This may be a fungal infection that can be easily treated.

Other side effects not listed above can also occur in some patients.
Tell your doctor or nurse if you develop any problems.

FDA Approval: Yes

cefepime

Trade Name:
Maxipime

Type of Drug:
Cefepime is an antibiotic that belongs to the class of drugs called cephalosporins. Cefepime is used to treat gram-negative and gram-positive bacteria, especially those causing infections in the lungs, kidneys, bladder, skin, and abdomen. It is active against some bacteria that are resistant to other antibiotics.

How Drug Works:
Cefepime stops bacteria from making their cell wall, so the bacteria die. Enzymes in the bacteria are not able to break down cefepime so that resistance does not develop easily.

How Drug Is Given:
Cefepime is given by injection in a vein over 30 minutes, 2 to 3 times a day for 7 to 10 days. The dose depends on the type of infection and how well your kidneys are working. Cefepime can also be given by an injection in the muscle.

 Read the following information. If you do not understand it or if any of it causes you special concern, check with your doctor.

Before taking this drug, tell your doctor if you are taking any other prescription or over-the-counter drugs, including vitamins and herbals.

Should I avoid any other medicines, foods, alcohol, and/or activities?
Your prescription and nonprescription medicines may interact with other drugs, causing harm. Certain foods or alcohol can also interact with drug products. Never begin taking a new medicine—prescription or non-prescription—without asking your doctor or nurse if it will interact with alcohol, food, or other medicines. Some drugs can cause drowsiness and affect activities such as driving.

Precautions:
Tell your doctor if you are allergic to any drugs, especially to cephalosporins, penicillins, or other antibiotics.

All antibiotics can cause allergic reactions. Stop the drug and tell your doctor or nurse right away if you develop a rash, hives, fever and chills, red blotches on your skin, swelling of face or lips, or difficulty breathing.

If you use a clinitest to test your urine for sugar, cefepime may cause a false-positive. Clinistix or Testape will not be affected by cefepime.

Taking antibiotics can change the normal organisms in your body. Women are at risk for fungal infections. Tell your nurse or doctor if you develop vaginal itching or discharge.

Tell all the doctors, dentists, and pharmacists you visit that you are taking this drug.

- Most of the following side effects probably will not occur.
- Your doctor or nurse will want to discuss specific care instructions with you.
- They can help you understand these side effects and help you deal with them.

Side Effects:

More Common Side Effects
Nausea
Diarrhea

Less Common Side Effects
Vomiting
Constipation
Abdominal pain
Heartburn
Vaginal itching

Rare Side Effects
Diarrhea related to infection of the intestinal lining (pseudomembranous colitis)
Itching
Muscle aches
Swelling
Redness of skin
Allergic reaction with fever, chills, rash, hives, swelling of face or throat
Severe rash followed by peeling of the skin
Decreased white blood cell count with increased risk of infection
Decreased red blood cell count with increased risk of anemia and tiredness (fatigue)
Decreased clotting ability of the blood with risk of bleeding
Dizziness
Headache
Sleepiness

Side Effects / Symptoms of the Drug
Stop taking the drug and call your doctor or nurse if you develop a rash, fever, chills, or swelling in your face or throat.

Other side effects not listed above can also occur in some patients.
Tell your doctor or nurse if you develop any problems.

FDA Approval: Yes

cefixime

Trade Name:
Suprax

Type of Drug:
Cefixime is an antibiotic that belongs to a group of drugs called cephalosporins.

How Drug Works:
Cefixime stops bacteria from making their protein cell wall, so the bacteria die. Cefixime is used to treat gram-negative bacteria, especially those causing infections of the urinary tract. It is also used for certain streptococcal infections and the flu (influenza virus) related to bronchitis.

How Drug Is Given:
Cefixime is given by mouth once or twice a day (morning and night) with or without food. Take the pill with a large glass of water, and at the same time each day for 5 to 14 days as directed. The dose and number of days you take the medicine depends on the type of infection and how your kidneys are working. Keep the medicine in a tightly closed container and out of the reach of children and pets.

How Should I Take This Drug?
Take this drug exactly as directed by your doctor. If you do not understand the instructions, ask your doctor or nurse to explain them to you.

 Read the following information. If you do not understand it or if any of it causes you special concern, check with your doctor.

Before taking this drug, tell your doctor if you are taking any other prescription or over-the-counter drugs, including vitamins and herbals.

Should I avoid any other medicines, foods, alcohol, and/or activities?
Your prescription and nonprescription medicines may interact with other drugs, causing harm. Certain foods or alcohol can also interact with drug products. Never begin taking a new medicine—prescription or nonprescription—without asking your doctor or nurse if it will interact with alcohol, food, or other medicines. Some drugs can cause drowsiness and affect activities such as driving.

Precautions:
Tell your doctor if you have any drug allergies, especially to antibiotic drugs. All antibiotics can cause allergic reactions. Stop the drug and tell your doctor or nurse right away if you develop a rash, hives, red blotches on your skin, difficulty breathing, or chest pain.

Use of antibiotics can change the normal organisms in your body. Women are at risk of getting fungal infections. Tell your nurse or doctor if you get vaginal itching or discharge.

This drug should be used with caution in patients with kidney problems or with a history of colitis (colon inflammation).

Tell all the doctors, dentists, and pharmacists you visit that you are taking this drug.
- Most of the following side effects probably will not occur.
- Your doctor or nurse will want to discuss specific care instructions with you.
- They can help you understand these side effects and help you deal with them.

Side Effects:

More Common Side Effects
Nausea
Vomiting
Diarrhea
Loss of appetite

Less Common Side Effects
Vaginal itching
Vaginal candidiasis (fungal infection)

Rare Side Effects
Diarrhea related to infection of the intestinal lining (pseudomembranous colitis)
Rash
Hives
Itching
Decreased white blood cell count with increased risk of infection
Fever, chills
Decreased red blood cell count with increased risk of anemia and tiredness (fatigue)
Dizziness
Headache
Sleepiness

Side Effects / Symptoms of the Drug
Stop the drug and call your doctor or nurse right away if you develop a rash, fever, muscle aches, or blood in your urine. This can be a serious reaction and needs to be treated right away.

Stop the drug and call your doctor or nurse right away if you get diarrhea that does not stop, abdominal cramping, and blood and/or pus in the stool. This needs to be treated right away.

Other side effects not listed above can also occur in some patients.
Tell your doctor or nurse if you develop any problems.

FDA Approval: Yes

cefoperazone sodium

Trade Name:
Cefobid

Type of Drug:
Cefoperazone sodium is an antibiotic that belongs to a group of drugs called cephalosporins.

How Drug Works:
Cefoperazone sodium stops bacteria from making their cell wall, so the bacteria die. Cefoperazone sodium is used to treat infections of the lungs, kidneys, bladder, skin and soft tissues, and infections in the blood (septicemia).

How Drug Is Given:
Cefoperazone sodium is given by an injection in the vein over 30 minutes, 2 to 4 times a day. Cefoperazone sodium can also be given by an injection into a muscle. The dose depends upon the type of infection and how well your kidneys are working.

 Read the following information. If you do not understand it or if any of it causes you special concern, check with your doctor.

Before taking this drug, tell your doctor if you are taking any other prescription or over-the-counter drugs, including vitamins and herbals.

Should I avoid any other medicines, foods, alcohol, and/or activities?
Your prescription and nonprescription medicines may interact with other drugs, causing harm. Certain foods or alcohol can also interact with drug products. Never begin taking a new medicine—prescription or non-prescription—without asking your doctor or nurse if it will interact with alcohol, food, or other medicines. Some drugs can cause drowsiness and affect activities such as driving.

Precautions:
If you have had an allergic reaction to other antibiotics, such as cephalosporins or penicillin, talk with your doctor before taking this medicine.

All antibiotics can cause allergic reactions. Stop the drug and tell your doctor or nurse right away if you develop a rash, fever and chills, swelling of your face or throat, hives, red blotches on your skin, or difficulty breathing.

Use of antibiotics can change the normal organisms in your body. Women are at risk of getting fungal infections. Tell your doctor or nurse right away if you get vaginal itching or discharge.

Cefoperazone sodium can prolong blood clotting. Talk to your doctor before taking this drug if you are also taking blood thinning medicines such as Coumadin or warfarin.

The drug dose must be reduced if you have kidney failure.

Tell all the doctors, dentists, and pharmacists you visit that you are taking this drug.
- Most of the following side effects probably will not occur.
- Your doctor or nurse will want to discuss specific care instructions with you.
- They can help you understand these side effects and help you deal with them.

Side Effects:

More Common Side Effects
Diarrhea
Loss of appetite

Less Common Side Effects
Vaginal itching
Vaginal candidiasis (fungal infection)

Rare Side Effects
Diarrhea related to infection of the intestinal lining (pseudomembranous colitis)
Severe allergic reaction with rash, hives, fever and chills, swelling of face and lips, and difficulty
    breathing
Itching
Prolonged bleeding time
Pain at injection site

Side Effects / Symptoms of the Drug
Stop the drug and call your doctor or nurse right away if you develop a rash, hives, fever and chills,
swelling of face and lips, or difficulty breathing.

Other side effects not listed above can also occur in some patients.
Tell your doctor or nurse if you develop any problems.

FDA Approval: Yes

cefotaxime sodium

Trade Name:
Claforan

Type of Drug:
Cefotaxime sodium is an antibiotic that belongs to a group of drugs called cephalosporins.

How Drug Works:
Cefotaxime sodium stops bacteria from making their cell wall, so the bacteria die. Cefotaxime sodium is used to treat serious lower respiratory tract and urinary tract infections, gynecologic infections, and infections of the blood, skin, and central nervous system.

How Drug Is Given:
Cefotaxime sodium is given by an injection in the vein over 30 minutes, 3 times a day. Cefotaxime sodium can also be given by an injection into a muscle. The dose depends upon the type of infection and how well your kidneys are working.

 Read the following information. If you do not understand it or if any of it causes you special concern, check with your doctor.

Before taking this drug, tell your doctor if you are taking any other prescription or over-the-counter drugs, including vitamins and herbals.

Should I avoid any other medicines, foods, alcohol, and/or activities?
Your prescription and nonprescription medicines may interact with other drugs, causing harm. Certain foods or alcohol can also interact with drug products. Never begin taking a new medicine—prescription or non-prescription—without asking your doctor or nurse if it will interact with alcohol, food, or other medicines. Some drugs can cause drowsiness and affect activities such as driving.

Precautions:
Tell your doctor if you have any drug allergies, especially to antibiotic drugs. All antibiotics can cause allergic reactions. Stop the drug and tell your doctor or nurse right away if you develop a rash, hives, red blotches on your skin, difficulty breathing, or chest pain.

Use of antibiotics can change the normal organisms in your body. Women are at risk of getting fungal infections. Tell your nurse or doctor if you get vaginal itching or discharge.

This drug should be used with caution in patients with kidney problems or with a history of colitis (colon inflammation).

Tell all the doctors, dentists, and pharmacists you visit that you are taking this drug.
- Most of the following side effects probably will not occur.
- Your doctor or nurse will want to discuss specific care instructions with you.
- They can help you understand these side effects and help you deal with them.

Side Effects:

More Common Side Effects
Nausea
Vomiting
Diarrhea
Loss of appetite

Less Common Side Effects
Vaginal itching
Pain at place of injection
Hardening of vein used for giving the drug
Vaginal candidiasis (fungal infection)

Rare Side Effects
Diarrhea related to infection of the intestinal lining (pseudomembranous colitis)
Rash
Hives
Itching
Decreased white blood cell count with increased risk of infection
Fever, chills
Decreased red blood cell count with increased risk of anemia and tiredness (fatigue)
Dizziness
Headache
Sleepiness

Side Effects / Symptoms of the Drug
Stop the drug and call your doctor or nurse right away if you develop a rash, fever, muscle aches, or blood in your urine. This can be a serious reaction and needs to be treated right away.

Stop the drug and call your doctor or nurse right away if you get diarrhea that does not stop, abdominal cramping, and blood and/or pus in the stool. This needs to be treated right away.

Other side effects not listed above can also occur in some patients.
Tell your doctor or nurse if you develop any problems.

FDA Approval: Yes

cefoxitin sodium

Trade Name:
Mefoxin

Type of Drug:
Cefoxitin sodium is an antibiotic that belongs to a group of drugs called cephalosporins.

How Drug Works:
Cefoxitin sodium stops bacteria from making their cell wall, so the bacteria die. Cefoxitin sodium is used to treat sensitive gram-negative infections and some gram-positive infections.

How Drug Is Given:
Cefoxitin sodium is given by an injection in the vein over 30 minutes, 2 to 4 times a day. Cefoxitin sodium can also be given by an injection into muscle. The dose depends upon the type of infection and how well your kidneys are working.

 Read the following information. If you do not understand it or if any of it causes you special concern, check with your doctor.

Before taking this drug, tell your doctor if you are taking any other prescription or over-the-counter drugs, including vitamins and herbals.

Should I avoid any other medicines, foods, alcohol, and/or activities?
Your prescription and nonprescription medicines may interact with other drugs, causing harm. Certain foods or alcohol can also interact with drug products. Never begin taking a new medicine—prescription or non-prescription—without asking your doctor or nurse if it will interact with alcohol, food, or other medicines. Some drugs can cause drowsiness and affect activities such as driving.

Precautions:
Tell your doctor if you have any drug allergies, especially to antibiotic drugs. All antibiotics can cause allergic reactions. Stop the drug and tell your doctor or nurse right away if you develop a rash, hives, red blotches on your skin, difficulty breathing, or chest pain.

Use of antibiotics can change the normal organisms in your body. Women are at risk of getting fungal infections. Tell your nurse or doctor if you get vaginal itching or discharge.

This drug should be used with caution in patients with kidney problems or a history of colitis (colon inflammation).

DO NOT drink alcohol until 3 days after this drug is stopped. It can have a dangerous drug interaction (flushing, throbbing headache, shortness of breath, nausea, vomiting, sweating, chest pain, increased blood pressure, increased heart rate, "black out," weakness, and blurred vision).

Tell all the doctors, dentists, and pharmacists you visit that you are taking this drug.

- Most of the following side effects probably will not occur.
- Your doctor or nurse will want to discuss specific care instructions with you.
- They can help you understand these side effects and help you deal with them.

Side Effects:

More Common Side Effects
Nausea
Vomiting
Diarrhea
Loss of appetite

Less Common Side Effects
Vaginal itching
Pain at place of injection
Hardening of vein used for giving the drug
Vaginal candidiasis (fungal infection)

Rare Side Effects
Diarrhea related to infection of the intestinal lining (pseudomembranous colitis)
Rash
Hives
Itching
Decreased white blood cell count with increased risk of infection
Decreased red blood cell count with increased risk of anemia and tiredness (fatigue)
Dizziness
Headache
Sleepiness
Prolonged bleeding time

Side Effects / Symptoms of the Drug
Stop the drug and call your doctor or nurse right away if you develop a rash, fever, muscle aches, or blood in your urine. This can be a serious reaction and needs to be treated right away.

Stop the drug and call your doctor or nurse right away if you get diarrhea that does not stop, abdominal cramping, and blood and/or pus in the stool. This needs to be treated right away.

Other side effects not listed above can also occur in some patients.
Tell your doctor or nurse if you develop any problems.

FDA Approval: Yes

cefpodoxime proxetin

Trade Name:
Vantin

Type of Drug:
Cefpodoxime proxetin is an antibiotic that belongs to a group of drugs called cephalosporins.

How Drug Works:
Cefpodoxime proxetin stops bacteria from making their cell wall, so the bacteria die. Cefpodoxime proxetin is used to treat infections of the lungs, kidneys, bladder, skin and soft tissues, and infections in the blood (septicemia).

How Drug Is Given:
Cefpodoxime proxetin is given by mouth as a pill or liquid usually twice a day (morning and night) with food. Take the pill with a large glass of water and preferably at the same time each day for 5 to 14 days as directed. Swallow the pill whole and do not crush it. Shake the liquid well before pouring the dose. The dose and number of days you take the medicine depends on the type of infection and how well your kidneys are working. Keep the medicine in a tightly closed container away from heat and moisture and out of the reach of children and pets.

How Should I Take This Drug?
Take this drug exactly as directed by your doctor. If you do not understand the instructions, ask your doctor or nurse to explain them to you.

 Read the following information. If you do not understand it or if any of it causes you special concern, check with your doctor.

Before taking this drug, tell your doctor if you are taking any other prescription or over-the-counter drugs, including vitamins and herbals.

Should I avoid any other medicines, foods, alcohol, and/or activities?
Your prescription and nonprescription medicines may interact with other drugs, causing harm. Certain foods or alcohol can also interact with drug products. Never begin taking a new medicine—prescription or nonprescription—without asking your doctor or nurse if it will interact with alcohol, food, or other medicines. Some drugs can cause drowsiness and affect activities such as driving.

Precautions:
Tell your doctor if you have any allergies to antibiotics. All antibiotics can cause allergic reactions. Stop the drug and tell your doctor or nurse right away if you develop a rash, fever and chills, swelling of your face or throat, hives, red blotches on your skin, or difficulty breathing.

Use of antibiotics can change the normal organisms in your body. Women are at risk of getting fungal infections. Tell your doctor or nurse right away if you get vaginal itching or discharge.

Tell all the doctors, dentists, and pharmacists you visit that you are taking this drug.

- Most of the following side effects probably will not occur.
- Your doctor or nurse will want to discuss specific care instructions with you.
- They can help you understand these side effects and help you deal with them.

Side Effects:

More Common Side Effects
Nausea
Vomiting
Diarrhea
Loss of appetite

Less Common Side Effects
Vaginal itching
Vaginal candidiasis (fungal infection)

Rare Side Effects
Diarrhea related to infection of the intestinal lining (pseudomembranous colitis)
Severe allergic reaction with rash, hives, fever and chills, difficulty breathing, or swelling of face and lips
Itching

Side Effects / Symptoms of the Drug
Stop the drug and call your doctor or nurse right away if you develop a rash, hives, fever and chills, difficulty breathing, or swelling in your face. This can be a serious reaction and needs to be treated right away.

Stop the drug and call your doctor or nurse right away if you get diarrhea that does not stop, abdominal cramping, and blood and/or pus in the stool. This needs to be treated right away.

Other side effects not listed above can also occur in some patients.
Tell your doctor or nurse if you develop any problems.

FDA Approval: Yes

cefprozil

Trade Name:
Cefzil

Type of Drug:
Cefprozil is an antibiotic that belongs to a group of drugs called cephalosporins.

How Drug Works:
Cefprozil stops bacteria from making their cell wall, so the bacteria die. Cefprozil is used to treat infections of the lungs, kidneys, bladder, skin and soft tissues, and infections in the blood (septicemia).

How Drug Is Given:
Cefprozil is given by mouth as a pill or liquid usually once or twice a day with or without food. Take the pill or liquid with a large glass of water, preferably at the same time each day for 7 to 14 days as directed. Swallow the pill whole; do not crush it. Shake the liquid well before pouring the dose. The dose and number of days you take the medicine depend on the type of infection and how well your kidneys are working. Keep the medicine in a tightly closed container away from heat and moisture and out of the reach of children and pets.

How Should I Take This Drug?
Take this drug exactly as directed by your doctor. If you do not understand the instructions, ask your doctor or nurse to explain them to you.

 Read the following information. If you do not understand it or if any of it causes you special concern, check with your doctor.

Before taking this drug, tell your doctor if you are taking any other prescription or over-the-counter drugs, including vitamins and herbals.

Should I avoid any other medicines, foods, alcohol, and/or activities?
Your prescription and nonprescription medicines may interact with other drugs, causing harm. Certain foods or alcohol can also interact with drug products. Never begin taking a new medicine—prescription or nonprescription—without asking your doctor or nurse if it will interact with alcohol, food, or other medicines. Some drugs can cause drowsiness and affect activities such as driving.

Precautions:
If you have had an allergic reaction to an antibiotic before, be sure to tell your doctor or nurse. All antibiotics can cause allergic reactions. Stop the drug and tell your doctor or nurse right away if you develop a rash, hives, fever and chills, red blotches on your skin, or difficulty breathing.

Use of antibiotics can change the normal organisms in your body. Women are at risk of getting fungal infections. Tell your doctor or nurse right away if you have vaginal itching or discharge.

This drug should be used with caution in patients with kidney problems.

Tell all the doctors, dentists, and pharmacists you visit that you are taking this drug.

- Most of the following side effects probably will not occur.
- Your doctor or nurse will want to discuss specific care instructions with you.
- They can help you understand these side effects and help you deal with them.

Side Effects:

More Common Side Effects
Nausea
Vomiting
Diarrhea
Loss of Appetite

Less Common Side Effects
Vaginal itching
Vaginal candidiasis (fungal infection)

Rare Side Effects
Diarrhea related to infection of the intestinal lining (pseudomembranous colitis)
Itching
Allergic reaction with fever and chills, rash, hives, difficulty breathing, and swelling of face or lips
Muscle aches

Side Effects / Symptoms of the Drug
Stop the drug and call your doctor or nurse right away if you develop a rash, fever, hives, difficulty breathing, or swelling of face or lips. This can be a serious reaction and needs to be treated right away.

Stop the drug and call your doctor or nurse right away if you get diarrhea that does not stop, abdominal cramping, and blood and/or pus in the stool. This needs to be treated right away.

Other side effects not listed above can also occur in some patients.
Tell your doctor or nurse if you develop any problems.

FDA Approval: Yes

ceftazidime

Trade Names:
Fortaz, Tazicef, Tazidime

Type of Drug:
Ceftazidime is an antibiotic that belongs to the group of drugs called cephalosporins.

How Drug Works:
Ceftazidime stops bacteria from making their cell wall, so the bacteria die. Ceftazidime is used to treat bacterial infections of the lower respiratory tract, urinary tract, skin, bone and joint, pelvis, and abdomen.

How Drug Is Given:
Ceftazidime is given by an injection in the vein over 30 minutes, 2 or 3 times a day. Ceftazidime can also be given by an injection into a muscle. The dose depends upon the type of infection and how well your kidneys are working.

 Read the following information. If you do not understand it or if any of it causes you special concern, check with your doctor.

Before taking this drug, tell your doctor if you are taking any other prescription or over-the-counter drugs, including vitamins and herbals.

Should I avoid any other medicines, foods, alcohol, and/or activities?
Your prescription and nonprescription medicines may interact with other drugs, causing harm. Certain foods or alcohol can also interact with drug products. Never begin taking a new medicine—prescription or nonprescription—without asking your doctor or nurse if it will interact with alcohol, food, or other medicines. Some drugs can cause drowsiness and affect activities such as driving.

Precautions:
Tell your doctor if you have any drug allergies, especially to antibiotic drugs. All antibiotics can cause allergic reactions. Stop the drug and tell your doctor or nurse right away if you develop a rash, hives, red blotches on your skin, difficulty breathing, or chest pain.

Use of antibiotics can change the normal organisms in your body. Women are at risk of getting fungal infections. Tell your nurse or doctor if you get vaginal itching or discharge.

This drug should be used with caution in patients with kidney problems or a history of colitis (colon inflammation).

Tell all the doctors, dentists, and pharmacists you visit that you are taking this drug.
- -
- Most of the following side effects probably will not occur.
- Your doctor or nurse will want to discuss specific care instructions with you.
- They can help you understand these side effects and help you deal with them.

Side Effects:

More Common Side Effects
Nausea
Vomiting
Diarrhea
Loss of appetite

Less Common Side Effects
Vaginal itching
Pain at place of injection
Hardening of vein used for giving the drug
Vaginal candidiasis (fungal infection)

Rare Side Effects
Diarrhea related to infection of the intestinal lining (psuedomembranous colitis)
Rash
Hives
Itching
Decreased white blood cell count with increased risk of infection
Fever, chills
Decreased red blood cell count with increased risk of anemia and tiredness (fatigue)
Dizziness
Headache
Sleepiness
Prolonged bleeding time

Side Effects / Symptoms of the Drug
Stop the drug and call your doctor or nurse right away if you develop a rash, fever, muscle aches, or blood in your urine. This can be a serious reaction and needs to be treated right away.

Stop the drug and call your doctor or nurse right away if you get diarrhea that does not stop, abdominal cramping, and blood and/or pus in the stool. This needs to be treated right away.

Other side effects not listed above can also occur in some patients.
Tell your doctor or nurse if you develop any problems.

FDA Approval: Yes

ceftibuten

Trade Name:
Cedax

Type of Drug:
Ceftibuten is an antibiotic that belongs to a group of drugs called cephalosporins.

How Drug Works:
Ceftibuten stops bacteria from making their cell wall, so the bacteria die. Ceftibuten is used to treat infections of the lungs, kidneys, bladder, skin and soft tissues, and infections in the blood (septicemia).

How Drug Is Given:
Ceftibuten is given by mouth as a pill or liquid once a day without food. Take the pill or liquid with a large glass of water, 1 hour before or 2 hours after a meal. Swallow the pill whole and do not crush it. Shake the liquid well before pouring the dose. Try to take the medicine at the same time each day for 10 days as directed. The dose is the same for all adults but is lower if your kidneys are not working well. Keep the medicine in a tightly closed container away from heat and moisture and out of the reach of children and pets.

How Should I Take This Drug?
Take this drug exactly as directed by your doctor. If you do not understand the instructions, ask your doctor or nurse to explain them to you.

 Read the following information. If you do not understand it or if any of it causes you special concern, check with your doctor.

Before taking this drug, tell your doctor if you are taking any other prescription or over-the-counter drugs, including vitamins and herbals.

Should I avoid any other medicines, foods, alcohol, and/or activities?
Your prescription and nonprescription medicines may interact with other drugs, causing harm. Certain foods or alcohol can also interact with drug products. Never begin taking a new medicine—prescription or nonprescription—without asking your doctor or nurse if it will interact with alcohol, food, or other medicines. Some drugs can cause drowsiness and affect activities such as driving.

Precautions:
Tell your doctor if you have any allergies to antibiotics. All antibiotics can cause allergic reactions. Stop the drug and tell your doctor or nurse right away if you develop a rash, fever and chills, swelling of your face or throat, hives, red blotches on your skin, or difficulty breathing.

Use of antibiotics can change the normal organisms of your body. Women are at risk of getting fungal infections. Tell your doctor or nurse right away if you get vaginal itching or discharge.

Tell all the doctors, dentists, and pharmacists you visit that you are taking this drug.

- Most of the following side effects probably will not occur.
- Your doctor or nurse will want to discuss specific care instructions with you.
- They can help you understand these side effects and help you deal with them.

Side Effects:

More Common Side Effects
Nausea
Vomiting
Diarrhea
Loss of appetite

Less Common Side Effects
Vaginal itching
Vaginal candidiasis (fungal infection)

Rare Side Effects
Diarrhea related to infection of the intestinal lining (pseudomembranous colitis)
Itching
Severe allergic reaction with fever and chills, rash, hives, difficulty breathing, or swelling of face
   and lips

Side Effects / Symptoms of the Drug
Stop the drug and call your doctor or nurse right away if you develop a rash, fever, hives, difficulty breathing, or swelling of face or lips. This can be a serious reaction and needs to be treated right away.

Stop the drug and call your doctor or nurse right away if you get diarrhea that does not stop, abdominal cramping, and blood and/or pus in the stool. This needs to be treated right away.

Other side effects not listed above can also occur in some patients.
Tell your doctor or nurse if you develop any problems.

FDA Approval: Yes

ceftriaxone sodium

Trade Name:
Rocephin

Type of Drug:
Ceftriaxone sodium is an antibiotic that belongs to a group of drugs called cephalosporins.

How Drug Works:
Ceftriaxone sodium stops bacteria from making their cell wall, so the bacteria die. Ceftriaxone sodium is used to treat bacterial infections of the lower respiratory tract, urinary tract, skin, bone and joint, pelvis, and abdomen.

How Drug Is Given:
Ceftriaxone sodium is given by an injection in the vein over 30 minutes, once or twice a day, for 4 to 14 days as directed. Ceftriaxone sodium can also be given by an injection into muscle. The dose and number of doses depends upon the type of infection.

 Read the following information. If you do not understand it or if any of it causes you special concern, check with your doctor.

Before taking this drug, tell your doctor if you are taking any other prescription or over-the-counter drugs, including vitamins and herbals.

Should I avoid any other medicines, foods, alcohol, and/or activities?
Your prescription and nonprescription medicines may interact with other drugs, causing harm. Certain foods or alcohol can also interact with drug products. Never begin taking a new medicine—prescription or non-prescription—without asking your doctor or nurse if it will interact with alcohol, food, or other medicines. Some drugs can cause drowsiness and affect activities such as driving.

Precautions:
Tell your doctor if you have allergies to any antibiotics. All antibiotics can cause allergic reactions. Stop the drug and tell your doctor or nurse right away if you develop a rash, hives, red blotches on your skin, difficulty breathing, or chest pain.

Use of antibiotics can change the normal organisms in your body. Women are at risk of getting fungal infections. Tell your nurse or doctor if you get vaginal itching or discharge.

This drug should be used with caution in patients with a history of colitis (colon inflammation).

Tell all the doctors, dentists, and pharmacists you visit that you are taking this drug.
- Most of the following side effects probably will not occur.
- Your doctor or nurse will want to discuss specific care instructions with you.
- They can help you understand these side effects and help you deal with them.

Side Effects:

More Common Side Effects
Nausea
Vomiting
Diarrhea
Loss of appetite

Less Common Side Effects
Vaginal itching
Pain at place of injection
Hardening of vein used for giving the drug
Vaginal candidiasis (fungal infection)

Rare Side Effects
Diarrhea related to infection of the intestinal lining (pseudomembranous colitis)
Rash
Hives
Itching
Decreased white blood cell count with increased risk of infection
Fever, chills
Decreased red blood cell count with increased risk of anemia and tiredness (fatigue)
Dizziness
Headache
Sleepiness
Prolonged bleeding time

Side Effects / Symptoms of the Drug
Stop the drug and call your doctor or nurse right away if you develop a rash, fever, muscle aches, or blood in your urine. This can be a serious reaction and needs to be treated right away.

Stop the drug and call your doctor or nurse right away if you get diarrhea that does not stop, abdominal cramping, and blood and/or pus in the stool. This needs to be treated right away.

Other side effects not listed above can also occur in some patients.
Tell your doctor or nurse if you develop any problems.

FDA Approval: Yes

celecoxib

Trade Name:
Celebrex

Type of Drug:
Celecoxib is a nonopioid analgesic that belongs to the general class of drugs called nonsteroidal anti-inflammatory drugs (NSAIDs).

How Drug Works:
Celecoxib blocks prostaglandins (natural substances in the body that cause pain) from being produced. This prevents pain receptors from passing the pain message to the brain so that the perception of pain is decreased. It also reduces inflammation and reduces fever. Celecoxib also has been shown to reduce the number of polyps in the colon in people with a family history of familial adenomatous polyposis (FAP). Often these polyps can become cancerous. Celecoxib is used to treat osteoarthritis, rheumatoid arthritis, and to prevent colon polyps in families with a history of FAP.

How Drug Is Given:
Celecoxib is taken by mouth 1 to 2 times a day as directed by your doctor. It can be taken with or without food. If it causes any stomach irritation, try taking the capsule with food. Take the capsule whole with a glass of water, and do not open it. The dose depends on the reason you are taking the medicine, and the number of capsules that you take depends on the amount of medicine in each capsule. Keep the medicine in a tightly closed container away from heat and moisture and out of the reach of children and pets.

How Should I Take This Drug?
Take this drug exactly as directed by your doctor. If you do not understand the instructions, ask your doctor or nurse to explain them to you.

 Read the following information. If you do not understand it or if any of it causes you special concern, check with your doctor.

Precautions:
Tell your doctor if you have liver or kidney problems. Your dose may need to be decreased.

Drug or blood-clotting levels may need to be checked more frequently if you are also taking Coumadin, a blood-thinning medicine, or lithium.

Do not take this drug if you are pregnant or breastfeeding.

Celecoxib may decrease the effect of your diuretic if you are taking Lasix or a thiazide diuretic; it may also decrease the blood pressure–lowering effect of angiotensin-converting enzyme (ACE) inhibitors such as lisinopril. Doses of these drugs may need to be increased while taking celecoxib. Talk to your doctor about this.

Bleeding of the gastrointestinal tract occurs rarely, especially in people who smoke, drink alcohol, take aspirin or steroid pills, take pills such as Coumadin to stop blood from clotting, or have taken nonsteroidal pills for a long time.

Tell all the doctors, dentists, and pharmacists you visit that you are taking this drug.

- Most of the following side effects probably will not occur.
- Your doctor or nurse will want to discuss specific care instructions with you.
- They can help you understand these side effects and help you deal with them.

Side Effects:

More Common Side Effects
Headache
Increase in blood liver function values

Less Common Side Effects
Fluid weight gain
Heartburn
Diarrhea
Abdominal pain

Rare Side Effects
Diverticulitis
Burping
Dry mouth
Vomiting
Rupture of stomach or duodenal ulcers
Bleeding in the esophagus, stomach, or intestines
Difficulty sleeping
Dizziness
Urinary tract infections
Decreased kidney function
Severe allergic reaction with hives, itching, rash, and difficulty breathing
Kidney failure

Side Effects / Symptoms of the Drug
Stop the drug and call your doctor or nurse right away if you get gnawing or burning stomach pain, black or tarry stools, or vomiting.

Report unexplained weight gain or swelling of the feet (edema).

Stop the drug and report signs and symptoms of liver failure right away: nausea; increased fatigue; feeling sleepy or drowsy; itching; flu-like symptoms of fever, headache, malaise (generally not feeling well); jaundice or yellowing of the skin and whites of the eyes; and pain in the right upper part of the abdomen.

Stop the drug and call your doctor or nurse right away if you get hives, or itching of the skin; call an ambulance to go to the emergency room if you have difficulty breathing.

Other side effects not listed above can also occur in some patients.
Tell your doctor or nurse if you develop any problems.

FDA Approval: Yes

cephradine

Trade Names:
Anspor, Velosef

Type of Drug:
Cephradine is an antibiotic that belongs to a group of drugs called cephalosporins.

How Drug Works:
Cephradine stops bacteria from making their cell wall, so the bacteria die. Cephradine is used to treat bacterial infections of the respiratory tract, urinary tract, skin, and bone and joint, blood, and in treating meningitis.

How Drug Is Given:
Cephradine is given as an injection in the vein over 30 minutes 4 to 6 times a day. It can also be given as an injection into the muscle. The dose and number of days you take the medicine depends on the type of infection and how well your kidneys are working.

 Read the following information. If you do not understand it or if any of it causes you special concern, check with your doctor.

Before taking this drug, tell your doctor if you are taking any other prescription or over-the-counter drugs, including vitamins and herbals.

Should I avoid any other medicines, foods, alcohol, and/or activities?
Your prescription and nonprescription medicines may interact with other drugs, causing harm. Certain foods or alcohol can also interact with drug products. Never begin taking a new medicine—prescription or nonprescription—without asking your doctor or nurse if it will interact with alcohol, food, or other medicines. Some drugs can cause drowsiness and affect activities such as driving.

Precautions:
Tell your doctor if you have allergies to any antibiotics. All antibiotics can cause allergic reactions. Stop the drug and tell your doctor or nurse right away if you develop a rash, hives, red blotches on your skin, difficulty breathing, or chest pain.

Use of antibiotics can change the normal organisms in your body. Women are at risk of getting fungal infections. Tell your nurse or doctor if you get vaginal itching or discharge.

Patients with kidney problems or with a history of colitis (colon inflammation) should use this drug with caution.

Tell all the doctors, dentists, and pharmacists you visit that you are taking this drug.

- Most of the following side effects probably will not occur.
- Your doctor or nurse will want to discuss specific care instructions with you.
- They can help you understand these side effects and help you deal with them.

Side Effects:

More Common Side Effects
Nausea
Vomiting
Diarrhea
Loss of appetite

Less Common Side Effects
Vaginal itching
Pain at place of injection
Hardening of vein used for giving the drug
Vaginal candidiasis (fungal infection)

Rare Side Effects
Diarrhea related to infection of the intestinal lining (pseudomembranous colitis)
Rash
Hives
Itching
Decreased white blood cell count with increased risk of infection
Decreased red blood cell count with increased risk of anemia and tiredness (fatigue)
Dizziness
Headache
Sleepiness
Prolonged bleeding time

Side Effects / Symptoms of the Drug
Stop the drug and call your doctor or nurse right away if you develop a rash, fever, muscle aches, or blood in your urine. This can be a serious reaction and needs to be treated right away.

Stop the drug and call your doctor or nurse right away if you get diarrhea that does not stop, abdominal cramping, and blood and/or pus in the stool. This needs to be treated right away.

Other side effects not listed above can also occur in some patients.
Tell your doctor or nurse if you develop any problems.

FDA Approval: Yes

choline magnesium trisalicylate

Trade Name:
Trilisate

Type of Drug:
Choline magnesium trisalicylate is a nonopioid analgesic that belongs to a general class of drugs called salicylates, which fall within a larger category called nonsteroidal anti-inflammatory drugs (NSAIDs).

How Drug Works:
Choline magnesium trisalicylate blocks the synthesis of prostaglandins. This prevents pain receptors from passing the pain message to the brain so that pain perception is decreased. Choline magnesium trisalicylate is also an anti-inflammatory drug that relieves pain and reduces fever.

How Drug Is Given:
Choline magnesium trisalicylate is taken by mouth with food or milk 3 times a day as needed. If you are taking an antacid, take the choline magnesium trisalicylate at least 1 hour before or 2 hours after your antacid. Usually the first time you try the medicine, you start with the lowest dose and increase it if needed. Keep the medicine in a tightly closed container away from heat and moisture and out of the reach of children and pets.

How Should I Take This Drug?
Take this drug exactly as directed by your doctor. If you do not understand the instructions, ask your doctor or nurse to explain them to you.

 Read the following information. If you do not understand it or if any of it causes you special concern, check with your doctor.

Before taking this drug, tell your doctor if you are taking any other prescription or over-the-counter drugs, including vitamins and herbals.

Should I avoid any other medicines, foods, alcohol, and/or activities?
Your prescription and nonprescription medicines may interact with other drugs, causing harm. Certain foods or alcohol can also interact with drug products. Never begin taking a new medicine—prescription or nonprescription—without asking your doctor or nurse if it will interact with alcohol, food, or other medicines. Some drugs can cause drowsiness and affect activities such as driving.

Precautions:
Tell your doctor if you are allergic to aspirin. Choline magnesium trisalicylate is similar to aspirin.

If you take too much choline magnesium trisalicylate, you can have dizziness, ringing in the ears (tinnitus), decreased hearing, nausea, vomiting, diarrhea, mental confusion, headache, sweating, fast breathing, and sleepiness or drowsiness. Be careful not to take more than the recommended dosages.

If you have stomach irritation (gastritis) or chronic renal failure (kidney damage), talk to your doctor before taking this drug.

Choline magnesium trisalicylate can make peptic ulcer disease worse.

Tell all the doctors, dentists, and pharmacists you visit that you are taking this drug.

- Most of the following side effects probably will not occur.
- Your doctor or nurse will want to discuss specific care instructions with you.
- They can help you understand these side effects and help you deal with them.

Side Effects:

Less Common Side Effects
Flushing
Dizziness
Decreased hearing
Ringing in the ears (tinnitus)

Rare Side Effects
Nausea
Vomiting
Diarrhea
Mental confusion
Headache
Increased rate of breathing
Heartburn
Loss of appetite
Liver damage (reversible)
Increase in blood kidney values

Other side effects not listed above can also occur in some patients.
Tell your doctor or nurse if you develop any problems.

FDA Approval: Yes

cidofovir

Trade Name:
Vistide

Type of Drug:
Cidofovir belongs to the general class of drugs called antivirals.

How Drug Works:
Cidofovir stops cytomegalovirus (CMV) growth and prevents the virus from reproducing.

How Drug Is Given:
Cidofovir is given by an injection into the vein over 1 hour. The treatment is given weekly for 2 weeks, then every other week. You will be given another medicine called probenecid to take with each dose of cidofovir. This helps to ensure you get the most out of the medicine. The dose depends upon your weight and the reason you are getting the medicine. Usually, the dose the first 2 weeks is higher than the weeks after. You may also get fluids given into the vein, as well as medicine to stop any nausea and vomiting. You should drink 1 to 2 quarts of fluid the night before the treatment, and 2 to 3 quarts the day after getting the medicine. It is very important to talk to your doctor or nurse if you have any problems during or after the treatments.

 Read the following information. If you do not understand it or if any of it causes you special concern, check with your doctor.

Before taking this drug, tell your doctor if you are taking any other prescription or over-the-counter drugs, including vitamins and herbals.

Should I avoid any other medicines, foods, alcohol, and/or activities?
Your prescription and nonprescription medicines may interact with other drugs, causing harm. Certain foods or alcohol can also interact with drug products. Never begin taking a new medicine—prescription or nonprescription—without asking your doctor or nurse if it will interact with alcohol, food, or other medicines. Some drugs can cause drowsiness and affect activities such as driving.

Precautions:
Cidofovir can lower your white blood cell count, which can increase your risk of getting an infection. Report fever of 100.5°F or higher, or signs of infection such as pain in passing your urine, or coughing and bringing up sputum.

Cidofovir can cause nausea and vomiting. Ask your doctor or nurse to give you medicines to prevent this or lessen it.

You will be given the drug probenecid before getting the cidofovir and at the end of the infusion for 2 doses. You will also get intravenous fluids with salt water to protect your kidneys. Your doctor will monitor your kidney function before and after each treatment. Drink 2 to 3 quarts of fluid the night before and the day following your treatment.

Potential side effects from probenecid include fever, rash, headache, and chills. Your doctor may give you medicines to prevent these effects. Talk with your doctor about this.

Cidofovir can cause decreased vision. Your doctor will ask you to see an eye doctor to watch for any changes.

Tell all the doctors, dentists, and pharmacists you visit that you are taking this drug.

- Most of the following side effects probably will not occur.
- Your doctor or nurse will want to discuss specific care instructions with you.
- They can help you understand these side effects and help you deal with them.

Side Effects:

More Common Side Effects
Nausea
Vomiting
Decreased white blood cell count with increased risk of infection
Fever
Rash
Headache
Chills
Feeling "blah"
Diarrhea
Decreased appetite
Difficulty breathing

Less Common Side Effects
Decreased red blood cell count with increased risk of anemia and tiredness (fatigue)
Abdominal pain
Increase in kidney function tests

Rare Side Effects
Visual changes
Decrease in blood bicarbonate level

Side Effects / Symptoms of the Drug
Stop the drug and call your doctor or nurse right away if you develop rash, fever, or chills. This can be a serious reaction and needs to be treated right away.

Report any changes in your vision immediately.

Other side effects not listed above can also occur in some patients.
Tell your doctor or nurse if you develop any problems.

FDA Approval: Yes

ciprofloxacin

Trade Name:
Cipro

Type of Drug:
Ciprofloxacin is an antibiotic that belongs to a group of drugs called fluoroquinolones.

How Drug Works:
Ciprofloxacin prevents bacteria from making more DNA, so the cells cannot continue to grow. Ciprofloxacin is used to treat some gram-negative and gram-positive bacteria and some mycobacteria.

How Drug Is Given:
Ciprofloxacin can be given by an injection or by mouth. As an injection, the medicine is given into a vein over 30 minutes twice a day for 7 to 14 days. As a pill, ciprofloxacin is given by mouth twice a day for 7 to 14 days as directed by your doctor. Take the pill with a full glass of water 1 hour before or 2 hours after eating. Swallow the pill whole and do not crush it. If you are taking an antacid, take the pill at least 2 hours after or before the antacid. The dose and number of days you take the medicine depend on the type of infection and how well your kidneys are working. Keep the medicine in a tightly closed container away from heat and moisture and out of the reach of children and pets.

How Should I Take This Drug?
Take this drug exactly as directed by your doctor. If you do not understand the instructions, ask your doctor or nurse to explain them to you.

 Read the following information. If you do not understand it or if any of it causes you special concern, check with your doctor.

Before taking this drug, tell your doctor if you are taking any other prescription or over-the-counter drugs, including vitamins and herbals.

Should I avoid any other medicines, foods, alcohol, and/or activities?
Your prescription and nonprescription medicines may interact with other drugs, causing harm. Certain foods or alcohol can also interact with drug products. Never begin taking a new medicine—prescription or nonprescription—without asking your doctor or nurse if it will interact with alcohol, food, or other medicines. Some drugs can cause drowsiness and affect activities such as driving.

Precautions:
Tell your doctor if you have allergies to any antibiotics.

Tell your doctor if you are also taking theophylline, as ciprofloxacin can increase your blood theophylline levels, sometimes to dangerous levels.

If you are also taking antacids, take them 2 hours before or after your ciprofloxacin doses.

All antibiotics can cause allergic reactions. Stop the drug and tell your doctor or nurse right away if you develop a rash, hives, red blotches on your skin, difficulty breathing, or chest pain.

Use of antibiotics can change the normal organisms in your body. Women are at risk of getting fungal infections. Tell your nurse or doctor if you get vaginal itching or discharge.

This drug should not be used by women who are pregnant or breastfeeding. It should be used cautiously in patients with seizure disorder.

Ciprofloxacin delays the excretion of caffeine from the body in those who drink coffee, tea, or soft drinks. Side effects such as headache, restlessness, dizziness, hallucinations, and seizures are increased in frequency if you drink a lot of caffeine. You should limit caffeine when taking this drug.

Take ciprofloxacin tablet(s) with 8 oz of water, and try to drink at least 2 to 3 quarts of fluid throughout the day while taking this medicine.

Tell all the doctors, dentists, and pharmacists you visit that you are taking this drug.

- Most of the following side effects probably will not occur.
- Your doctor or nurse will want to discuss specific care instructions with you.
- They can help you understand these side effects and help you deal with them.

Side Effects:

More Common Side Effects
Vaginal itching
Vaginal candidiasis (fungal infection)

Less Common Side Effects
Nausea
Vomiting
Abdominal pain
Diarrhea
Loss of appetite
Increase in blood tests for kidney function
Irritation of vein used for giving the drug

Rare Side Effects
Headache
Restlessness
Dizziness
Hallucinations
Seizures
Rash
Hives
Flushing
Fever
Chills
Increased sensitivity to sunlight
Diarrhea related to infection of the intestinal lining (pseudomembranous colitis)

Side Effects / Symptoms of the Drug
Stop the drug and call your doctor or nurse right away if you develop a rash, fever, muscle aches, or blood in your urine. Your doctor will give you another effective antibiotic.

Stop the drug and call your doctor or nurse right away if you get diarrhea that does not go away, abdominal cramping, and blood and/or pus in the stool. This needs to be treated right away.

Other side effects not listed above can also occur in some patients.
Tell your doctor or nurse if you develop any problems.

FDA Approval: Yes

citalopram hydrobromide

Trade Name:
Celexa

Type of Drug:
Citalopram hydrobromide belongs to a general class of antianxiety and antidepressant drugs.

How Drug Works:
Citalopram hydrobromide appears to increase activity in the brain and central nervous system. It does this by stopping the uptake of serotonin by the brain cells. This relieves the depression.

How Drug Is Given:
Citalopram hydrobromide is given by mouth once a day, with or without food. Take with a glass of water at about the same time every day. It may take 4 weeks before you feel any better, so make sure you don't stop the medicine until you talk to your doctor. The dose is determined by how much of the medicine you need and your age. Usually the dose is small at first, and then it is gradually increased until you feel better (to a maximum dose). If you are over 60 years old, the dose is started at the same amount, but it cannot be increased as much as in younger people. This is because the same higher doses can cause more side effects in older people. Keep the medicine in a tightly closed container away from heat and moisture and out of the reach of children and pets.

How Should I Take This Drug?
Take this drug exactly as directed by your doctor. If you do not understand the instructions, ask your doctor or nurse to explain them to you.

 Read the following information. If you do not understand it or if any of it causes you special concern, check with your doctor.

Before taking this drug, tell your doctor if you are taking any other prescription or over-the-counter drugs, including vitamins and herbals.

Should I avoid any other medicines, foods, alcohol, and/or activities?
Your prescription and nonprescription medicines may interact with other drugs, causing harm. Certain foods or alcohol can also interact with drug products. Never begin taking a new medicine—prescription or non-prescription—without asking your doctor or nurse if it will interact with alcohol, food, or other medicines. Some drugs can cause drowsiness and affect activities such as driving.

Precautions:
The dose may be lowered in an elderly person who has liver problems.

This drug interacts with many other drugs. Make sure you tell your doctor about all the medicines you are taking, including over-the-counter medicines. If you have been taking an antidepressant of the monamine oxidase inhibitor family, you must stop it and be off it for at least 14 days before starting citalopram hydrobromide.

Tell your doctor if you are taking any of the following drugs, as they may have serious interactions with citalopram hydrobromide: warfarin (Coumadin), cimetidine, lithium, metoprolol, ketoconazole, erythromycin, or other trycyclic antidepressants.

If you have a seizure disorder, tell your doctor. You will need to be watched closely while taking citalopram hydrobromide.

You will usually feel an effect within 1 to 4 weeks, but it may take longer. You should keep taking the medicine as directed by your doctor. If you get side effects that do not go away or get worse, call your doctor.

Do not drink alcohol while taking this medicine. It may worsen the depression.

Tell all the doctors, dentists, and pharmacists you visit that you are taking this drug.
- -
- Most of the following side effects probably will not occur.
- Your doctor or nurse will want to discuss specific care instructions with you.
- They can help you understand these side effects and help you deal with them.

Side Effects:

More Common Side Effects
Nausea
Dry mouth
Increased heart rate
Dizziness when standing from a lying or sitting position
Low blood pressure
Frequent urination

Less Common Side Effects
Stomach irritation
Diarrhea
Heartburn
Vomiting
Abdominal pain
Mouth sores
Burping
High blood pressure
Slow heart rate
Swelling of the hands or feet
Heart pain
Irregular heartbeat
Flushing of the face
Sleepiness
Difficulty sleeping
Rash
Itching
Urine retention
Difficulty urinating

Rare Side Effects
Gallbladder irritation
Hiccups
Heart damage
Difficulty concentrating
Changes in emotion
Acne
Changes in sexual functioning
Blood in the urine

Irritation or inflammation of the colon
Irritation of veins
Agitation
Confusion
Increased sensitivity to sunlight
Dry skin
Kidney stones

Side Effects / Symptoms of the Drug
Stop taking the drug and call your doctor if you develop blood in the urine or back pain.

Other side effects not listed above can also occur in some patients.
Tell your doctor or nurse if you develop any problems.

FDA Approval: Yes

clindamycin phosphate

Trade Name:
Cleocin

Type of Drug:
Clindamycin phosphate is an antibiotic used to treat bacterial infections.

How Drug Works:
Clindamycin phosphate prevents the bacterial cell from making protein so the cell dies. Clindamycin phosphate is used to treat gram-positive and gram-negative bacteria.

How Drug Is Given:
Clindamycin phosphate can be given by mouth as a capsule or liquid 4 times a day, or as an injection into the vein or muscle 2 to 4 times a day. The dose and route depend upon your size and type of infection. When taking the capsule or liquid, drink a full glass of water after each dose. Shake the liquid before pouring the dose. Try to take the medicine at the same time each day. Keep the medicine in a tightly closed container away from heat and moisture and out of the reach of children and pets.

How Should I Take This Drug?
Take this drug exactly as directed by your doctor. If you do not understand the instructions, ask your doctor or nurse to explain them to you.

 Read the following information. If you do not understand it or if any of it causes you special concern, check with your doctor.

Before taking this drug, tell your doctor if you are taking any other prescription or over-the-counter drugs, including vitamins and herbals.

Should I avoid any other medicines, foods, alcohol, and/or activities?
Your prescription and nonprescription medicines may interact with other drugs, causing harm. Certain foods or alcohol can also interact with drug products. Never begin taking a new medicine—prescription or nonprescription—without asking your doctor or nurse if it will interact with alcohol, food, or other medicines. Some drugs can cause drowsiness and affect activities such as driving.

Precautions:
Tell your doctor if you have any allergies, especially to antibiotic drugs. All antibiotics can cause allergic reactions. Stop the drug and tell your doctor or nurse right away if you develop a rash, hives, red blotches on your skin, difficulty breathing, or chest pain.

Use of antibiotics can change the normal organisms in your body. Women are at risk of getting fungal infections. Tell your nurse or doctor if you get vaginal itching or discharge.

This drug should not be used by women who are pregnant or breastfeeding or by patients with a history of colitis (colon inflammation).

Take oral form of clindamycin phosphate with at least 8 oz of water to prevent esophageal irritation. You may take the drug with food to decrease stomach upset.

Tell all the doctors, dentists, and pharmacists you visit that you are taking this drug.
- Most of the following side effects probably will not occur.
- Your doctor or nurse will want to discuss specific care instructions with you.
- They can help you understand these side effects and help you deal with them.

Side Effects:

More Common Side Effects
Nausea
Diarrhea

Less Common Side Effects
Vomiting
Abdominal pain
Bloated feeling
Decreased appetite
Pain at place of injection
Vaginal itching
Vaginal candidiasis (fungal infection)

Rare Side Effects
Rash
Hives
Diarrhea related to infection of the intestinal lining (pseudomembranous colitis)

Side Effects / Symptoms of the Drug
If you develop diarrhea with abdominal cramping or blood in your stool, call your doctor or nurse right away.

Stop the drug and call your doctor or nurse right away if you develop a rash, fever, muscle aches, or blood in your urine. This can be a serious reaction and needs to be treated right away.

> *Other side effects not listed above can also occur in some patients.*
> **Tell your doctor or nurse if you develop any problems.**

FDA Approval: Yes

clonazepam

Trade Name:
Klonopin

Type of Drug:
Clonazepam is an antianxiety agent that belongs to a class of drugs called benzodiazepines.

How Drug Works:
Clonazepam appears to indirectly stop neurotransmitter activity in the brain. It is used to manage panic attacks and seizures.

How Drug Is Given:
Clonazepam is given as a pill by mouth 3 times a day, with the last dose at bedtime. Take the pill with or without food, and try to take it at the same times each day. The dose depends upon your size and the reason the medicine is being taken. Do not stop taking the medicine all at once; it needs to be stopped gradually. Talk to your doctor first. Keep the medicine in a tightly closed container away from heat and moisture and out of the reach of children and pets.

How Should I Take This Drug?
Take this drug exactly as directed by your doctor. If you do not understand the instructions, ask your doctor or nurse to explain them to you.

 Read the following information. If you do not understand it or if any of it causes you special concern, check with your doctor.

Before taking this drug, tell your doctor if you are taking any other prescription or over-the-counter drugs, including vitamins and herbals.

Should I avoid any other medicines, foods, alcohol, and/or activities?
Your prescription and nonprescription medicines may interact with other drugs, causing harm. Certain foods or alcohol can also interact with drug products. Never begin taking a new medicine—prescription or non-prescription—without asking your doctor or nurse if it will interact with alcohol, food, or other medicines. Some drugs can cause drowsiness and affect activities such as driving.

Precautions:
DO NOT drink alcohol while taking clonazepam.

Take clonazepam only as directed by your doctor. Clonazepam may cause psychological dependence (addiction) and physical dependence (body goes into withdrawal if drug is suddenly stopped). When taken as directed by your doctor or nurse, this will not be a problem.

Clonazepam may cause you to feel drowsy or dizzy. This is more likely to occur if you are taking other drugs that depress the nervous system such as opioids, antianxiety drugs, or some antinausea medicines. Do not drive or operate heavy machinery until you know the effect the drug will have. Talk to your doctor or nurse if you feel too drowsy or have dizziness that does not go away.

Abruptly stopping the drug can cause anxiety, dizziness, nausea and vomiting, and tiredness. The drug should be gradually stopped.

Women who are pregnant, breastfeeding mothers, or patients with severe liver disease or glaucoma should not use this drug.

Tell all the doctors, dentists, and pharmacists you visit that you are taking this drug.
- Most of the following side effects probably will not occur.
- Your doctor or nurse will want to discuss specific care instructions with you.
- They can help you understand these side effects and help you deal with them.

Side Effects:

More Common Side Effects
Drowsiness

Less Common Side Effects
Decrease in blood pressure when changing position
Decreased mental alertness
Dizziness

Rare Side Effects
Lack of coordination
Difficulty walking
Difficulty speaking
Depression
Problems with memory
Nervousness
Mood changes
Confusion
Tremors
Change in activity level
Constipation
Decreased appetite
Heartburn
Heart palpitations
Chest pain
Swelling in feet
Acne flare-ups
Itching
Change in sexual interest

Side Effects / Symptoms of the Drug
Tell your doctor or nurse if you feel too sleepy or if dizziness does not go away.

Other side effects not listed above can also occur in some patients.
Tell your doctor or nurse if you develop any problems.

FDA Approval: Yes

clonidine hydrochloride

Trade Name:
Duraclon

Type of Drug:
Clonidine hydrochloride is a nonopioid analgesic that belongs to a general class of drugs called antiadrenergic agents.

How Drug Works:
Clonidine hydrochloride is given via the epidural space in the spinal cord where it stimulates adrenergic receptors. When given together with opioid analgesics, it increases the pain-relieving effect. The drug is especially useful for neuropathic pain.

How Drug Is Given:
Clonidine hydrochloride is given as a continuous infusion into the spinal canal via an epidural catheter with other medicines to stop pain. The catheter will remain in place as long as you are receiving this medicine into the spine. The dose depends upon the type of pain and the relief you get.

 Read the following information. If you do not understand it or if any of it causes you special concern, check with your doctor.

Before taking this drug, tell your doctor if you are taking any other prescription or over-the-counter drugs, including vitamins and herbals.

Should I avoid any other medicines, foods, alcohol, and/or activities?
Your prescription and nonprescription medicines may interact with other drugs, causing harm. Certain foods or alcohol can also interact with drug products. Never begin taking a new medicine—prescription or nonprescription—without asking your doctor or nurse if it will interact with alcohol, food, or other medicines. Some drugs can cause drowsiness and affect activities such as driving.

Precautions:
Since clonidine hydrochloride affects the central nervous system (CNS), it is important not to take other drugs or substances that are known CNS depressants, such as alcohol, sedatives, and hypnotics.

You will have your blood pressure taken frequently during the first 2 days of using the drug, as it can cause your blood pressure to drop. Tell your doctor or nurse if you feel dizzy when you stand up or feel differently.

Tell your doctor if you are taking any medicines for your heart, as some may interact with clonidine hydrochloride.

Abruptly stopping the drug can cause anxiety, nervousness, headache, tremors, and an increase in blood pressure. The drug should be gradually stopped.

Make sure that you tell your doctor or nurse right away if you develop any problems with the epidural catheter or skin site where the catheter goes into your body.

Tell all the doctors, dentists, and pharmacists you visit that you are taking this drug.

- Most of the following side effects probably will not occur.
- Your doctor or nurse will want to discuss specific care instructions with you.
- They can help you understand these side effects and help you deal with them.

Side Effects:

More Common Side Effects
Decreased blood pressure
Decreased heart rate

Less Common Side Effects
If drug is stopped suddenly, increased blood pressure, nervousness, agitation, headache, and tremors

Rare Side Effects
If drug is stopped suddenly, stroke, brain damage, or death in rare cases

Other side effects not listed above can also occur in some patients.
Tell your doctor or nurse if you develop any problems.

FDA Approval: Yes

codeine

Trade Names:
Capital and codeine, Codaphen, Codeine as a sulfate or phosphate, Empirin with codeine, Fiorinal with codeine, Odalan, Phenaphen with codeine, Soma Compound with codeine, Tylenol with codeine.

Type of Drug:
Codeine is an opioid analgesic that resembles morphine.

How Drug Works:
Codeine relieves mild to moderate pain. It binds to the opiate receptors in the central nervous system, altering the perception of pain as well as the emotional response to pain.

How Drug Is Given:
Codeine is given as a pill, or it can be given as an injection in the vein, muscle, or under the skin. It is often given with acetaminophen to make it work better. Take the medicine every 3 to 4 hours as needed for pain. Your doctor may suggest that you take the codeine with a laxative so that you don't get constipated. Keep the medicine in a tightly closed container away from heat and moisture and out of the reach of children and pets.

How Should I Take This Drug?
Take this drug exactly as directed by your doctor. If you do not understand the instructions, ask your doctor or nurse to explain them to you.

 Read the following information. If you do not understand it or if any of it causes you special concern, check with your doctor.

Before taking this drug, tell your doctor if you are taking any other prescription or over-the-counter drugs, including vitamins and herbals.

Should I avoid any other medicines, foods, alcohol, and/or activities?
Your prescription and nonprescription medicines may interact with other drugs, causing harm. Certain foods or alcohol can also interact with drug products. Never begin taking a new medicine—prescription or non-prescription—without asking your doctor or nurse if it will interact with alcohol, food, or other medicines. Some drugs can cause drowsiness and affect activities such as driving.

Precautions:
Take the smallest effective dose to prevent development of tolerance (larger doses needed to give the same effect) and physical dependence (body goes into withdrawal if drug is suddenly stopped). This is different from addiction, which is psychological dependence (take drug for psychological effect, not for relief of pain). Tell your doctor or nurse if you still have pain even though you are taking the medicine as directed.

Since codeine affects the central nervous system, it is important not to take other drugs or substances that are known CNS depressants such as alcohol, sedatives, and hypnotics.

Acetaminophen or aspirin may be combined with codeine to increase the pain relief action.

The oral dose given for pain relief is more than its equivalent SQ (subcutaneous) or IM (intramuscular) dose for the same pain relief.

Patients with liver or kidney problems, hypothyroidism, head injury, or increased intrcranial pressure should use codeine cautiously.

Opioid analgesics often cause constipation. Your doctor may suggest that you take a laxative. Talk to your nurse or doctor about this.

Tell all the doctors, dentists, and pharmacists you visit that you are taking this drug.

• Most of the following side effects probably will not occur.
• Your doctor or nurse will want to discuss specific care instructions with you.
• They can help you understand these side effects and help you deal with them.

Side Effects:

More Common Side Effects
Drowsiness
Sedation
Mood changes
Dizziness
Constipation
Dry mouth

Less Common Side Effects
Euphoria
Depression
Mental clouding
Nausea
Vomiting
Dizziness when changing position
Flushing
Itching
Sweating
Decreased heart rate
Difficulty urinating

Rare Side Effects
Seizures
Tiny pupils in eyes
Decreased breathing rate
Ruptured bowel from constipation
Decreased sexual ability
Decreased sexual interest

Side Effects / Symptoms of the Drug
Drink fluids (8 oz every hour in sips) to prevent constipation. Also, try to eat foods high in fiber such as bran. You may need to take a stool softener, bulk forming agent, and/or laxative to help keep your bowels movements regular. Call your doctor or nurse right away if you have not moved your bowels in 2 days.

Other side effects not listed above can also occur in some patients.
Tell your doctor or nurse if you develop any problems.

FDA Approval: Yes

co-trimoxazole; trimethoprim and sulfamethoxazole

Trade Names:
Bactrim, Bactrim DS, Cotrim, Septra, SMX-TMP, Sulfamethoxazole-Trimethoprim, TMP-SMX, Trimethoprim-Sulfamethoxazole

Type of Drug:
Co-trimoxazole (trimethoprim and sulfamethoxazole) is an antibiotic of the sulfonamide group, commonly called a "sulfa drug."

How Drug Works:
Co-trimoxazole stops folic acid synthesis, which is needed for cell growth. This prevents bacteria from dividing (reproducing). This drug is active against gram-positive and gram-negative bacteria and some protozoa. It is the first line treatment for *P. carinii* pneumonia.

How Drug Is Given:
This medicine is given by mouth or as an injection in the vein. The pill should be taken with an 8 oz glass of water twice a day for 7 to 14 days as directed. The shot form is given 3 to 4 times a day for up to 21 days. The dose and number of doses depends upon your size and the type of infection being treated. Keep the medicine in a tightly closed container away from heat and moisture and out of the reach of children and pets.

How Should I Take This Drug?
Take this drug exactly as directed by your doctor. If you do not understand the instructions, ask your doctor or nurse to explain them to you.

 Read the following information. If you do not understand it or if any of it causes you special concern, check with your doctor.

Before taking this drug, tell your doctor if you are taking any other prescription or over-the-counter drugs, including vitamins and herbals.

Should I avoid any other medicines, foods, alcohol, and/or activities?
Your prescription and nonprescription medicines may interact with other drugs, causing harm. Certain foods or alcohol can also interact with drug products. Never begin taking a new medicine—prescription or nonprescription—without asking your doctor or nurse if it will interact with alcohol, food, or other medicines. Some drugs can cause drowsiness and affect activities such as driving.

Precautions:
Tell your doctor if you have any allergies, especially to antibiotic drugs. If you have an allergy to sulfites, you should not take this drug.

All antibiotics can cause allergic reactions. Stop the drug and tell your doctor or nurse right away if you develop a rash, hives, red blotches on your skin, difficulty breathing, or chest tightness.

Tell your doctor if you are taking warfarin (Coumadin), oral hypoglycemic agents (for diabetes mellitus), phenytoin (Dilantin), thiazide diuretics, cyclosporine, methotrexate, or vitamin C. Talk with your doctor about drug interactions.

Use of antibiotics can change the normal organisms in your body. Women are at risk of getting fungal infections. Tell your nurse or doctor if you get vaginal itching or discharge.

Try to drink at least 2 to 3 quarts of fluid throughout the day.

Co-trimoxazole or trimethoprim and sulfamethoxazole can decrease the effectiveness of oral contraceptives. Women should use a barrier contraceptive in addition to "the pill" during the course of antibiotic therapy.

This drug should not be used by women who are pregnant or breastfeeding or by patients who have severe kidney disease.

Tell all the doctors, dentists, and pharmacists you visit that you are taking this drug.
- Most of the following side effects probably will not occur.
- Your doctor or nurse will want to discuss specific care instructions with you.
- They can help you understand these side effects and help you deal with them.

Side Effects:

More Common Side Effects
Nausea
Loss of appetite

Less Common Side Effects
Vomiting
Soreness of tongue
Abdominal pain
Diarrhea
Increase in blood tests for kidney function
Irritation of vein used for giving the drug

Rare Side Effects
Diarrhea related to infection of the intestinal lining (pseudomembranous colitis)
Rash
Hives
Itching
Decreased white blood cell count with increased risk of infection
Decreased platelet count with increased risk of bleeding
Decreased red blood cell count with increased risk of anemia and tiredness (fatigue)
Fever
Headache
Dizziness when standing
Difficulty sleeping
Tiredness (fatigue)
Feeling weak
Depression
Hallucinations

Side Effects / Symptoms of the Drug
Call your doctor or nurse right away if you have a sore tongue or have irritation of the lining of the mouth. The doctor may add a vitamin (folinic acid) to decrease this side effect.

Stop the drug and call your doctor or nurse right away if you develop a rash, fever, muscle aches, or blood in your urine. This can be a serious reaction and needs to be treated right away.

Other side effects not listed above can also occur in some patients.
Tell your doctor or nurse if you develop any problems.

FDA Approval: Yes

darbapoetin alfa

Trade Name:
Aranesp

Type of Drug:
Darbapoetin alfa belongs to a general class of man-made substances called biological response modifiers. It is used to prevent or treat anemia (low red blood cell count) after chemotherapy.

How Drug Works:
Darbapoetin alfa is similar to a hormone in your body called erythropoietin that makes the body's bone marrow produce more red blood cells.

How Drug Is Given:
Darbapoetin alfa is given as an injection under the skin every 1 to 2 weeks. You or a family member may be taught to give the injection. Keep the syringes, needles, and supplies in a safe place, out of the reach of children and pets. The medicine should be kept in its original container in the refrigerator, but do not let it freeze; you should take it out 1 hour before the shot is due. Do not shake the drug. The dose may be increased or decreased depending upon your response. Your blood counts will be checked at regular intervals. Keep the used syringes and needles in a special container. Ask your nurse or doctor about this and when you should bring the filled container back to the office.

How Should I Take This Drug?
Take this drug exactly as directed by your doctor. If you do not understand the instructions, ask your doctor or nurse to explain them to you.

 Read the following information. If you do not understand it or if any of it causes you special concern, check with your doctor.

Before taking this drug, tell your doctor if you are taking any other prescription or over-the-counter drugs, including vitamins and herbals.

Should I avoid any other medicines, foods, alcohol, and/or activities?
Your prescription and nonprescription medicines may interact with other drugs, causing harm. Certain foods or alcohol can also interact with drug products. Never begin taking a new medicine—prescription or nonprescription—without asking your doctor or nurse if it will interact with alcohol, food, or other medicines. Some drugs can cause drowsiness and affect activities such as driving.

Precautions:
This drug can cause an allergic reaction. You will be watched closely for signs and symptoms of a reaction when you first start receiving this drug. Symptoms can include rash, hives, flushing, and difficulty breathing. Symptoms of anemia (fatigue, low energy level, headaches) will go away once the red blood cell count goes back to a higher level.

You should not take darbapoetin alfa if you have uncontrolled hypertension (high blood pressure).

Your doctor will check your iron level in the blood. You may need to take iron pills to help your body make more red blood cells.

Tell all the doctors, dentists, and pharmacists you visit that you are taking this drug.
- -
- Most of the following side effects probably will not occur.
- Your doctor or nurse will want to discuss specific care instructions with you.
- They can help you understand these side effects and help you deal with them.

Side Effects:

Less Common Side Effects
Diarrhea
Swelling in legs or feet
Fever
Fatigue
Headache
Muscle aches

Rare Side Effects
Blood clots in the lungs or blood vessels
Rash
Hives
Difficulty breathing

Side Effects / Symptoms of the Drug
Call your doctor or nurse right away if you get a rash, hives, or difficulty breathing.

Report swelling of your feet or legs, bad pain in your legs, and/or fever if it occurs.

> *Other side effects not listed above can also occur in some patients.*
> ***Tell your doctor or nurse if you develop any problems.***

FDA Approval: Yes

demeclocycline hydrochloride

Trade Name:
Declomycin

Type of Drug:
Demeclocycline hydrochloride is an antibiotic that belongs to a class of drugs called tetracyclines.

How Drug Works:
Demeclocycline hydrochloride interferes with protein synthesis so that the bacteria are unable to reproduce. This drug is used to treat many gram-positive and gram-negative bacteria and some protozoa.

How Drug Is Given:
Demeclocycline hydrochloride is a pill given by mouth, usually 2 to 4 times a day. Take the pill on an empty stomach with a full glass of water, 1 hour before or 2 hours after eating a meal or dairy products like milk, yogurt, and ice cream. If you have nausea when taking the medicine, take it with a cracker but no dairy products. If you are also taking iron pills, take the iron pills 2 hours before or 3 hours after the demeclocycline hydrochloride pill. Keep the medicine in a tightly closed container away from heat and moisture and out of the reach of children and pets.

How Should I Take This Drug?
Take this drug exactly as directed by your doctor. If you do not understand the instructions, ask your doctor or nurse to explain them to you.

 Read the following information. If you do not understand it or if any of it causes you special concern, check with your doctor.

Before taking this drug, tell your doctor if you are taking any other prescription or over-the-counter drugs, including vitamins and herbals.

Should I avoid any other medicines, foods, alcohol, and/or activities?
Your prescription and nonprescription medicines may interact with other drugs, causing harm. Certain foods or alcohol can also interact with drug products. Never begin taking a new medicine—prescription or nonprescription—without asking your doctor or nurse if it will interact with alcohol, food, or other medicines. Some drugs can cause drowsiness and affect activities such as driving.

Precautions:
Tell your doctor if you are also taking anticoagulants such as warfarin (Coumadin), kaopectate, methoxyflurane, or lithium. There may be serious drug interactions. Talk to your doctor about this.

Demeclocycline hydrochloride can decrease the effectiveness of oral contraceptives. Women taking oral contraceptives should also use a barrier contraception.

Tell your doctor if you have any allergies, especially to antibiotic drugs.

All antibiotics can cause allergic reactions. Stop the drug and tell your doctor or nurse right away if you develop a rash, hives, red blotches on your skin, difficulty breathing, or chest pain.

Use of antibiotics can change the normal organisms in your body. Women are at risk of getting fungal infections. Tell your nurse or doctor if you get vaginal itching or discharge.

Demeclocycline hydrochloride can increase your sensitivity to direct sunlight. Try to avoid direct sunlight, and keep your head, arms, and legs covered when outside.

This drug should not be used in women who are pregnant or breastfeeding.

Tell all the doctors, dentists, and pharmacists you visit that you are taking this drug.
- Most of the following side effects probably will not occur.
- Your doctor or nurse will want to discuss specific care instructions with you.
- They can help you understand these side effects and help you deal with them.

Side Effects:

More Common Side Effects
Nausea
Increased sensitivity to sunlight

Less Common Side Effects
Vomiting
Diarrhea
Loss of appetite
Abdominal discomfort
Heartburn
Irritated tongue
Vaginal itching or discharge
Vaginal candidiasis (fungal infection)

Rare Side Effects
Rash
Darkening of nail beds
Fever
Hives
Muscle aches
Decreased white blood cell count with increased risk of infection
Decreased platelet count with increased risk of bleeding
Decreased red blood cell count with increased risk of anemia and tiredness (fatigue)
Diarrhea related to infection of the intestinal lining (pseudomembranous colitis)
Lightheadedness
Dizziness
Headache

Side Effects / Symptoms of the Drug
Do not drive a car or operate heavy machinery until you know the effect that demeclocycline hydrochloride has on you. If you are dizzy, lightheaded, or feel tired, you should not drive or operate heavy machinery.

Stop the drug and call your doctor or nurse right away if you develop a rash, fever, muscle aches, diarrhea with abdominal cramping, or blood or pus in your stool. This can be a serious reaction and needs to be treated right away.

Other side effects not listed above can also occur in some patients.
Tell your doctor or nurse if you develop any problems.

FDA Approval: Yes

deodorized tincture of opium

Trade Names:
DTO, Laudanum

Type of Drug:
Deodorized tincture of opium is an opiate used to control diarrhea.

How Drug Works:
Deodorized tincture of opium increases the tone of the smooth muscle in the intestines. It stops the normal movement and slows down the passage of intestinal contents. This allows water to be absorbed from the liquid stool, decreasing diarrhea.

How Drug Is Given:
Deodorized tincture of opium is taken by mouth, mixed in water or juice. Your doctor will tell you how often to take it, usually 1 to 4 times a day or after each loose stool (bowel movement), but not more than 6 times a day. Do not take more than your doctor tells you. The medicine should be stored in a closed container and protected from light. Keep it out of the reach of children and pets.

How Should I Take This Drug?
Take this drug exactly as directed by your doctor. If you do not understand the instructions, ask your doctor or nurse to explain them to you.

 Read the following information. If you do not understand it or if any of it causes you special concern, check with your doctor.

Before taking this drug, tell your doctor if you are taking any other prescription or over-the-counter drugs, including vitamins and herbals.

Should I avoid any other medicines, foods, alcohol, and/or activities?
Your prescription and nonprescription medicines may interact with other drugs, causing harm. Certain foods or alcohol can also interact with drug products. Never begin taking a new medicine—prescription or nonprescription—without asking your doctor or nurse if it will interact with alcohol, food, or other medicines. Some drugs can cause drowsiness and affect activities such as driving.

Precautions:
If deodorized tincture of opium is used for a long time, physical dependence may develop (body goes into withdrawal if drug is stopped abruptly). It is a controlled substance and is stronger than paragoric.

To help decrease the diarrhea, change your diet. Try to eat small, frequent meals that are warm or at room temperature. Avoid foods that cause gas (such as broccoli or beans), fatty foods (such as bacon or cheeses), citrus fruits and juices, and high lactose-foods (such as milk or ice cream). Eat foods high in sodium and potassium (such as soups, sports drinks, and bananas). Eat foods high in soluble fiber (such as rice or bananas). Avoid foods high in insoluble fiber (such as cereal or nuts). Try to drink at least eight oz glasses of water a day. To add calories, dilute with fruit juice.

Tell all the doctors, dentists, and pharmacists you visit that you are taking this drug.
- Most of the following side effects probably will not occur.
- Your doctor or nurse will want to discuss specific care instructions with you.
- They can help you understand these side effects and help you deal with them.

Side Effects:

More Common Side Effects
Nausea

Less Common Side Effects
Vomiting

Other side effects not listed above can also occur in some patients.
Tell your doctor or nurse if you develop any problems.

FDA Approval: Yes

desipramine hydrochloride

Trade Names:
Norpramin, Pertofrane

Type of Drug:
Desipramine hydrochloride is used to reduce anxiety and depression and belongs to a general class of drugs called tricyclic antidepressants.

How Drug Works:
Desipramine hydrochloride works by increasing the amount of serotonin and norepinephrine in the brain so that the feeling of depression is prevented or relieved. By a separate mechanism, desipramine hydrochloride may also reduce pain related to peripheral neuropathy.

How Drug Is Given:
Desipramine hydrochloride is a pill given by mouth. Often, you can take it as a single dose at bedtime. Take with juice if needed to cover the taste in your mouth. Try to take it at about the same time every day. It may take 4 weeks before you feel any better, so make sure you do not stop the medicine until you talk to your doctor. The dose is determined by how much of the medicine you need and your age. Usually the dose is small at first, and then it is gradually increased until you feel better (to a maximum dose). If you are over 60 years old, the dose is started at the same amount, but it cannot be increased as much as in younger people. This is because the same higher doses can cause more side effects in older people. Keep the medicine in a tightly closed container away from heat and moisture and out of the reach of children and pets.

How Should I Take This Drug?
Take this drug exactly as directed by your doctor. If you do not understand the instructions, ask your doctor or nurse to explain them to you.

 Read the following information. If you do not understand it or if any of it causes you special concern, check with your doctor.

Before taking this drug, tell your doctor if you are taking any other prescription or over-the-counter drugs, including vitamins and herbals.

Should I avoid any other medicines, foods, alcohol, and/or activities?
Your prescription and nonprescription medicines may interact with other drugs, causing harm. Certain foods or alcohol can also interact with drug products. Never begin taking a new medicine—prescription or non-prescription—without asking your doctor or nurse if it will interact with alcohol, food, or other medicines. Some drugs can cause drowsiness and affect activities such as driving.

Precautions:
Tell your doctor if you are taking any of the following drugs as they may have serious interactions with desipramine hydrochloride: warfarin (Coumadin), monoamine oxidase inhibitors or other antidepressant drugs, or amphetamines.

Once you start taking desipramine hydrochloride, it may take 2 weeks or longer for the antidepressant effect to work. This drug can be used to help you get to sleep at night, and this effect starts right away. If you are taking it to help relieve pain, relief usually starts right away as well.

Tell your doctor if you have had a heart attack, have a seizure disorder, or have benign prostatic hypertrophy (BPH). You should not take desipramine hydrochloride.

Tell your doctor if you have urine retention, narrow-angle glaucoma, hyperthyroidism, liver problems, or thoughts of suicide. This drug should be used very cautiously if you have any of these conditions.

Try to take your dose of the medicine at bedtime so it will help you sleep better.

The drug should not be given to women who are pregnant or breastfeeding.

Since desipramine hydrochloride affects the central nervous system (CNS), it is important not to take other drugs or substances that are known CNS depressants such as alcohol, sedatives, and hypnotics.

Tell all the doctors, dentists, and pharmacists you visit that you are taking this drug.
- Most of the following side effects probably will not occur.
- Your doctor or nurse will want to discuss specific care instructions with you.
- They can help you understand these side effects and help you deal with them.

Side Effects:

More Common Side Effects

Drowsiness

Weakness

Dry mouth

Dizziness

Tiredness (fatigue)

Less Common Side Effects

Confusion (especially in the elderly)

Disorientation

Hallucinations

Decrease in blood pressure when changing positions

Increased heart rate

Loss of appetite

Urinary retention

Rare Side Effects

Fine tremors

Difficulty speaking

Numbness and tingling in hands and/or feet related to irritation of nerves

Changes in the electrical activity of the heart (EKG)

Abdominal cramping

Hives

Rigidity

Difficulty swallowing

Blurred vision

Increase in blood pressure

Nausea

Vomiting

Diarrhea

Rash

Increased sensitivity to sunlight

Side Effects / Symptoms of the Drug

The drowsiness and/or dizziness usually goes away in 1 to 2 weeks. Do not drive or operate heavy machinery if you feel drowsy or dizzy.

Be careful walking around or changing position if you are drowsy. Stop the drug and call your doctor or nurse if the drowsiness does not go away or if you have trouble walking or moving because of it.

Tell your doctor or nurse if you get fine tremors, feel like your body is rigid, or have difficulty speaking or swallowing. You can be given another medicine to take away these problems.

Other side effects not listed above can also occur in some patients.
Tell your doctor or nurse if you develop any problems.

FDA Approval: Yes

dexamethasone

Trade Name:
Decadron

Type of Drug:
Dexamethasone belongs to a general class of drugs called glucocorticoid steroids.

How Drug Works:
Dexamethasone interferes with the pathways responsible for nausea and vomiting related to chemotherapy. The drug has other uses such as part of a chemotherapy regime or to reduce swelling of the brain (see page 72).

How Drug Is Given:
Dexamethasone can be given as a pill or as an injection in a vein over 5 minutes. Take the pill with food or milk to protect the stomach from irritation. When it is given as an injection in the vein, you may be given special medicine to stop the acid in your stomach. The dose and how often you take dexamethasone depends on the reason you are taking it. Make sure you tell your doctor if you have a history of ulcers, as dexamethasone can make them bleed or rupture. Keep the medicine in a tightly closed container away from heat and moisture and out of the reach of children and pets.

How Should I Take This Drug?
Take this drug exactly as directed by your doctor. If you do not understand the instructions, ask your doctor or nurse to explain them to you.

 Read the following information. If you do not understand it or if any of it causes you special concern, check with your doctor.

Before taking this drug, tell your doctor if you are taking any other prescription or over-the-counter drugs, including vitamins and herbals.

Should I avoid any other medicines, foods, alcohol, and/or activities?
Your prescription and nonprescription medicines may interact with other drugs, causing harm. Certain foods or alcohol can also interact with drug products. Never begin taking a new medicine—prescription or nonprescription—without asking your doctor or nurse if it will interact with alcohol, food, or other medicines. Some drugs can cause drowsiness and affect activities such as driving.

Precautions:
Dexamethasone can irritate the stomach, so the pill form must be taken with food. If you develop stomach pain or vomit any blood, tell your doctor immediately. If you have a stomach ulcer, you may not be able to take this drug without extra protective medicines.

This drug suppresses the immune system so it can increase susceptibility to infections. In addition, the drug may mask the signs of infections, such as fever.

When you are taking dexamethasone, do not have any immunizations (vaccinations) without your doctor's okay. Try to avoid contact with people who have recently taken the oral polio vaccine or who have had chickenpox or measles. Check with your doctor about this.

If you take dexamethasone for a long time, do not stop the medicine abruptly as this can cause a decrease in the steroid hormones your body makes (adrenal insufficiency). Symptoms of this are nausea, loss of appetite, fatigue, dizziness, difficulty breathing, joint pain, depression, low blood sugar, and low blood pressure. The drug should be stopped gradually.

If you are a diabetic, this medicine will raise your blood sugar levels, and you may need to take extra diabetes medicine. Talk to your doctor about this.

When this drug is taken for a long time, some side effects may not occur until months after the drug is used.

Tell all the doctors, dentists, and pharmacists you visit that you are taking this drug.

- Most of the following side effects probably will not occur.
- Your doctor or nurse will want to discuss specific care instructions with you.
- They can help you understand these side effects and help you deal with them.

Side Effects:

More Common Side Effects
Increased appetite with weight gain
Sodium and fluid retention with swelling of ankles, increased blood pressure, congestive heart failure
Depression
Increased blood sugar
Sleep disturbance
Increased risk of infection
Bruising of the skin
Mood changes
Delayed wound healing

Less Common Side Effects
Decrease in serum potassium (symptoms are loss of appetite, muscle twitching, increased thirst, frequent urination)
Fracture of weak bones
Fungal infections (white patches in mouth, vagina)
Sweating
Diarrhea
Nausea
Headache
Increased heart rate
Loss of calcium from bones

Rare Side Effects
Cataracts
Personality changes
Blurred vision
Stomach ulcer, which may bleed (hemorrhage)

Side Effects / Symptoms of the Drug
Tell your doctor or nurse immediately if you develop any of the following: stomach pain or vomiting blood; new bone pain; signs of infection such as fever, bad cough, and bringing up sputum; or burning when you pass urine.

Always take the pill form with food or milk.

Other side effects not listed above can also occur in some patients.
Tell your doctor or nurse if you develop any problems.

FDA Approval: Yes

diazepam

Trade Name:
Valium

Type of Drug:
Diazepam belongs to a general class of antianxiety drugs called benzodiazepines.

How Drug Works:
Diazepam binds to certain receptors in the brain and spinal cord to reduce anxiety, cause muscle relaxation, and prevent seizures.

How Drug Is Given:
Diazepam is given in pill form by mouth, or as an injection in a vein or muscle. The dose and how often the dose is given depends on the reason it is given and your size. Keep the medicine in a tightly closed container away from heat and moisture and out of the reach of children and pets.

How Should I Take This Drug?
Take this drug exactly as directed by your doctor. If you do not understand the instructions, ask your doctor or nurse to explain them to you.

 Read the following information. If you do not understand it or if any of it causes you special concern, check with your doctor.

Before taking this drug, tell your doctor if you are taking any other prescription or over-the-counter drugs, including vitamins and herbals.

Should I avoid any other medicines, foods, alcohol, and/or activities?
Your prescription and nonprescription medicines may interact with other drugs, causing harm. Certain foods or alcohol can also interact with drug products. Never begin taking a new medicine—prescription or nonprescription—without asking your doctor or nurse if it will interact with alcohol, food, or other medicines. Some drugs can cause drowsiness and affect activities such as driving.

Precautions:
Tell your doctor if you are taking any of the following drugs as they may have serious interactions with diazepam: oral contraceptives, isoniazid, ketoconazole, cimetidine, digoxin, levodopa, or a tricyclic antidepressant drug.

You should not take this drug if you have acute angle closure glaucoma.

Take diazepam only as directed by your doctor. Diazepam may cause psychological dependence (addiction) and physical dependence (body goes into withdrawal if drug is suddenly stopped). When taken as directed by your doctor or nurse, this will not be a problem.

Abruptly stopping the drug can cause anxiety, dizziness, nausea and vomiting, and tiredness. The drug should be gradually discontinued.

When you start taking the drug, you may feel drowsy, dizzy, confused, weak, or have a headache. This should go away after a few days of taking the drug. If not, talk to your doctor, and your dose may need to be reduced.

The drug should not be used by women who are pregnant or breastfeeding.

Since diazepam affects the central nervous system (CNS), do not take other drugs or substances that are known CNS depressants such as alcohol, sedatives, and hypnotics.

Tell all the doctors, dentists, and pharmacists you visit that you are taking this drug.

- Most of the following side effects probably will not occur.
- Your doctor or nurse will want to discuss specific care instructions with you.
- They can help you understand these side effects and help you deal with them.

Side Effects:

More Common Side Effects
Drowsiness (when first starting the drug)
Tiredness (when first starting the drug)
Confusion (when first starting the drug)
Headache (when first starting the drug)

Less Common Side Effects
Feeling "hung over" the next day
Decreased coordination
Decreased mental alertness
Decreased blood pressure
Decreased heart rate

Rare Side Effects
Vivid dreams
Slurred speech
Bizarre behavior
Nausea
Vomiting
Abdominal discomfort
Decreased breathing rate
Rash
Hives
Pain at place of injection

Side Effects / Symptoms of the Drug
Be careful walking around or changing position if you are drowsy. Stop the drug and call your doctor or nurse if the drowsiness does not go away, or if you have trouble walking or moving because of it.

Do not drive a vehicle when feeling drowsy.

Other side effects not listed above can also occur in some patients.
Tell your doctor or nurse if you develop any problems.

FDA Approval: Yes

dicloxacillin sodium

Trade Names:
Dycill, Dynapen, Pathocil

Type of Drug:
Dicloxacillin sodium is an antibiotic drug that belongs to the group called penicillins.

How Drug Works:
Dicloxacillin sodium prevents bacteria from making their cell wall, so the bacteria cells die. It is used to treat infections of the upper and lower respiratory tracts and skin.

How Drug Is Given:
Dicloxacillin sodium is given by mouth as a capsule or liquid 4 times a day for up to 14 days as directed. Take the capsule with a full glass of water on an empty stomach, 1 hour before or 2 hours after eating. Make sure to swallow the capsule whole; do not open or crush it. Shake the liquid well before pouring the dose. The dose and length of time you take the medicine depends on the type and severity of your infection. Keep the medicine in a tightly closed container away from heat and moisture and out of the reach of children and pets.

How Should I Take This Drug?
Take this drug exactly as directed by your doctor. If you do not understand the instructions, ask your doctor or nurse to explain them to you.

 Read the following information. If you do not understand it or if any of it causes you special concern, check with your doctor.

Before taking this drug, tell your doctor if you are taking any other prescription or over-the-counter drugs, including vitamins and herbals.

Should I avoid any other medicines, foods, alcohol, and/or activities?
Your prescription and nonprescription medicines may interact with other drugs, causing harm. Certain foods or alcohol can also interact with drug products. Never begin taking a new medicine—prescription or non-prescription—without asking your doctor or nurse if it will interact with alcohol, food, or other medicines. Some drugs can cause drowsiness and affect activities such as driving.

Precautions:
Tell your doctor if you have any allergies, especially to antibiotic drugs.

All antibiotics can cause allergic reactions. Stop the drug and tell your doctor or nurse right away if you develop a rash, hives, red blotches on your skin, difficulty breathing, or chest pain.

Use of antibiotics can change the normal organisms in your body. Women are at risk of getting fungal infections. Tell your nurse or doctor if you get vaginal itching or discharge.

This drug should be used with caution in women who are pregnant or breastfeeding.

Side Effects:

More Common Side Effects
Nausea

Less Common Side Effects
Vomiting
Diarrhea
Loss of appetite
Vaginal candidiasis (fungal infection)

Rare Side Effects
Diarrhea related to infection of the intestinal lining (pseudomembranous colitis)
Rash
Hives
Itching
Fever
Chills
Muscle aches
Swelling of hands and/or feet
Peeling of skin

Side Effects / Symptoms of the Drug
Stop the drug and call your doctor or nurse right away if you develop a rash, hives, fever, chills, muscle aches, and/or peeling of your skin. This can be a serious reaction and needs to be treated right away.

Stop the drug and call your doctor or nurse right away if you get diarrhea that does not stop, abdominal cramping, and blood and/or pus in the stool. This needs to be treated right away.

Other side effects not listed above can also occur in some patients.
Tell your doctor or nurse if you develop any problems.

FDA Approval: Yes

diphenhydramine hydrochloride

Trade Name:
Benadryl

Type of Drug:
Diphenhydramine hydrochloride belongs to the general class of drugs called antihistamines.

How Drug Works:
Diphenhydramine hydrochloride has slight activity in preventing nausea and vomiting caused by chemotherapy. It also prevents or can stop some side effects from other antinausea medicines. Diphenhydramine hydrochloride may be prescribed for sleep. The drug decreases allergic response by blocking histamine.

How Drug Is Given:
Diphenhydramine hydrochloride is given as a capsule, pill, or liquid by mouth, or as an injection in a vein or muscle. The dose, how often you take it, and for how long depends on why you are taking the medicine. Keep the medicine in a tightly closed container away from heat and moisture and out of the reach of children and pets.

How Should I Take This Drug?
Take this drug exactly as directed by your doctor. If you do not understand the instructions, ask your doctor or nurse to explain them to you.

 Read the following information. If you do not understand it or if any of it causes you special concern, check with your doctor.

Before taking this drug, tell your doctor if you are taking any other prescription or over-the-counter drugs, including vitamins and herbals.

Should I avoid any other medicines, foods, alcohol, and/or activities?
Your prescription and nonprescription medicines may interact with other drugs, causing harm. Certain foods or alcohol can also interact with drug products. Never begin taking a new medicine—prescription or nonprescription—without asking your doctor or nurse if it will interact with alcohol, food, or other medicines. Some drugs can cause drowsiness and affect activities such as driving.

Precautions:
Diphenhydramine hydrochloride, an antinausea drug, is usually given before chemotherapy. It usually causes sleepiness. Do not drive or operate heavy machinery when you are drowsy.

Tell all the doctors, dentists, and pharmacists you visit that you are taking this drug.
- Most of the following side effects probably will not occur.
- Your doctor or nurse will want to discuss specific care instructions with you.
- They can help you understand these side effects and help you deal with them.

Side Effects:

More Common Side Effects
Sedation
Drowsiness
Dry mouth

Less Common Side Effects
Dizziness
Confusion
Increased ability to get excited
Decreased blood pressure

Rare Side Effects
Blurred vision
Double vision
Ringing in the ears (tinnitus)
Inability to fully empty bladder
Difficulty with urination
Frequent urination
Rash
Hives
Increased sensitivity to light
Increased heart rate
Decreased white blood cell count with increased risk of infection
Decreased platelet count with increased risk of bleeding
Decreased red blood cell count with increased risk of anemia and tiredness (fatigue)

Other side effects not listed above can also occur in some patients.
Tell your doctor or nurse if you develop any problems.

FDA Approval: Yes

diphenoxylate hydrochloride with atropine

Trade Name:
Lomotil

Type of Drug:
Diphenoxylate hydrochloride with atropine is a drug used to control diarrhea.

How Drug Works:
Diphenoxylate hydrochloride with atropine combination is a synthetic opiate-like drug that slows intestinal smooth muscle. This slows the normal forward movement of the intestines (peristalsis), so that water is absorbed from the liquid stool, decreasing diarrhea.

How Drug Is Given:
Diphenoxylate hydrochloride with atropine is given as a pill or liquid by mouth. The liquid comes in a bottle with a special dropper. Make sure you use the dropper to measure the dose exactly. The dose and how often it is given depends on how severe the diarrhea is. Usually the medicine is given after each loose stool but no more than 4 doses a day. Your doctor will tell you exactly how to take it. Talk to your doctor or nurse if you still have diarrhea after taking the medicine as directed. Keep the medicine in a tightly closed container away from heat and moisture and out of the reach of children and pets.

How Should I Take This Drug?
Take this drug exactly as directed by your doctor. If you do not understand the instructions, ask your doctor or nurse to explain them to you.

 Read the following information. If you do not understand it or if any of it causes you special concern, check with your doctor.

Before taking this drug, tell your doctor if you are taking any other prescription or over-the-counter drugs, including vitamins and herbals.

Should I avoid any other medicines, foods, alcohol, and/or activities?
Your prescription and nonprescription medicines may interact with other drugs, causing harm. Certain foods or alcohol can also interact with drug products. Never begin taking a new medicine—prescription or nonprescription—without asking your doctor or nurse if it will interact with alcohol, food, or other medicines. Some drugs can cause drowsiness and affect activities such as driving.

Precautions:
If diphenoxylate hydrochloride with atropine is used for a long time, physical dependence may develop (body goes into withdrawal if drug is stopped abruptly). It is a controlled substance.

This drug should not be used if you have jaundice, diarrhea from poisoning, or an infection in your intestines caused by antibiotics (pseudomembranous colitis). Talk with your doctor or nurse about this.

To help decrease the diarrhea, change your diet. Try to eat small, frequent meals that are warm or at room temperature. Avoid foods that cause gas (such as broccoli or beans), fatty foods (such as bacon or cheeses), citrus fruits and juices, and high-lactose foods (such as milk or ice cream). Eat foods high in sodium and potassium (such as soups or sports drinks). Eat foods high in soluble fiber (such as rice or bananas). Avoid foods high in insoluble fiber (such as cereal or nuts). Try to drink at least eight 8 oz glasses of water a day. To add calories, dilute with fruit juice.

Tell your doctor if you drink alcohol or take barbiturates or monoamine oxidase inhibitors (a type of antidepressant drug). Talk with your doctor about possible drug interactions.

Tell all the doctors, dentists, and pharmacists you visit that you are taking this drug.
- • Most of the following side effects probably will not occur.
- • Your doctor or nurse will want to discuss specific care instructions with you.
- • They can help you understand these side effects and help you deal with them.

Side Effects:

More Common Side Effects
Nausea
Dry mouth
Sleepiness

Less Common Side Effects
Vomiting
Restlessness
Abdominal bloating
Loss of appetite
Dizziness
Tiredness (fatigue)
Difficulty sleeping

Rare Side Effects
Intestines stop moving (paralytic ileus)
Headache
Numbness and tingling in hands and/or feet
Blurred vision
Rash
Itching
Facial swelling

Side Effects / Symptoms of the Drug
Stop the drug and tell your doctor or nurse right away if you get a rash and/or swelling of the face. This may be an allergic reaction.

Other side effects not listed above can also occur in some patients.
Tell your doctor or nurse if you develop any problems.

FDA Approval: Yes

docusate calcium, docusate potassium, docusate sodium

Trade Names:
Colace, Diocto-K, Dioctyl Calcium Sulfosuccinate, Dioctyl Potassium Sulfosuccinate, Dioctyl Sodium Sulfosuccinate, Diosuccin, DOK-250, Doxinate, Duosol, Laxinate 100, Regular SS, Stulex

Type of Drug:
Docusate calcium, docusate potassium, and docusate sodium belong to a class of drugs called stool softeners. They are used to treat constipation.

How Drug Works:
Docusate calcium, docusate potassium, and docusate sodium work to increase the amount of water that the stool absorbs as it passes through the intestines. This softens the stool.

How Drug Is Given:
Docusate calcium/potassium/sodium are soft-gel caps that are given by mouth. The dose is usually standard, but if you still have trouble with hard stools, your doctor may increase the dose or give you a different medicine. Do not take mineral oil if you are taking docusate calcium/potassium/sodium. It may cause the mineral oil to be absorbed into your body. Keep the medicine in a tightly closed container away from heat and moisture and out of the reach of children and pets.

How Should I Take This Drug?
Take this drug exactly as directed by your doctor. If you do not understand the instructions, ask your doctor or nurse to explain them to you.

 Read the following information. If you do not understand it or if any of it causes you special concern, check with your doctor.

Before taking this drug, tell your doctor if you are taking any other prescription or over-the-counter drugs, including vitamins and herbals.

Should I avoid any other medicines, foods, alcohol, and/or activities?
Your prescription and nonprescription medicines may interact with other drugs, causing harm. Certain foods or alcohol can also interact with drug products. Never begin taking a new medicine—prescription or nonprescription—without asking your doctor or nurse if it will interact with alcohol, food, or other medicines. Some drugs can cause drowsiness and affect activities such as driving.

Precautions:
To prevent constipation, try to drink 2 to 3 quarts of fluid a day, increase the amount of bran, fruits, and vegetables in your diet (try to eat 5 servings of fruits and vegetables daily), eat vegetable fiber or cereal, and do light exercise as much as you can.

Docusate calcium, docusate potassium, and docusate sodium are not absorbed into the body, so there are no side effects.

Take with full glass of water, or with juice if you do not like the taste.

Docusate calcium, docusate potassium, and docusate sodium may take up to 3 days to soften the stool.

Docusate calcium is useful in preventing straining-at-stool and useful in preventing constipation, but it is not effective as treatment once constipation has occurred.

Stop drug if abdominal cramping occurs.

Tell all the doctors, dentists, and pharmacists you visit that you are taking this drug.

- Most of the following side effects probably will not occur.
- Your doctor or nurse will want to discuss specific care instructions with you.
- They can help you understand these side effects and help you deal with them.

Side effects can occur in some patients.
Tell your doctor or nurse if you develop any problems.

FDA Approval: Yes

dolasetron mesylate

Trade Name:
Anzamet

Type of Drug:
Dolasetron mesylate belongs to a general class of drugs called serotonin antagonists. It is an antinausea medicine.

How Drug Works:
Dolasetron mesylate blocks the serotonin pathway by which chemotherapy stimulates the vomiting center in the brain.

How Drug Is Given:
Dolasetron mesylate is given as a tablet by mouth or as an injection into the vein over 1 to 15 minutes. It is given before chemotherapy or surgery. The dose can be a standard dose or based on your weight.

How Should I Take This Drug?
Take this drug exactly as directed by your doctor. If you do not understand the instructions, ask your doctor or nurse to explain them to you.

 Read the following information. If you do not understand it or if any of it causes you special concern, check with your doctor.

Before taking this drug, tell your doctor if you are taking any other prescription or over-the-counter drugs, including vitamins and herbals.

Should I avoid any other medicines, foods, alcohol, and/or activities?
Your prescription and nonprescription medicines may interact with other drugs, causing harm. Certain foods or alcohol can also interact with drug products. Never begin taking a new medicine—prescription or nonprescription—without asking your doctor or nurse if it will interact with alcohol, food, or other medicines. Some drugs can cause drowsiness and affect activities such as driving.

Precautions:
Do not use if pregnant or breastfeeding.

Tell all the doctors, dentists, and pharmacists you visit that you are taking this drug.

- Most of the following side effects probably will not occur.
- Your doctor or nurse will want to discuss specific care instructions with you.
- They can help you understand these side effects and help you deal with them.

Side Effects:

Less Common Side Effects
Headache

Rare Side Effects
Fever
Tiredness (fatigue)
Bone pain
Muscle aches
Constipation
Heartburn
Loss of appetite
Inflammation of the pancreas
Changes in electrical activity of heart
Flushing
Vivid dreams
Sleep problems
Confusion
Anxiety
Anaphylaxis
Swelling in the face
Itching

Other side effects not listed above can also occur in some patients.
Tell your doctor or nurse if you develop any problems.

FDA Approval: Yes

doxepin hydrochloride

Trade Name:
Sinequan

Type of Drug:
Doxepin hydrochloride is a drug used to treat anxiety and depression. It is related to the tricyclic antidepressants.

How Drug Works:
Doxepin hydrochloride exerts its effect at the nerve endings, where it encourages the availability of norepinephrine, which decreases or stops the feeling of depression.

How Drug Is Given:
Doxepin hydrochloride is a capsule or liquid taken by mouth 1 to 3 times a day as directed. You can take it with or without food. The liquid comes with a special dropper to measure out the dose. This should be mixed with water or juice but not carbonated beverages. Take your last dose (or your single dose if taking the medicine once a day) at bedtime to help you sleep. Keep the medicine in a tightly closed container away from heat and moisture and out of the reach of children and pets.

How Should I Take This Drug?
Take this drug exactly as directed by your doctor. If you do not understand the instructions, ask your doctor or nurse to explain them to you.

 Read the following information. If you do not understand it or if any of it causes you special concern, check with your doctor.

Before taking this drug, tell your doctor if you are taking any other prescription or over-the-counter drugs, including vitamins and herbals.

Should I avoid any other medicines, foods, alcohol, and/or activities?
Your prescription and nonprescription medicines may interact with other drugs, causing harm. Certain foods or alcohol can also interact with drug products. Never begin taking a new medicine—prescription or nonprescription—without asking your doctor or nurse if it will interact with alcohol, food, or other medicines. Some drugs can cause drowsiness and affect activities such as driving.

Precautions:
Doxepin hydrochloride reduces anxiety as well. This effect occurs before the antidepressant effect, which can take up to 2 to 3 weeks.

DO NOT drink alcohol while taking doxepin hydrochloride.

Tell your doctor if you are taking other antidepressants (monoamine oxidase inhibitors), or have glaucoma or urinary retention. You should NOT take doxepin hydrochloride.

Tell your doctor if you are taking cimetidine or tolazamide. They may have serious interactions with doxepin hydrochloride.

Drowsiness may occur at first but usually goes away after a few days. If the drowsiness does not go away, talk to your doctor about lowering the dose or changing to another drug.

Tell all the doctors, dentists, and pharmacists you visit that you are taking this drug.

- Most of the following side effects probably will not occur.
- Your doctor or nurse will want to discuss specific care instructions with you.
- They can help you understand these side effects and help you deal with them.

Side Effects:

More Common Side Effects
Drowsiness

Less Common Side Effects
Dry mouth
Decreased appetite
Indigestion
Changes in taste including metallic taste of foods
Urinary retention

Rare Side Effects
Dizziness
Confusion
Disorientation
Hallucinations
Numbness and tingling in hands and/or feet
Tremors
Blurred vision
Difficulty walking
Change in blood pressure
Increased heart rate
Nausea
Vomiting
Diarrhea
Rash
Hives
Increased sensitivity to sunlight
Changes in sexual desire

Side Effects / Symptoms of the Drug
The drowsiness and/or dizziness usually goes away within 1 to 2 weeks. Do not drive or operate heavy machinery if you feel drowsy or dizzy.

Be careful walking around or changing position if you are drowsy. Stop the drug and call your doctor or nurse if the drowsiness does not go away, or if you have trouble walking or moving because of it.

Tell your doctor or nurse if you get fine tremors, feel like your body is rigid, or have difficulty speaking or swallowing. You can be given another medicine to take away these problems.

Other side effects not listed above can also occur in some patients.
Tell your doctor or nurse if you develop any problems.

FDA Approval: Yes

dronabinol

Trade Name:
Marinol

Type of Drug:
Dronabinol belongs to a general class of drugs called cannabinoids that are used to treat nausea and vomiting.

How Drug Works:
Dronabinol is useful for some patients in preventing nausea and vomiting following chemotherapy when the usual antinausea agents are ineffective. It is also used to stimulate appetite. Its exact mechanism is not known.

How Drug Is Given:
Dronabinol is a soft-gel capsule given by mouth. It is taken 1 to 3 hours before chemotherapy, then again 2 to 4 hours after chemotherapy as directed. The dose depends upon your size and whether you have any side effects. If you do not have any side effects but still have some nausea, the dose will be increased by your doctor. Keep the medicine in a tightly closed container away from heat and moisture and out of the reach of children and pets.

How Should I Take This Drug?
Take this drug exactly as directed by your doctor. If you do not understand the instructions, ask your doctor or nurse to explain them to you.

 Read the following information. If you do not understand it or if any of it causes you special concern, check with your doctor.

Before taking this drug, tell your doctor if you are taking any other prescription or over-the-counter drugs, including vitamins and herbals.

Should I avoid any other medicines, foods, alcohol, and/or activities?
Your prescription and nonprescription medicines may interact with other drugs, causing harm. Certain foods or alcohol can also interact with drug products. Never begin taking a new medicine—prescription or nonprescription—without asking your doctor or nurse if it will interact with alcohol, food, or other medicines. Some drugs can cause drowsiness and affect activities such as driving.

Precautions:
Dronabinol can produce a physical and psychological dependency. Take only as directed by your doctor.

Dronabinol may cause changes in thought processes or mood, especially in the elderly. It should be used cautiously, if at all, in the elderly.

Tell all the doctors, dentists, and pharmacists you visit that you are taking this drug.
- -
- Most of the following side effects probably will not occur.
- Your doctor or nurse will want to discuss specific care instructions with you.
- They can help you understand these side effects and help you deal with them.

Side Effects:

More Common Side Effects
Mood changes
Disorientation
Drowsiness
Muddled thinking
Dizziness
Change in ability to perceive surroundings
Decreased coordination
Dry mouth
Increased appetite

Less Common Side Effects
Increased heart rate
Decreased blood pressure when changing position

Side Effects / Symptoms of the Drug
Be careful getting up, changing position, or when walking.

Report any problems in thinking, movement, or dizziness.

Other side effects not listed above can also occur in some patients.
Tell your doctor or nurse if you develop any problems.

FDA Approval: Yes

droperidol

Trade Name:
Inapsine

Type of Drug:
Droperidol belongs to a general class of drugs called butyrophenones that are used to treat nausea and vomiting.

How Drug Works:
Droperidol is useful in preventing nausea and vomiting resulting from chemotherapy. It blocks messages to the part of the brain responsible for nausea and vomiting. Its main use is before surgery and as a person is being put to sleep for surgery.

How Drug Is Given:
Droperidol is given as an injection in a vein or muscle. It can be used before surgery to help you relax and sleep. The dose depends on your size.

 Read the following information. If you do not understand it or if any of it causes you special concern, check with your doctor.

Before taking this drug, tell your doctor if you are taking any other prescription or over-the-counter drugs, including vitamins and herbals.

Should I avoid any other medicines, foods, alcohol, and/or activities?
Your prescription and nonprescription medicines may interact with other drugs, causing harm. Certain foods or alcohol can also interact with drug products. Never begin taking a new medicine—prescription or non-prescription—without asking your doctor or nurse if it will interact with alcohol, food, or other medicines. Some drugs can cause drowsiness and affect activities such as driving.

Precautions:
Droperidol will make you feel very sleepy. Do not drive or operate heavy machinery when you are drowsy.

Droperidol can cause extrapyramidal side effects. These include restlessness, tongue protrusion, and involuntary movements. These side effects stop when you are given diphenhydramine hydrochloride.

Tell all the doctors, dentists, and pharmacists you visit that you are taking this drug.
- -
- Most of the following side effects probably will not occur.
- Your doctor or nurse will want to discuss specific care instructions with you.
- They can help you understand these side effects and help you deal with them.

Side Effects:

More Common Side Effects
Feeling sedated
Sleepiness
Decreased blood pressure

Less Common Side Effects
Decreased breathing rate
Increased heart rate

Rare Side Effects
Cough
Chills
Facial sweating
Shivering

Side Effects / Symptoms of the Drug
Be careful getting up, changing position, or walking. Do not drive a motor vehicle when taking this drug.

Other side effects not listed above can also occur in some patients.
Tell your doctor or nurse if you develop any problems.

FDA Approval: Yes

erythromycin

Trade Names:
ERYC, E-mycin, Erythrocin, Illotycin

Type of Drug:
Erythromycin is an antibiotic belonging to the general class of macrolide antibiotics. It is active against gram-positive and gram-negative bacteria, as well as other organisms.

How Drug Works:
Erythromycin causes bacteria to stop growing and dividing. At higher doses, erythromycin can kill the bacteria.

How Drug Is Given:
Erythromycin can be given by injection or by mouth. As an injection, the medicine is given into a vein over 60 minutes 4 times a day for 7 to 10 days. Do not drink alcohol when taking erythromycin by vein. By mouth, erythromycin is available as a capsule, pill, chewable tablet, or liquid. Take erythromycin by mouth 3 to 4 times a day for 10 days as directed by your doctor. Take it with a full glass of water. Be sure to ask if you can take it with food; some types can be and others need to be taken 1 hour before or 2 hours after eating. Swallow the pill or capsule whole and do not crush it. Make sure you shake the liquid well before pouring the dose. The dose and number of days you take the medicine depends on the type of infection, how well your liver is working, and whether you have any hearing problems. Keep the medicine in a tightly closed container away from heat and moisture and out of the reach of children and pets.

How Should I Take This Drug?
Take this drug exactly as directed by your doctor. If you do not understand the instructions, ask your doctor or nurse to explain them to you.

 Read the following information. If you do not understand it or if any of it causes you special concern, check with your doctor.

Before taking this drug, tell your doctor if you are taking any other prescription or over-the-counter drugs, including vitamins and herbals.

Should I avoid any other medicines, foods, alcohol, and/or activities?
Your prescription and nonprescription medicines may interact with other drugs, causing harm. Certain foods or alcohol can also interact with drug products. Never begin taking a new medicine—prescription or nonprescription—without asking your doctor or nurse if it will interact with alcohol, food, or other medicines. Some drugs can cause drowsiness and affect activities such as driving.

Precautions:
Tell your doctor if you have any drug allergies, especially to antibiotic drugs.

All antibiotics can cause allergic reactions. Stop the drug and tell your doctor or nurse right away if you develop a rash, hives, red blotches on your skin, difficulty breathing, or chest tightness.

Use of antibiotics can change the normal organisms in your body. Women are at risk for fungal infections. Tell your nurse or doctor if you have vaginal itching or discharge.

Erythromycin can interact with other medicines. Be sure to tell your doctor about all the medicines you are taking, especially if you are taking warfarin (Coumadin), seizure medicines, aminophylline, or theophylline.

Tell your doctor if you have any hearing loss, as erythromycin may cause further loss of hearing.

Tell all the doctors, dentists, and pharmacists you visit that you are taking this drug.
- -
- Most of the following side effects probably will not occur.
- Your doctor or nurse will want to discuss specific care instructions with you.
- They can help you understand these side effects and help you deal with them.

Side Effects:

More Common Side Effects
Nausea

Diarrhea

Loss of appetite

Irritation of the vein used for intravenous injection

Pain at the intravenous injection site

Less Common Side Effects
Vomiting

Liver problems with fever, nausea, skin rash, stomach pain, weakness, yellow eyes or skin, and vomiting

Rare Side Effects
Inflammation of the pancreas with severe abdominal pain

Muscle aches

Severe allergic reaction with fever, chills, rash, swelling of face or throat, and difficulty breathing

Diarrhea related to infection of the intestinal lining (pseudomembranous colitis)

Irregular heartbeat

Loss of hearing (high frequency sounds)

Dizziness

Unsteady gait

Ringing in the ears (tinnitus)

Side Effects / Symptoms of the Drug
Stop the drug and call your doctor or nurse right away if you have severe diarrhea, vomiting, or swelling of the face or throat.

Stop the drug and tell your doctor or nurse right away if you develop a rash, hives, fever, chills, red blotches on skin, difficulty breathing, or swelling.

Other side effects not listed above can also occur in some patients.
Tell your doctor or nurse if you develop any problems.

FDA Approval: Yes

etidronate disodium

Trade Name:
Didronel

Type of Drug:
Etidronate disodium belongs to a class of calcium-lowering drugs called biphosphonates. It is used to treat high calcium blood levels in patients with metastatic disease.

How Drug Works:
Etidronate disodium prevents bone from breaking down, so calcium is not released into the blood.

How Drug Is Given:
Etidronate disodium can be given by an injection in a vein or as a pill. The injection is given over 2 hours. The pill is given by mouth once a day, or in divided doses if you feel sick to your stomach. Take the pill with a large glass of juice or water 2 hours before a meal. Do not take with milk or milk products as this can lessen the effect. The dose depends on your size and weight, and your doctor may change the dose based on how you respond. Keep the medicine in a tightly closed container away from heat and moisture and out of the reach of children and pets.

How Should I Take This Drug?
Take this drug exactly as directed by your doctor. If you do not understand the instructions, ask your doctor or nurse to explain them to you.

 Read the following information. If you do not understand it or if any of it causes you special concern, check with your doctor.

Before taking this drug, tell your doctor if you are taking any other prescription or over-the-counter drugs, including vitamins and herbals.

Should I avoid any other medicines, foods, alcohol, and/or activities?
Your prescription and nonprescription medicines may interact with other drugs, causing harm. Certain foods or alcohol can also interact with drug products. Never begin taking a new medicine—prescription or nonprescription—without asking your doctor or nurse if it will interact with alcohol, food, or other medicines. Some drugs can cause drowsiness and affect activities such as driving.

Precautions:
You will probably also receive intravenous fluids, as it is important for your kidneys to make a lot of urine.

Tell all the doctors, dentists, and pharmacists you visit that you are taking this drug.

- Most of the following side effects probably will not occur.
- Your doctor or nurse will want to discuss specific care instructions with you.
- They can help you understand these side effects and help you deal with them.

Side Effects:

More Common Side Effects
Decreased blood level of magnesium and phosphorus

Less Common Side Effects
Increase in kidney function blood tests

Rare Side Effects
Diarrhea
Nausea
Vomiting
Abdominal pain
Rash

Other side effects not listed above can also occur in some patients.
Tell your doctor or nurse if you develop any problems.

FDA Approval: Yes

famciclovir

Trade Name:
Famvir

Type of Drug:
Famciclovir belongs to the general class of drugs called antivirals.

How Drug Works:
Famciclovir prevents viral DNA from being made. It is used in the treatment of a variety of herpes viruses.

How Drug Is Given:
Famciclovir is a tablet taken by mouth 2 to 3 times a day for 5 to 7 days as directed by your doctor. Take with a full glass of water, with or without food. The dose depends on how well your kidneys are working and on the infection being treated. Keep the medicine in a tightly closed container away from heat and moisture and out of the reach of children and pets.

How Should I Take This Drug?
Take this drug exactly as directed by your doctor. If you do not understand the instructions, ask your doctor or nurse to explain them to you.

 Read the following information. If you do not understand it or if any of it causes you special concern, check with your doctor.

Before taking this drug, tell your doctor if you are taking any other prescription or over-the-counter drugs, including vitamins and herbals.

Should I avoid any other medicines, foods, alcohol, and/or activities?
Your prescription and nonprescription medicines may interact with other drugs, causing harm. Certain foods or alcohol can also interact with drug products. Never begin taking a new medicine—prescription or non-prescription—without asking your doctor or nurse if it will interact with alcohol, food, or other medicines. Some drugs can cause drowsiness and affect activities such as driving.

Precautions:
Famciclovir is very well tolerated with few side effects.

Doses will likely be reduced if you have kidney disease.

Tell all the doctors, dentists, and pharmacists you visit that you are taking this drug.
- Most of the following side effects probably will not occur.
- Your doctor or nurse will want to discuss specific care instructions with you.
- They can help you understand these side effects and help you deal with them.

Side Effects:

More Common Side Effects
Headache

Less Common Side Effects
Nausea

Other side effects not listed above can also occur in some patients.
Tell your doctor or nurse if you develop any problems.

FDA Approval: Yes

fentanyl citrate

Trade Names:
Actiq, Oral Transmucosal Fentanyl

Type of Drug:
Fentanyl citrate is an opioid analgesic.

How Drug Works:
Fentanyl citrate relieves moderate to severe breakthrough pain; the pain relief is quick (onset within 5 minutes) with the maximum effect in 25 to 30 minutes. Fentanyl citrate binds to opioid receptors in the brain and central nervous system (CNS). It alters the perception of pain as well as the emotional response to it. The oral transmucosal fentanyl looks like a flat tablet attached to a handle. It is placed against the lining of the mouth (mucosa) where it is sucked, and the drug is absorbed into the blood.

How Drug Is Given:
Remove the medicine from its foil pouch right before you are going to use it. Put it in your mouth between the cheek and the lower gum. Suck the medicine from the handle over 15 minutes. You can move the medicine from one side of the mouth to the other, but don't chew or swallow it. If you feel better before the 15 minutes is up or if you feel dizzy or unwell, stop and take the medicine out of your mouth. Take the medicine off its stick, wrap it in toilet tissue, and flush it down the toilet. The strengths are color coded and the color of the wrapper tells you the dose of the medicine. The dose depends on the relief you get. If you need more than 3 doses, then your long-acting pain medicine dose needs to be increased. Keep the medicine in a tightly closed container away from heat and moisture and out of the reach of children and pets. Children and pets have died from taking the medicine by accident.

How Should I Take This Drug?
Take this drug exactly as directed by your doctor. If you do not understand these instructions, ask your doctor or nurse to explain them to you.

 Read the following information. If you do not understand it or if any of it causes you special concern, check with your doctor.

Before taking this drug, tell your doctor if you are taking any other prescription or over-the-counter drugs, including vitamins and herbals.

Should I avoid any other medicines, foods, alcohol, and/or activities?
Your prescription and nonprescription medicines may interact with other drugs, causing harm. Certain foods or alcohol can also interact with drug products. Never begin taking a new medicine—prescription or non-prescription—without asking your doctor or nurse if it will interact with alcohol, food, or other medicines. Some drugs can cause drowsiness and affect activities such as driving.

Precautions:
Fentanyl citrate is an effective and safe drug when used correctly. However, it can be dangerous, and the relevant safety points should be remembered. This drug is only for people who have taken opioid analgesic drugs before and have some tolerance to this type of medicine. Otherwise, it can cause breathing problems (slow breathing or breathing may stop).

Fentanyl citrate should not be used by people with head injury or increased pressure in the head, or by nursing mothers. The drug should be used cautiously in people with liver disease, kidney problems, chronic lung disease, heart disease (slow pulse), and the elderly. This drug MUST be kept out of the reach of children or pets, as it may be lethal to them.

Keep the medicine away from the eyes, skin, or other mucous membranes when not sucking the medication. Wash your hands after discarding any unused portion of the medicine.

Call your nurse or doctor if you take 4 of the same tablet within 60 minutes without relief, or if you find you have to take the drug more than 4 times a day to control your pain. The dose should probably be increased, and your doctor or nurse will tell you how to do this.

Since fentanyl citrate affects the central nervous system (CNS), it is important not to take other drugs or substances that are known CNS depressants such as alcohol, sedatives, and hypnotics.

You should be on a bowel regimen to prevent constipation while you are taking opioid pain relievers. Talk to your nurse or doctor about this.

Take the smallest effective dose to prevent the development of tolerance and physical dependence. Tolerance can develop (larger doses needed to give the same effect) as well as physical dependence (body goes into withdrawal if drug is suddenly stopped). This is different from addiction, which is psychological dependence (take drug for psychological effect not for the relief of pain). Tell your doctor or nurse if you still have pain even though you are taking the medicine as directed.

 Tell all the doctors, dentists, and pharmacists you visit that you are taking this drug.

- Most of the following side effects probably will not occur.
- Your doctor or nurse will want to discuss specific care instructions with you.
- They can help you understand these side effects and help you deal with them.

Side Effects:

More Common Side Effects

Sleepiness

Vomiting

Nausea

Dizziness

Constipation

Less Common Side Effects

Difficulty walking

Confusion

Nervousness

Headache

Feeling tired

Flushing

Decreased breathing rate

Depression

Difficulty sleeping

Fever

Changes in vision

Rare Side Effects

Muscle aches

Cough

Swelling of feet

Itching

Dehydration

Sore throat

Loss of appetite

Diarrhea

Rash

Stomach upset

Side Effects / Symptoms of the Drug

Stop taking the medicine and call your doctor or nurse right away if you have any difficulty breathing or walking.

Tell your doctor or nurse right away if the dose of the drug does not take away the pain, if you need to take the drug more than 4 times a day, or if you are constipated and have not moved your bowels in 2 or more days.

Other side effects not listed above can also occur in some patients.
Tell your doctor or nurse if you develop any problems.

FDA Approval: Yes

fentanyl transdermal system

Trade Name:
Duragesic

Type of Drug:
Fentanyl transdermal system is an opioid analgesic.

How Drug Works:
Fentanyl transdermal system relieves moderate to severe pain. Fentanyl binds to opioid receptors in the brain and central nervous system, altering the perception of pain as well as the emotional response to pain. Fentanyl transdermal system is a patch. The patch is placed on the skin, and the drug is absorbed through the skin.

How Drug Is Given:
Fentanyl transdermal system is a patch that has the medicine inside it. When you first start the patch, you will not feel its effect for 17 to 20 hours, so you need to take other pain medicine until the patch starts working. The patch is put firmly on the skin. First, find a good place on your body to put the patch; it should be clean, flat, and without any skin injury, bumps, etc. The best sites to apply the patch are on the chest below the collar bones, on your back, or on the tops of your arms. Choose sites that will not bend or wrinkle a lot. Avoid skin that is irritated or has been radiated. You can clip any of the hair at the site but do not shave it. Then, press the patch firmly to the skin, and keep the palm of your hand pressed on the patch for at least 30 to 60 seconds. Make sure that all the edges stick to your skin. Some people like to tape the patch to the skin with paper tape or put a film dressing over it. If it is very hot and you sweat a lot, you may need to use a sticky solution like Skin Prep or benzoin. Ask your nurse or doctor about this. Write the date and time on the white sticker that comes with the patch. When you shower, you can cover the patch with plastic wrap lightly taped over it, or you may not have to use anything. The patch should be left on for 3 days. Try to change the patch at about the same time of the day. Sometimes, especially if you have high fevers, you may need to change the patch every 2 days. When you remove the old patch, gently pull it off the skin and then fold it in half back on itself. Flush it down the toilet in case there is some drug left in it. Keep the box of unopened patches in a safe place and out of the reach of children or pets. The dose depends on how much opioid medicine you needed before to control your pain. If you did not get good control with the other medicine, the patch dose should be higher than the pill dose; the right dose is the dose that controls your pain.

How Should I Take This Drug?
Take this drug exactly as directed by your doctor. If you do not understand these instructions, ask your doctor or nurse to explain them to you.

 Read the following information. If you do not understand it or if any of it causes you special concern, check with your doctor.

Before taking this drug, tell your doctor if you are taking any other prescription or over-the-counter drugs, including vitamins and herbals.

Should I avoid any other medicines, foods, alcohol, and/or activities?
Your prescription and nonprescription medicines may interact with other drugs, causing harm. Certain foods or alcohol can also interact with drug products. Never begin taking a new medicine—prescription or nonprescription—without asking your doctor or nurse if it will interact with alcohol, food, or other medicines. Some drugs can cause drowsiness and affect activities such as driving.

Precautions:
If you have never taken opioid pain relievers before, your doctor will start you at the lowest dose. Keep a record of the pain relievers you are taking so that you can show it to your doctor or nurse. This will help in determining the best dosage for you.

Since fentanyl transdermal system affects the central nervous system (CNS), it is important not to take other drugs or substances that are known CNS depressants such as alcohol, sedatives, and hypnotics.

You should be on a bowel regimen to prevent constipation while you are taking opioid pain relievers. Talk to your nurse or doctor about this.

Acetaminophen or aspirin may be combined with fentanyl transdermal system to increase the pain relief action.

Take the smallest effective dose to prevent development of tolerance and physical dependence. Tolerance can develop (larger doses are needed to give the same effect) as well as physical dependence (body goes into withdrawal if drug is suddenly stopped). This is different from addiction, which is psychological dependence (taking drug for psychological effect, not for relief of pain). Tell your doctor or nurse if you still have pain even though you are taking the medicine as directed.

Tell all the doctors, dentists, and pharmacists you visit that you are taking this drug.

- Most of the following side effects probably will not occur.
- Your doctor or nurse will want to discuss specific care instructions with you.
- They can help you understand these side effects and help you deal with them.

Side Effects:

More Common Side Effects
Sleepiness   Dizziness
Constipation   Nausea

Less Common Side Effects
Difficulty breathing   Decreased breathing rate
Confusion   Depression
Tremors   Lack of coordination
Euphoria   Difficulty speaking
Vomiting   Chest pain
Decreased blood pressure   Sweating
   when changing positions Rash
Difficulty urinating   Itching

Rare Side Effects
Blood-tinged sputum   Sore throat
Hiccups   Asthma
Hallucinations   Headache

Side Effects / Symptoms of the Drug
Tell your doctor or nurse right away if you have any difficulty breathing, in passing your urine, or walking. Report any other problems.

Tell your doctor or nurse if you have skin problems where you apply the patch. They will tell you ways to prevent this.

Other side effects not listed above can also occur in some patients.
Tell your doctor or nurse if you develop any problems.

FDA Approval: Yes

fluconazole

Trade Name:
Diflucan

Type of Drug:
Fluconazole is an antifungal drug that belongs to the azole class.

How Drug Works:
Fluconazole prevents fungi from reproducing. It also injures the cell wall, so the cell cannot get the nutrients it needs to live.

How Drug Is Given:
Fluconazole can be given by an injection in the vein, or as a pill or liquid by mouth. When given as an injection, it is given once a day, as an infusion over a few hours (not more than about 7 oz an hour). The pill or liquid is taken once a day with a large glass of water. Make sure to shake the liquid before pouring the dose. The dose depends on the type of infection being treated and how well your kidneys are working. The first dose is usually 2 times the daily dose to get the blood level up quickly. Keep the medicine in a tightly closed container away from heat and moisture and out of the reach of children and pets.

How Should I Take This Drug?
Take this drug exactly as directed by your doctor. If you do not understand the instructions, ask your doctor or nurse to explain them to you.

 Read the following information. If you do not understand it or if any of it causes you special concern, check with your doctor.

Before taking this drug, tell your doctor if you are taking any other prescription or over-the-counter drugs, including vitamins and herbals.

Should I avoid any other medicines, foods, alcohol, and/or activities?
Your prescription and nonprescription medicines may interact with other drugs, causing harm. Certain foods or alcohol can also interact with drug products. Never begin taking a new medicine—prescription or nonprescription—without asking your doctor or nurse if it will interact with alcohol, food, or other medicines. Some drugs can cause drowsiness and affect activities such as driving.

Precautions:
Your dose may need to be reduced if you have kidney problems.

Tell your doctor if you are also taking warfarin (Coumadin), phenytoin (Dilantin), cyclosporine, rifampin, sulfonylurea antidiabetic agents, or thiazide diuretics. Talk to your doctor about possible drug interactions.

All drugs used to fight microorganisms can cause allergic reactions. Stop the drug and tell your nurse or doctor right away if you develop a rash, hives, red blotches on your skin, difficulty breathing, or chest pain.

Tell all the doctors, dentists, and pharmacists you visit that you are taking this drug.

- Most of the following side effects probably will not occur.
- Your doctor or nurse will want to discuss specific care instructions with you.
- They can help you understand these side effects and help you deal with them.

Side Effects:

Less Common Side Effects
Mild nausea
Mild vomiting
Diarrhea
Abdominal pain
Abnormal liver function blood tests
Dizziness
Headache

Rare Side Effects
Loss of appetite
Heartburn
Dry mouth
Abdominal bloating
Rash
Itching
Darkening and peeling of skin
Sleepiness
Feeling "blah"
Tiredness (fatigue)
Seizure
Psychiatric disturbances
Liver problems

Side Effects / Symptoms of the Drug
Call your doctor or nurse if you develop rash, fever, or chills. Your doctor needs to evaluate you.

Other side effects not listed above can also occur in some patients.
Tell your doctor or nurse if you develop any problems.

FDA Approval: Yes

flucytosine

Trade Name:
Ancobon

Type of Drug:
Flucytosine is an antifungal drug used to treat fungus infections.

How Drug Works:
Flucytosine interferes with cell division and prevents fungus from reproducing.

How Drug Is Given:
Flucytosine is given as a capsule by mouth in 4 divided doses a day. Take with a full glass of water. Do not crush or open the capsule. If you get sick to your stomach and if you are taking more than 1 capsule at a time, try spacing them out over 15 minutes. Also, remember to take your antinausea medicine 1 hour before the dose. The dose depends on the infection being treated and how well your kidneys are working. Keep the medicine in a tightly closed container away from heat and moisture and out of the reach of children and pets.

How Should I Take This Drug?
Take this drug exactly as directed by your doctor. If you do not understand the instructions, ask your doctor or nurse to explain them to you.

 Read the following information. If you do not understand it or if any of it causes you special concern, check with your doctor.

Before taking this drug, tell your doctor if you are taking any other prescription or over-the-counter drugs, including vitamins and herbals.

Should I avoid any other medicines, foods, alcohol, and/or activities?
Your prescription and nonprescription medicines may interact with other drugs, causing harm. Certain foods or alcohol can also interact with drug products. Never begin taking a new medicine—prescription or non-prescription—without asking your doctor or nurse if it will interact with alcohol, food, or other medicines. Some drugs can cause drowsiness and affect activities such as driving.

Precautions:
All drugs used to fight microorganisms can cause allergic reactions. Stop the drug and tell your nurse or doctor right away if you develop a rash, hives, red blotches on your skin, difficulty breathing, or chest tightness.

The risks and benefits of the drug should be carefully considered before using it in women who are pregnant.

Tell all the doctors, dentists, and pharmacists you visit that you are taking this drug.

- Most of the following side effects probably will not occur.
- Your doctor or nurse will want to discuss specific care instructions with you.
- They can help you understand these side effects and help you deal with them.

Side Effects:

More Common Side Effects
Sore throat
Sores in mouth or on lips
Diarrhea
Nausea

Less Common Side Effects
Decreased white blood cell count with increased risk of infection
Decreased platelet count with increased risk of bleeding
Decreased red blood cell count with increased risk of anemia and tiredness (fatigue)
Vomiting
Loss of appetite
Abdominal bloating
Increase in liver function blood tests

Rare Side Effects
Aplastic anemia
Bowel rupture following severe diarrhea
Redness of skin
Itching
Abdominal pain
Confusion
Sleepiness
Headache
Fever

Side Effects / Symptoms of the Drug
Stop the drug and call your doctor or nurse right away if you get redness of the skin, itching, fever, increased heart rate, dizziness, and/or abdominal pain. Your doctor needs to evaluate you.

Other side effects not listed above can also occur in some patients.
Tell your doctor or nurse if you develop any problems.

FDA Approval: Yes

fluoxetine hydrochloride

Trade Name:
Prozac

Type of Drug:
Fluoxetine hydrochloride belongs to a general class of drugs called antidepressants. It is used to treat anxiety or depression.

How Drug Works:
Fluoxetine hydrochloride stops the uptake of serotonin at the nerve endings in the brain. This decreases the feeling of depression.

How Drug Is Given:
Fluoxetine hydrochloride is taken by mouth once in the morning, or in 2 divided doses in the morning and at noontime. The medicine comes as a pill or liquid that should be taken with a glass of water, with or without food. Do not drink alcohol while taking this drug. The dose depends on your age, how well your liver is working, and other medicines you are taking. Keep the medicine in a tightly closed container away from heat and moisture and out of the reach of children and pets.

How Should I Take This Drug?
Take this drug exactly as directed by your doctor. If you do not understand the instructions, ask your doctor or nurse to explain them to you.

 Read the following information. If you do not understand it or if any of it causes you special concern, check with your doctor.

Before taking this drug, tell your doctor if you are taking any other prescription or over-the-counter drugs, including vitamins and herbals.

Should I avoid any other medicines, foods, alcohol, and/or activities?
Your prescription and nonprescription medicines may interact with other drugs, causing harm. Certain foods or alcohol can also interact with drug products. Never begin taking a new medicine—prescription or nonprescription—without asking your doctor or nurse if it will interact with alcohol, food, or other medicines. Some drugs can cause drowsiness and affect activities such as driving.

Precautions:
DO NOT drink alcohol while taking this drug.

Tell your doctor if you are taking any of the following drugs as they may have serious interactions with fluoxetine hydrochloride: other antidepressant drugs, carbamazepine (Tegretol), dextromethorphan, diazepam, digoxin, lithium, phenytoin (Dilantin), tryptophan, or warfarin (Coumadin).

Once you start taking fluoxetine hydrochloride, it may take up to 4 weeks before you feel the full effect of the drug.

The drug should not be given to women who are pregnant or breastfeeding.

It is very important that you wait 2 weeks between stopping antidepressants classified as monoamine oxidase inhibitors and starting fluoxetine hydrochloride. Talk to your doctor or nurse about this. If you stop fluoxetine hydrochloride and are going to start a monoamine oxidase inhibitor, you must wait 5 weeks.

Tell all the doctors, dentists, and pharmacists you visit that you are taking this drug.
- Most of the following side effects probably will not occur.
- Your doctor or nurse will want to discuss specific care instructions with you.
- They can help you understand these side effects and help you deal with them.

Side Effects:

More Common Side Effects
Headache

Less Common Side Effects
Difficulty sleeping
Anxiety
Decreased ability to concentrate
Tremors
Dizziness
Nausea
Loss of appetite
Weight loss in underweight individuals
Muscle or bone pain

Rare Side Effects
Rash
Hives
Abnormal dreams
Tiredness (fatigue)
Blurred vision
Seizures
Vomiting
Constipation
Dry mouth
Changes in taste
Decreased coordination
Decreased mental alertness
Decreased sexual ability
Difficulty breathing
Chest or arm pain
Nasal congestion
Pain in muscles, joints, and/or back
Flu-like symptoms

Other side effects not listed above can also occur in some patients.
Tell your doctor or nurse if you develop any problems.

FDA Approval: Yes

foscarnet sodium

Trade Name:
Foscavir

Type of Drug:
Foscarnet sodium belongs to the general class of drugs called antivirals.

How Drug Works:
Foscarnet sodium prevents reproduction of viruses. Foscarnet sodium is used for herpes viruses that do not respond to other treatment and viral eye infection (CMV retinitis).

How Drug Is Given:
Foscarnet sodium is given as an injection in the vein. When starting the treatment, foscarnet is given 3 times a day over at least 1 hour (induction) for 2 to 3 weeks; it is then given once a day over 2 hours. The dose depends on the infection being treated, your weight, and how well your kidneys are working.

 Read the following information. If you do not understand it or if any of it causes you special concern, check with your doctor.

Before taking this drug, tell your doctor if you are taking any other prescription or over-the-counter drugs, including vitamins and herbals.

Should I avoid any other medicines, foods, alcohol, and/or activities?
Your prescription and nonprescription medicines may interact with other drugs, causing harm. Certain foods or alcohol can also interact with drug products. Never begin taking a new medicine—prescription or non-prescription—without asking your doctor or nurse if it will interact with alcohol, food, or other medicines. Some drugs can cause drowsiness and affect activities such as driving.

Precautions:
Your doctor will check your kidney function before you get this drug and frequently during treatment.

Foscarnet sodium may decrease blood minerals. Tell your nurse or doctor if you notice tingling around your mouth, numbness, or a sensation of pins and needles.

Tell your doctor if you are also receiving pentamidine, amphotericin B, aminoglycoside antibiotics, or hypocalcemic agents, as you should not receive foscarnet sodium.

Tell all the doctors, dentists, and pharmacists you visit that you are taking this drug.
- Most of the following side effects probably will not occur.
- Your doctor or nurse will want to discuss specific care instructions with you.
- They can help you understand these side effects and help you deal with them.

Side Effects:

More Common Side Effects
Abnormal kidney function tests
Headache
Dizziness
Decreased red blood cell count with increased risk of anemia and tiredness (fatigue)
Nausea
Vomiting
Diarrhea

Less Common Side Effects
Numbness or tingling in hands and/or feet
Seizures
Loss of appetite
Abdominal pain
Decreased white blood cell count with increased risk of infection
Irritation of vein used for giving the drug
Rash
Sweating
Low calcium blood level

Rare Side Effects
Irritation of vagina
Irritation of skin of penis
Difficulty concentrating

Side Effects / Symptoms of the Drug
Tell your doctor or nurse right away if you think you have a temperature over 100.5°F or have chills.

Tell your doctor or nurse if you have nausea or vomiting. Other medicines to prevent this problem can be given.

Other side effects not listed above can also occur in some patients.
Tell your doctor or nurse if you develop any problems.

FDA Approval: Yes

furosemide

Trade Name:
Lasix

Type of Drug:
Furosemide belongs to a class of drugs called diuretics.

How Drug Works:
Furosemide prevents the kidneys from reabsorbing sodium and chloride to help control a buildup of fluid in the body and it increases the excretion of calcium to help treat hypercalcemia.

How Drug Is Given:
Furosemide can be given as a pill or an injection in a vein. The dose and how it is given depend on how much fluid the doctor wants to remove and how quickly. Keep the medicine in a tightly closed container away from heat and moisture and out of the reach of children and pets.

How Should I Take This Drug?
Take this drug exactly as directed by your doctor. If you do not understand the instructions, ask your doctor or nurse to explain them to you.

 Read the following information. If you do not understand it or if any of it causes you special concern, check with your doctor.

Before taking this drug, tell your doctor if you are taking any other prescription or over-the-counter drugs, including vitamins and herbals.

Should I avoid any other medicines, foods, alcohol, and/or activities?
Your prescription and nonprescription medicines may interact with other drugs, causing harm. Certain foods or alcohol can also interact with drug products. Never begin taking a new medicine—prescription or non-prescription—without asking your doctor or nurse if it will interact with alcohol, food, or other medicines. Some drugs can cause drowsiness and affect activities such as driving.

Precautions:
Furosemide often takes with it other electrolytes (potassium, chloride, magnesium), which your body needs. Thus, your doctor may add these electrolytes to your intravenous fluid, or give it to you separately to replace the lost electrolytes.

The drug should not be used in women who are pregnant or breastfeeding.

If you are taking furosemide to help remove calcium from the blood, you will receive an intravenous infusion of salt water (normal saline). Furosemide helps your kidneys excrete this salt water, and the water takes the calcium with it out of your body.

Tell all the doctors, dentists, and pharmacists you visit that you are taking this drug.
- -
- Most of the following side effects probably will not occur.
- Your doctor or nurse will want to discuss specific care instructions with you.
- They can help you understand these side effects and help you deal with them.

Side Effects:

More Common Side Effects
Loss of potassium from the blood (hypokalemia)
Loss of chloride from the blood (hypochloremia)
Increased uric acid in the blood
Loss of magnesium from the blood (hypomagnesemia)

Less Common Side Effects
Ringing in the ears (tinnitus), especially if high doses are used
Decreased hearing, especially if high doses are used
Headache

Rare Side Effects
Numbness and tingling in the hands and/or feet
Dizziness when standing
Increased sensitivity to sunlight
Hives
Rash
Itching

Side Effects / Symptoms of the Drug
Tell your doctor or nurse right away if you get ringing in your ears (tinnitus) or if you think your hearing is decreased.

Other side effects not listed above can also occur in some patients.
Tell your doctor or nurse if you develop any problems.

FDA Approval: Yes

gabapentin

Trade Name:
Neurontin

Type of Drug:
Gabapentin is a nonopioid analgesic that belongs to a general class of drugs called anticonvulsants.

How Drug Works:
It is not known how gabapentin works. It is useful in the treatment of neuropathic pain.

How Drug Is Given:
Gabapentin is a capsule taken by mouth 3 times a day. The dose depends on how much is needed to control the pain. Take with or without food, with a glass of water. Keep the medicine in a tightly closed container away from heat and moisture and out of the reach of children and pets.

How Should I Take This Drug?
Take this drug exactly as directed by your doctor. If you do not understand the instructions, ask your doctor or nurse to explain them to you.

 Read the following information. If you do not understand it or if any of it causes you special concern, check with your doctor.

Before taking this drug, tell your doctor if you are taking any other prescription or over-the-counter drugs, including vitamins and herbals.

Should I avoid any other medicines, foods, alcohol, and/or activities?
Your prescription and nonprescription medicines may interact with other drugs, causing harm. Certain foods or alcohol can also interact with drug products. Never begin taking a new medicine—prescription or nonprescription—without asking your doctor or nurse if it will interact with alcohol, food, or other medicines. Some drugs can cause drowsiness and affect activities such as driving.

Precautions:
The dose of gabapentin will need to be reduced if your kidney function decreases (renal insufficiency).

The dose will gradually be increased over about 3 days until an effective dose is reached.

Gabapentin can cause dizziness, tiredness, drowsiness, and difficulty walking. Until you know how the drug affects you, avoid driving or handling heavy machinery.

Tell all the doctors, dentists, and pharmacists you visit that you are taking this drug.
- Most of the following side effects probably will not occur.
- Your doctor or nurse will want to discuss specific care instructions with you.
- They can help you understand these side effects and help you deal with them.

Side Effects:

More Common Side Effects
Sleepiness
Dizziness
Tiredness (fatigue)

Less Common Side Effects
Difficulty walking
Tremors
Nervousness
Difficulty speaking
Amnesia
Depression
Headache
Confusion
Mood swings
Numbness in hands and/or feet
Decreased reflexes
Irritability
Heartburn
Nausea
Vomiting
Rash
Hair thinning

Rare Side Effects
Double vision
Increased sensitivity to sunlight
Constipation
Thirst
Increased saliva in the mouth
Cough
Nosebleeds
Changes in menstrual periods
Change in blood pressure
Chest pain

Dry eyes
Hearing loss
Change in appetite and taste
Sores in mouth or on lips
Runny nose
Difficulty breathing
Difficulty in passing your urine
Changes in sexual functioning
Increased heart rate

Side Effects / Symptoms of the Drug
Call your doctor or nurse right away if you have difficulty walking, difficulty in passing your urine, develop a rash, have changes in vision, or get any other problems taking the drug.

Other side effects not listed above can also occur in some patients.
Tell your doctor or nurse if you develop any problems.

FDA Approval: Yes

gallium nitrate

Trade Name:
Ganite

Type of Drug:
Gallium nitrate belongs to a general class of drugs called hypocalcemic agents.

How Drug Works:
Gallium nitrate stops the release of calcium from the bones by blocking bone breakdown.

How Drug Is Given:
Gallium nitrate is given as an injection in a vein continuously over 24 hours. The dose depends on your size, how well your kidneys are working, and how serious the high calcium is.

 Read the following information. If you do not understand it or if any of it causes you special concern, check with your doctor.

Before taking this drug, tell your doctor if you are taking any other prescription or over-the-counter drugs, including vitamins and herbals.

Should I avoid any other medicines, foods, alcohol, and/or activities?
Your prescription and nonprescription medicines may interact with other drugs, causing harm. Certain foods or alcohol can also interact with drug products. Never begin taking a new medicine—prescription or non-prescription—without asking your doctor or nurse if it will interact with alcohol, food, or other medicines. Some drugs can cause drowsiness and affect activities such as driving.

Precautions:
This drug should not be given to patients with severe kidney dysfunction.

Gallium nitrate may be given if your calcium level stays high after receiving intravenous salt water and furosemide.

Tell all the doctors, dentists, and pharmacists you visit that you are taking this drug.
- Most of the following side effects probably will not occur.
- Your doctor or nurse will want to discuss specific care instructions with you.
- They can help you understand these side effects and help you deal with them.

Side Effects:

More Common Side Effects
Temporary decrease in blood levels of phosphate and bicarbonate

Less Common Side Effects
Abnormal kidney function blood tests
Diarrhea
Nausea
Constipation

Rare Side Effects
Kidney damage
Vomiting

Other side effects not listed above can also occur in some patients.
Tell your doctor or nurse if you develop any problems.

FDA Approval: Yes

ganciclovir

Trade Name:
Cytovene

Type of Drug:
Ganciclovir belongs to the general class of drugs called antivirals.

How Drug Works:
Ganciclovir prevents viruses from reproducing. It is used to treat herpes viruses, Epstein Barr virus, and cytomegalovirus (CMV).

How Drug Is Given:
Ganciclovir is given as an injection in the vein over at least 1 hour, every 12 hours for 14 to 21 days to start, and then for "maintenance" once a day either 5 or 7 days a week. The dose depends upon your size and how well your kidneys are working. You need to drink lots of fluid to keep your kidneys flushed out. You may need to have fluids given intravenously. The dose may need to be steady if you have problems taking the drug (low white blood cell count, low platelet count, or high kidney blood tests).

 Read the following information. If you do not understand it or if any of it causes you special concern, check with your doctor.

Before taking this drug, tell your doctor if you are taking any other prescription or over-the-counter drugs, including vitamins and herbals.

Should I avoid any other medicines, foods, alcohol, and/or activities?
Your prescription and nonprescription medicines may interact with other drugs, causing harm. Certain foods or alcohol can also interact with drug products. Never begin taking a new medicine—prescription or non-prescription—without asking your doctor or nurse if it will interact with alcohol, food, or other medicines. Some drugs can cause drowsiness and affect activities such as driving.

Precautions:
If you are getting ganciclovir for an eye infection (CMV retinitis), tell your doctor or nurse right away if you have any changes in your vision. During treatment, you may be asked to see an eye doctor at regular intervals.

All drugs used to treat infections can cause allergic reactions. Stop the drug and tell your nurse or doctor right away if you develop a rash, hives, red blotches on your skin, difficulty breathing, or chest pain.

Ganciclovir can irritate the veins used for giving the drug. Your doctor or nurse may advise you to have a large catheter (central line) inserted to protect the veins in your arms and make it easier to give the drug.

It is important to have enough water in your body. Try to drink 2 to 3 quarts of fluid a day. It may be necessary to get IV fluids if you are not able to drink enough liquids.

This drug should not be used during pregnancy.

Ganciclovir can lower your blood counts (white blood cells, red blood cells, platelets). Your doctor will check your blood counts before and after each treatment to see its effect. Your doctor or nurse will give you specific instructions if they are low.

Tell all the doctors, dentists, and pharmacists you visit that you are taking this drug.

- Most of the following side effects probably will not occur.
- Your doctor or nurse will want to discuss specific care instructions with you.
- They can help you understand these side effects and help you deal with them.

Side Effects:

More Common Side Effects
Irritation of vein used for giving the drug
Decreased white blood cells with increased risk of infection
Decreased platelets with increased risk of bleeding
Detachment of the retina in the eye

Less Common Side Effects
Headache
Confusion
Abnormal dreams
Dizziness
Difficulty walking

Rare Side Effects
Nausea
Vomiting
Diarrhea
Loss of appetite
Increased kidney function tests
Change in blood pressure
Irregular heartbeat
Rash
Fever
Decreased red blood cell count with increased risk of anemia and tiredness (fatigue)
Infertility in males

Side Effects / Symptoms of the Drug
Tell your doctor nurse right away if you get a rash or fever.

Other side effects not listed above can also occur in some patients.
Tell your doctor or nurse if you develop any problems.

FDA Approval: Yes

gentamycin sulfate

Trade Names:
Garamycin, Gentamycin

Type of Drug:
Gentamycin sulfate is an antibiotic that belongs to the group of drugs called aminoglycosides.

How Drug Works:
Gentamycin sulfate appears to prevent bacteria from making their cell walls, causing the cells die. It is used to treat many sensitive gram-negative and some gram-positive bacteria.

How Drug Is Given:
Gentamycin sulfate is given as an injection in the muscle or in a vein over at least 1 hour. The dose depends on the level of the drug in your blood, how well your kidneys are working, and your weight.

 Read the following information. If you do not understand it or if any of it causes you special concern, check with your doctor.

Before taking this drug, tell your doctor if you are taking any other prescription or over-the-counter drugs, including vitamins and herbals.

Should I avoid any other medicines, foods, alcohol, and/or activities?
Your prescription and nonprescription medicines may interact with other drugs, causing harm. Certain foods or alcohol can also interact with drug products. Never begin taking a new medicine—prescription or nonprescription—without asking your doctor or nurse if it will interact with alcohol, food, or other medicines. Some drugs can cause drowsiness and affect activities such as driving.

Precautions:
Gentamycin sulfate may injure the nerve for hearing (eighth cranial nerve, auditory). Tell your doctor or nurse right away if you feel dizzy, have difficulty walking, ringing in your ears, a roaring sound in your ears, or any decrease in hearing. The drug should be stopped and changed to another effective drug without this problem.

Gentamycin sulfate may injure your kidneys. Your doctor will monitor blood tests to find this early if it occurs. Make sure you tell your doctor if you have ever had any kidney problems.

Tell your doctor if you have any allergies, especially to antibiotic drugs.

All antibiotics can cause allergic reactions. Stop the drug and tell your nurse or doctor right away if you develop a rash, hives, or red blotches on your skin. Stop the drug and tell your doctor or nurse right away if you have any difficulty breathing or have chest pain.

Use of antibiotics can change the normal organisms in your body. Women are at risk of getting fungal infections. Tell your nurse or doctor if you get vaginal itching or discharge.

This drug should be used during pregnancy only if infection is life-threatening and no safer drug exists.

Tell all the doctors, dentists, and pharmacists you visit that you are taking this drug.

- Most of the following side effects probably will not occur.
- Your doctor or nurse will want to discuss specific care instructions with you.
- They can help you understand these side effects and help you deal with them.

Side Effects:

More Common Side Effects
Nausea
Headache
Feeling drowsy or sleepy

Less Common Side Effects
Dizziness
Ringing in the ears (tinnitis)
Roaring sound in the ears
Difficulty walking
Decreased appetite
Kidney damage

Rare Side Effects
Diarrhea related to infection of the intestinal lining (pseudomembranous colitis)
Decreased hearing
Tingling of skin
Vomiting
Decreased blood counts (white blood cells, red blood cells, platelets)
Rash
Hives
Fever

Side Effects / Symptoms of the Drug
Stop the drug and call your doctor or nurse right away if you get a rash, hives, fever, chills, muscle aches, and/or peeling of your skin. This can be a serious reaction and needs to be treated right away.

Stop the drug and call your doctor or nurse right away if you get diarrhea that does not stop, abdominal cramping, and blood and/or pus in the stool. This needs to be treated right away.

Stop the drug and report immediately any ringing or roaring sounds in your ears or hearing loss.

Other side effects not listed above can also occur in some patients.
Tell your doctor or nurse if you develop any problems.

FDA Approval: Yes

glycerine suppository

Trade Names:
Fleet Babylax, Sani-Supp

Type of Drug:
Glycerine suppository is a laxative. It is used to treat constipation.

How Drug Works:
Glycerine suppository pulls water from the intestines into the stool and stimulates the intestines to expel the feces.

How Drug Is Given:
The glycerine suppository is inserted into the rectum and must stay there for at least 15 minutes. It will work 15 to 30 minutes later. To insert the suppository, open the package and dip the tip in water. If you are right-handed, lie down on your left side, bring your knees up near your chest, and insert the suppository in your rectum about an inch. Stay in this position for about 15 minutes, then get up and wash your hands well. Keep the suppositories in a safe place, often the refrigerator, out of the reach of children and pets.

How Should I Take This Drug?
Take this drug exactly as directed by your doctor. If you do not understand the instructions, ask your doctor or nurse to explain them to you.

 Read the following information. If you do not understand it or if any of it causes you special concern, check with your doctor.

Before taking this drug, tell your doctor if you are taking any other prescription or over-the-counter drugs, including vitamins and herbals.

Should I avoid any other medicines, foods, alcohol, and/or activities?
Your prescription and nonprescription medicines may interact with other drugs, causing harm. Certain foods or alcohol can also interact with drug products. Never begin taking a new medicine—prescription or nonprescription—without asking your doctor or nurse if it will interact with alcohol, food, or other medicines. Some drugs can cause drowsiness and affect activities such as driving.

Precautions:
To prevent constipation, try to drink 2 to 3 quarts of fluid daily, increase the amount of bran, fruits, and vegetables in your diet (try to eat 5 servings of fruits and vegetables daily), eat vegetable fiber or cereal, and do gentle exercise as tolerated.

Some laxatives can cause diarrhea, which can cause loss of fluids, nutrients, and electrolytes. It is important to replace the fluid that you lose through diarrhea. Try to drink 2 to 3 quarts of fluid daily. Fluids with electrolytes, such as chicken soup or sports drinks, are helpful in replacing potassium and salt that are lost in diarrhea. Take laxatives according to your prescribed schedule.

If you use laxatives all the time, your body will forget the normal process of moving your bowels. You then depend on the laxative for a bowel movement.

If you are taking opioid pain relievers, you will need to take a laxative regularly.

Tell all the doctors, dentists, and pharmacists you visit that you are taking this drug.

- Most of the following side effects probably will not occur.
- Your doctor or nurse will want to discuss specific care instructions with you.
- They can help you understand these side effects and help you deal with them.

Side Effects:

More Common Side Effects
Loss of normal reflexes to move bowels when laxatives are used on a long-term basis
Cramping pain
Rectal irritation

Less Common Side Effects
Dehydration due to fluid loss in diarrhea
Rectal inflammation
Rectal discomfort

Other side effects not listed above can also occur in some patients.
Tell your doctor or nurse if you develop any problems.

FDA Approval: Yes

granisetron hydrochloride

Trade Name:
Kytril

Type of Drug:
Granisetron hydrochloride belongs to a general class of drugs called serotonin antagonists. It is an antinausea medicine.

How Drug Works:
Granisetron hydrochloride blocks two pathways of serotonin release to prevent chemotherapy-related nausea and vomiting. It binds to the serotonin receptors in the gastrointestinal tract (lining of the stomach), thus preventing the stimulation of the vomiting center and chemoreceptor trigger zone in the brain. In addition, it responds to high levels of serotonin released from chemotherapy injury to the cells lining the stomach.

How Drug Is Given:
Granisetron hydrochloride is given as an injection in a vein over 5 minutes, or as a pill 1 hour before chemotherapy. The dose depends on your weight, or it can be a standard dose for all adults. Keep the medicine in a tightly closed container away from heat and moisture and out of the reach of children and pets.

How Should I Take This Drug?
Take this drug exactly as directed by your doctor. If you do not understand the instructions, ask your doctor or nurse to explain them to you.

 Read the following information. If you do not understand it or if any of it causes you special concern, check with your doctor.

Before taking this drug, tell your doctor if you are taking any other prescription or over-the-counter drugs, including vitamins and herbals.

Should I avoid any other medicines, foods, alcohol, and/or activities?
Your prescription and nonprescription medicines may interact with other drugs, causing harm. Certain foods or alcohol can also interact with drug products. Never begin taking a new medicine—prescription or nonprescription—without asking your doctor or nurse if it will interact with alcohol, food, or other medicines. Some drugs can cause drowsiness and affect activities such as driving.

Tell all the doctors, dentists, and pharmacists you visit that you are taking this drug.

- Most of the following side effects probably will not occur.
- Your doctor or nurse will want to discuss specific care instructions with you.
- They can help you understand these side effects and help you deal with them.

Side Effects:

More Common Side Effects
None

Less Common Side Effects
Headache
Constipation
Diarrhea

Rare Side Effects
Tiredness (fatigue)
Sleepiness

Other side effects not listed above can also occur in some patients.
Tell your doctor or nurse if you develop any problems.

FDA Approval: Yes

haloperidol

Trade Name:
Haldol

Type of Drug:
Haloperidol belongs to a general class of drugs called butyrophenones. It is used to treat nausea and vomiting.

How Drug Works:
Haloperidol is useful in preventing nausea and vomiting resulting from chemotherapy. It blocks the messages to the part of the brain responsible for nausea and vomiting. It may be used to decrease agitation, as well as other uses.

How Drug Is Given:
Haloperidol is given as an injection in a muscle or vein, or by mouth as a pill. The dose depends on your weight and how well you respond to the medicine. Keep the medicine in a tightly closed container away from heat and moisture and out of the reach of children and pets.

How Should I Take This Drug?
Take this drug exactly as directed by your doctor. If you do not understand the instructions, ask your doctor or nurse to explain them to you.

 Read the following information. If you do not understand it or if any of it causes you special concern, check with your doctor.

Before taking this drug, tell your doctor if you are taking any other prescription or over-the-counter drugs, including vitamins and herbals.

Should I avoid any other medicines, foods, alcohol, and/or activities?
Your prescription and nonprescription medicines may interact with other drugs, causing harm. Certain foods or alcohol can also interact with drug products. Never begin taking a new medicine—prescription or nonprescription—without asking your doctor or nurse if it will interact with alcohol, food, or other medicines. Some drugs can cause drowsiness and affect activities such as driving.

Precautions:
Haloperidol may make you feel very sleepy. Do not drive or operate heavy machinery when you are drowsy.

Haloperidol may cause extrapyramidal side effects. These include restlessness, tongue protrusion, and involuntary movements. These side effects stop immediately when you are given diphenhydramine.

Tell all the doctors, dentists, and pharmacists you visit that you are taking this drug.
- Most of the following side effects probably will not occur.
- Your doctor or nurse will want to discuss specific care instructions with you.
- They can help you understand these side effects and help you deal with them.

Side Effects:

More Common Side Effects
Feeling sedated
Sleepiness

Less Common Side Effects
Decreased breathing rate
Increased heart rate
Decrease in blood pressure when changing position

Rare Side Effects
Change in electrical activity of heart

Side Effects / Symptoms of the Drug
Take care in getting up, changing position, or when walking.

Other side effects not listed above can also occur in some patients.
Tell your doctor or nurse if you develop any problems.

FDA Approval: Yes

hydromorphone

Trade Name:
Dilaudid

Type of Drug:
Hydromorphone is an opioid analgesic.

How Drug Works:
Hydromorphone relieves moderate to severe pain and is similar to morphine. It binds to opioid receptors in the brain and central nervous system (CNS), altering the perception of pain as well as the emotional response to pain.

How Drug Is Given:
Hydromorphone is given in a number of ways. It can be given by mouth as a pill or a liquid. As an injection, it is given under the skin or in a vein as a short infusion or a continuous infusion with extra medicine that you can take when needed (patient controlled analgesia or PCA). It can also be given as a rectal suppository. Take the pill or liquid with a full glass of water, with or without food. Make sure to shake the liquid before pouring the dose. When taking a suppository, open the package and dip the tip in water. If you are right-handed, lie down on your left side, bring your knees up near your chest, and insert the suppository in your rectum about an inch. Stay in this position for about 15 minutes, then get up and wash your hands well. The dose depends on how well the medicine controls your pain. The medicine will cause constipation, so make sure you take a laxative regularly to prevent this. Keep the medicine in a tightly closed container away from heat and moisture and out of the reach of children and pets.

How Should I Take This Drug?
Take this drug exactly as directed by your doctor. If you do not understand the instructions, ask your doctor or nurse to explain them to you.

 Read the following information. If you do not understand it or if any of it causes you special concern, check with your doctor.

Before taking this drug, tell your doctor if you are taking any other prescription or over-the-counter drugs, including vitamins and herbals.

Should I avoid any other medicines, foods, alcohol, and/or activities?
Your prescription and nonprescription medicines may interact with other drugs, causing harm. Certain foods or alcohol can also interact with drug products. Never begin taking a new medicine—prescription or nonprescription—without asking your doctor or nurse if it will interact with alcohol, food, or other medicines. Some drugs can cause drowsiness and affect activities such as driving.

Precautions:
Take the smallest effective dose to prevent development of tolerance and physical dependence. Tolerance (larger doses needed to give the same effect) can develop as well as physical dependence (body goes into withdrawal if drug is suddenly stopped). This is different from addiction, which is psychological dependence (take drug for psychological effect, not for relief of pain). Tell your doctor or nurse if you still have pain even though you are taking the medicine as directed.

Since hydromorphone affects the central nervous system, it is important not to take other drugs or substances that are known CNS depressants such as alcohol, sedatives, and hypnotics.

Acetaminophen or aspirin may be combined with hydromorphone to increase the pain relief action.

You should be on a bowel regimen to prevent constipation while you are taking opioid pain relievers. Talk to your nurse or doctor about this.

Tell all the doctors, dentists, and pharmacists you visit that you are taking this drug.
- Most of the following side effects probably will not occur.
- Your doctor or nurse will want to discuss specific care instructions with you.
- They can help you understand these side effects and help you deal with them.

Side Effects:

More Common Side Effects
Constipation
Drowsiness
Sedation
Dizziness
Nausea
Dry mouth

Less Common Side Effects
Mood changes
Euphoria
Mental clouding
Decreased breathing rate
Vomiting
Delayed digestion
Decreased blood pressure when changing position
Decreased heart rate

Rare Side Effects
Small pupils in the eyes
Seizures
Difficulty urinating
Decreased sexual interest
Impotence
Bowel rupture due to constipation

Side Effects / Symptoms of the Drug
Drink fluids (8 oz every hour in sips) to prevent constipation. Also, try to eat foods high in fiber such as bran. You may need to take a stool softener, bulk-forming agent, and/or laxative to help keep your bowel movements regular.

Call your doctor or nurse right away if you have not moved your bowels in 2 days.

Abruptly stopping the drug can cause anxiety, dizziness, nausea and vomiting, and tiredness. The drug should be gradually discontinued.

Other side effects not listed above can also occur in some patients.
Tell your doctor or nurse if you develop any problems.

FDA Approval: Yes

ibuprofen

Trade Names:
Advil, Genpril, Haltran, Ibuprin, Midol 200, Nuprin, Rufen

Type of Drug:
Ibuprofen belongs to the general class of nonopioid analgesic drugs called nonsteroidal anti-inflammatory drugs (NSAIDs).

How Drug Works:
Ibuprofen blocks the synthesis of prostaglandins. This prevents pain receptors from passing the pain message to the brain so that pain perception is decreased. This drug reduces inflammation. It also reduces fever by helping the body to dilate blood vessels so that heat is lost from the body. Ibuprofen is especially helpful in relieving bone pain related to cancer.

How Drug Is Given:
Ibuprofen is a pill taken by mouth with milk, food, or an antacid to protect the stomach. Keep the medicine in a tightly closed container away from heat and moisture and out of the reach of children and pets.

How Should I Take This Drug?
Take this drug exactly as directed by your doctor. If you do not understand the instructions, ask your doctor or nurse to explain them to you.

 Read the following information. If you do not understand it or if any of it causes you special concern, check with your doctor.

Before taking this drug, tell your doctor if you are taking any other prescription or over-the-counter drugs, including vitamins and herbals.

Should I avoid any other medicines, foods, alcohol, and/or activities?
Your prescription and nonprescription medicines may interact with other drugs, causing harm. Certain foods or alcohol can also interact with drug products. Never begin taking a new medicine—prescription or nonprescription—without asking your doctor or nurse if it will interact with alcohol, food, or other medicines. Some drugs can cause drowsiness and affect activities such as driving.

Precautions:
DO NOT take aspirin or other nonsteroidal anti-inflammatory drugs with ibuprofen. This may increase the risk of bleeding or stomach irritation.

DO NOT take ibuprofen if you have a peptic or duodenal ulcer. Ibuprofen can cause rupture of the ulcer and life threatening bleeding. Talk to your doctor about this.

If you have asthma and nasal polyps, or if you have ever had breathing difficulty after taking aspirin or other anti-inflammatory drugs, DO NOT take ibuprofen. Also, if you have kidney problems, do not take ibuprofen as this may cause acute kidney failure.

Do not drink alcohol while taking ibuprofen, as this may increase the risk of bleeding.

Tell your doctor if you are taking medicine to decrease blood clotting such as Coumadin, or steroids such as prednisone. It is important to talk with your doctor about risk of bleeding.

Tell all the doctors, dentists, and pharmacists you visit that you are taking this drug.

- Most of the following side effects probably will not occur.
- Your doctor or nurse will want to discuss specific care instructions with you.
- They can help you understand these side effects and help you deal with them.

Side Effects:

More Common Side Effects
Heartburn
Nausea
Dizziness
Drowsiness

Less Common Side Effects
Vomiting
Diarrhea
Sores in mouth or on lips
Abdominal pain
Headache
Tiredness (fatigue)
Confusion
Mood swings
Loss of appetite
Constipation
Bloating
Bleeding from the gastrointestinal tract
Nervousness
Anxiety
Depression
Peptic ulcers

Rare Side Effects
Decreased hearing
Visual changes
Double vision
Jaundice
Hepatitis
Liver damage
Rash and itching
Decreased white blood cell count with increased risk of infection
Decreased platelet count with increased risk of bleeding
Decreased red blood cell count with increased risk of anemia and tiredness (fatigue)
Kidney failure
Blood in urine
Hair loss
Acne
Facial flushing

Side Effects / Symptoms of the Drug
Call your doctor or nurse right away if you are vomiting blood, or a coffee-ground material, notice blood in your stools, or stools appear tarry. Stop taking ibuprofen until after you talk with your doctor.

Call your doctor or nurse right away if your vision is blurred. Stop taking ibuprofen until you talk to your doctor or nurse.

> *Other side effects not listed above can also occur in some patients.*
> *Tell your doctor or nurse if you develop any problems.*

FDA Approval: Yes

imipenem/cilastatin sodium

Trade Name:
Primaxin

Type of Drug:
Imipenem/cilastatin sodium belongs to the general class of drugs called antibiotics.

How Drug Works:
Imipenem prevents bacteria from making their cell wall, so the cells die. Cilastin sodium is added to prevent an enzyme made by the kidneys from breaking down the antibiotic imipenem. The drug is used to treat gram-positive and gram-negative bacteria. It is used to treat infections of the lungs, urinary tract, abdomen, pelvis, skin, bones, and joints.

How Drug Is Given:
Imipenem/cilastin sodium is given as an injection in the vein over 1 hour, 3 to 4 times a day, or in the muscle twice a day. The dose depends on your weight and how well your kidneys are working.

 Read the following information. If you do not understand it or if any of it causes you special concern, check with your doctor.

Before taking this drug, tell your doctor if you are taking any other prescription or over-the-counter drugs, including vitamins and herbals.

Should I avoid any other medicines, foods, alcohol, and/or activities?
Your prescription and nonprescription medicines may interact with other drugs, causing harm. Certain foods or alcohol can also interact with drug products. Never begin taking a new medicine—prescription or nonprescription—without asking your doctor or nurse if it will interact with alcohol, food, or other medicines. Some drugs can cause drowsiness and affect activities such as driving.

Precautions:
Tell your doctor if you have any drug allergies, especially to antibiotic drugs.

All antibiotics can cause allergic reactions. Stop the drug and tell your doctor or nurse right away if you develop a rash, hives, red blotches on your skin, difficulty breathing, or chest pain.

Use of antibiotics can change the normal organisms in your body. Women are at risk of getting fungal infections. Tell your nurse or doctor if you get vaginal itching or discharge.

Tell all the doctors, dentists, and pharmacists you visit that you are taking this drug.
- Most of the following side effects probably will not occur.
- Your doctor or nurse will want to discuss specific care instructions with you.
- They can help you understand these side effects and help you deal with them.

Side Effects:

More Common Side Effects
Nausea
Vaginal itching
Vaginal candidiasis (fungal infection)

Less Common Side Effects
Vomiting
Diarrhea
Loss of appetite
Pain and redness at place of injection
Hardening of vein used for giving the drug

Rare Side Effects
Diarrhea related to infection of the intestinal lining (pseudomembranous colitis)
Rash
Hives
Fever
Chills
Muscle aches
Swelling of feet
Redness of skin
Decreased white blood cell count with increased risk of infection
Decreased red blood cell count with increased risk of anemia and tiredness (fatigue)
Dizziness
Headache
Sleepiness
Seizures

Side Effects / Symptoms of the Drug
Stop the drug and call your doctor or nurse right away if you get diarrhea that does not stop, abdominal cramping, and blood and/or pus in the stool. This needs to be treated right away.

Stop the drug and call your doctor or nurse right away if you develop a rash, hives, fever, chills, muscle aches, and/or peeling of your skin. This can be a serious reaction and needs to be treated right away.

Other side effects not listed above can also occur in some patients.
Tell your doctor or nurse if you develop any problems.

FDA Approval: Yes

imipramine pamoate

Trade Name:
Tofranil-PM

Type of Drug:
Imipramine pamoate belongs to a general class of drugs called tricyclic antidepressants.

How Drug Works:
Imipramine pamoate increases the amount of serotonin and norepinephrine at the nerve endings in the brain. This decreases or stops the feeling of depression. It is also useful for promoting sleep and in treating hiccups.

How Drug Is Given:
Imipramine pamoate is given as a pill, usually once a day at bedtime. If you take it more than once a day, take the last dose at bedtime to help you sleep. Take with a glass of water, with or without food. The dose depends on your age and how well the medicine works for you. Keep the medicine in a tightly closed container away from heat and moisture and out of the reach of children and pets. If needed, the medicine can also be given as an injection in a muscle.

How Should I Take This Drug?
Take this drug exactly as directed by your doctor. If you do not understand the instructions, ask your doctor or nurse to explain them to you.

 Read the following information. If you do not understand it or if any of it causes you special concern, check with your doctor.

Before taking this drug, tell your doctor if you are taking any other prescription or over-the-counter drugs, including vitamins and herbals.

Should I avoid any other medicines, foods, alcohol, and/or activities?
Your prescription and nonprescription medicines may interact with other drugs, causing harm. Certain foods or alcohol can also interact with drug products. Never begin taking a new medicine—prescription or nonprescription—without asking your doctor or nurse if it will interact with alcohol, food, or other medicines. Some drugs can cause drowsiness and affect activities such as driving.

Precautions:
DO NOT drink alcohol when taking imipramine pamoate.

Tell your doctor if you are taking any of the following drugs as they may have serious interactions with imipramine pamoate: other antidepressant drugs (monoamine oxidase inhibitors), sedatives, amphetamines, cimetidine, warfarin (Coumadin), or barbiturates.

Once you start taking imipramine pamoate, it may take up to 2 weeks before you feel the full effect of the drug.

Tell your doctor if you have had a heart attack (myocardial infarction), have a seizure disorder, or have benign prostatic hypertrophy. You should not take imipramine pamoate.

Tell your doctor if you have urinary retention, narrow-angle glaucoma, hyperthyroidism, liver problems, or have thoughts of suicide. Use this drug very cautiously if you have any of these conditions.

Abruptly stopping the drug can cause anxiety, dizziness, nausea and vomiting, and tiredness. The drug should be gradually discontinued.

Tell all the doctors, dentists, and pharmacists you visit that you are taking this drug.
- Most of the following side effects probably will not occur.
- Your doctor or nurse will want to discuss specific care instructions with you.
- They can help you understand these side effects and help you deal with them.

Side Effects:

More Common Side Effects
Drowsiness
Dizziness
Weakness
Tiredness (fatigue)

Less Common Side Effects
Confusion
Disorientation
Change in blood pressure when changing position
Increased heart rate
Dry mouth
Decreased appetite
Nausea
Urinary retention

Rare Side Effects
Fine tremors
Rigidity
Difficulty speaking
Difficulty swallowing
Numbness and tingling in hands and/or feet related to irritation of nerves
Blurred vision
Changes in electrical activity of heart (EKG)
Increase in blood pressure
Vomiting
Diarrhea
Abdominal cramping
Rash
Hives
Increased sensitivity to sunlight

Side Effects / Symptoms of the Drug
The drowsiness and/or dizziness usually goes away in 1 to 2 weeks. Do not drive or operate heavy machinery if you feel drowsy or dizzy.

Be careful walking around or changing position if you are drowsy. Stop the drug and call your doctor or nurse if the drowsiness does not go away, or if you have trouble walking or moving because of it.

Tell your doctor or nurse if you get fine tremors, feel like your body is rigid, or have difficulty speaking or swallowing. You can be given another medicine to lessen these problems.

Other side effects not listed above can also occur in some patients.
Tell your doctor or nurse if you develop any problems.

FDA Approval: Yes

indomethacin

Trade Names:
Indocin, Indocin SR, Indotech

Type of Drug:
Indomethacin is a nonopioid analgesic that belongs to the general class of drugs called nonsteroidal anti-inflammatory drugs (NSAIDs).

How Drug Works:
Indomethacin blocks the synthesis of prostaglandins. This prevents pain receptors from passing the pain message to the brain so that pain perception is decreased. This drug reduces inflammation. It also reduces fever by helping the body to dilate blood vessels so that heat is lost from the body. It is helpful in reducing fevers, but because the drug has serious side effects it is not commonly used for this purpose.

How Drug Is Given:
Indomethacin can be taken by mouth or as a rectal suppository. Indomethacin comes as a capsule, extended-release capsule, or liquid. Do not open or crush the extended release capsule. Shake the liquid before pouring the dose. Take the medicine 3 to 4 times a day as directed with food, milk, or antacid to protect your stomach. To take the rectal suppository, open the package and dip the tip in water. If you are right-handed, lie down on your left side, bring your knees up near your chest, and insert the suppository in your rectum about an inch. Stay in this position for about 15 minutes, then get up and wash your hands well. Keep the medicine in a tightly closed container away from heat and moisture and out of the reach of children and pets.

How Should I Take This Drug?
Take this drug exactly as directed by your doctor. If you do not understand the instructions, ask your doctor or nurse to explain them to you.

 Read the following information. If you do not understand it or if any of it causes you special concern, check with your doctor.

Before taking this drug, tell your doctor if you are taking any other prescription or over-the-counter drugs, including vitamins and herbals.

Should I avoid any other medicines, foods, alcohol, and/or activities?
Your prescription and nonprescription medicines may interact with other drugs, causing harm. Certain foods or alcohol can also interact with drug products. Never begin taking a new medicine—prescription or non-prescription—without asking your doctor or nurse if it will interact with alcohol, food, or other medicines. Some drugs can cause drowsiness and affect activities such as driving.

Precautions:
DO NOT take aspirin or other nonsteroidal anti-inflammatory drugs with indomethacin. This may increase the risk of stomach irritation and the occurrence of aplastic anemia.

DO NOT take indomethacin if you have a peptic or duodenal ulcer. Indomethacin can cause rupture of the ulcer and life-threatening bleeding. Do not take indomethacin if you are allergic to aspirin or have severe kidney or liver disease. Talk to your doctor about this.

Indomethacin has many drug interactions. DO NOT take indomethacin if you are also taking methotrexate (especially high dose), diflunisal, or triamterene.

Tell your doctor if you are taking medicine such as Coumadin to decrease blood clotting or steroids such as prednisone. It is important to talk with your doctor about your risk for bleeding.

Do not drink alcohol while taking indomethacin, as this may increase the risk of bleeding.

Tell all the doctors, dentists, and pharmacists you visit that you are taking this drug.

- Most of the following side effects probably will not occur.
- Your doctor or nurse will want to discuss specific care instructions with you.
- They can help you understand these side effects and help you deal with them.

Side Effects:

More Common Side Effects
Headache
Vomiting
Ringing in ears (tinnitus)
Tremors
Sleeplessness

Less Common Side Effects

Dizziness
Tiredness (fatigue)
Nausea
Heartburn, indigestion, epigastric pain

Depression
Numbness and tingling in hands and/or feet
Loss of appetite
Bleeding from gastrointestinal tract

Rare Side Effects
Kidney problems with blood or protein in urine
Increased heart rate
Palpitations
Increased blood pressure
Edema
Rash
Itching
Decreased white blood cell count with increased risk of infection
Decreased platelet count with increased risk of bleeding
Decreased red blood cell count with increased risk of anemia and tiredness (fatigue)
Allergic reaction with asthma, fever, difficulty breathing, anaphylaxis
Congestive heart failure
Chest pain
Nightmares
Confusion
Blurred vision
Hearing loss

Side Effects / Symptoms of the Drug
Call your doctor or nurse right away if you have bleeding from the stomach such as vomiting blood or a coffee-ground material, blood in your stool, or black, tarry stools. Stop taking indomethacin until after you talk with your doctor or nurse.

Call your doctor or nurse right away if you have changes in vision or neurologic side effects occur (numbness and tingling, confusion, nightmares, or depression). Stop taking indomethacin until you talk to your doctor or nurse.

Other side effects not listed above can also occur in some patients.
Tell your doctor or nurse if you develop any problems.

FDA Approval: Yes

itraconazole

Trade Name:
Sporanox

Type of Drug:
Itraconazole is an antifungal.

How Drug Works:
Itraconazole is an antifungal that stops fungi from reproducing and kills the organisms at higher doses.

How Drug Is Given:
Itraconazole can be taken by mouth as a pill or liquid, or given as an injection in a vein, 1 to 2 times a day. The pill should be taken with food. Take the liquid on an empty stomach 1 hour before or 2 hours after a meal. Shake well before pouring the dose. The dose and number of doses depend on the type of infection being treated. In severe infections, higher doses 3 times a day are used for the first 3 days. Keep the medicine in a tightly closed container away from heat and moisture and out of the reach of children and pets.

How Should I Take This Drug?
Take this drug exactly as directed by your doctor. If you do not understand the instructions, ask your doctor or nurse to explain them to you.

 Read the following information. If you do not understand it or if any of it causes you special concern, check with your doctor.

Before taking this drug, tell your doctor if you are taking any other prescription or over-the-counter drugs, including vitamins and herbals.

Should I avoid any other medicines, foods, alcohol, and/or activities?
Your prescription and nonprescription medicines may interact with other drugs, causing harm. Certain foods or alcohol can also interact with drug products. Never begin taking a new medicine—prescription or nonprescription—without asking your doctor or nurse if it will interact with alcohol, food, or other medicines. Some drugs can cause drowsiness and affect activities such as driving.

Precautions:
Tell your doctor if you are taking omeprazole, cimetidine, ranitidine, pepcid, oral antidiabetic agents, carbamazepine, digoxin, lovastatin, or simvastatin. Talk to your doctor about possible drug interactions.

Tell your doctor if you are taking astemizole, cisapride, or terfenadine. You must stop taking these drugs if you take itraconazole.

All drugs used to fight microorganisms can cause allergic reactions. Stop the drug and tell your nurse or doctor right away if you develop a rash, hives, red blotches on your skin, difficulty breathing, or chest pain.

Tell all the doctors, dentists, and pharmacists you visit that you are taking this drug.

- Most of the following side effects probably will not occur.
- Your doctor or nurse will want to discuss specific care instructions with you.
- They can help you understand these side effects and help you deal with them.

Side Effects:

More Common Side Effects
Mild nausea
Mild vomiting
Mild diarrhea

Less Common Side Effects
Rash
Itching
Hives
Increase in liver function blood tests

Rare Side Effects
Inflammation of liver
Fever
Chills

Side Effects / Symptoms of the Drug
Call your doctor or nurse if you develop rash, fever, or chills. Your doctor needs to evaluate you.

Other side effects not listed above can also occur in some patients.
Tell your doctor or nurse if you develop any problems.

FDA Approval: Yes

kanamycin sulfate

Trade Name:
Kantrex

Type of Drug:
Kanamycin sulfate is an antibiotic that belongs to the group of drugs called aminoglycosides.

How Drug Works:
Kanamycin sulfate appears to prevent bacteria from making their cell walls, so the cells die. It is used to treat many sensitive gram-negative and some gram-positive bacteria.

How Drug Is Given:
Kanamycin sulfate is usually given by an injection in a vein or muscle, but it can also be given by mouth. The dose is given 2 to 3 times a day. The dose depends on your weight, how well your kidneys are working, and the medicine level in your blood. If capsules are given by mouth, such as before bowel surgery, the dose and schedule is standard. Keep the medicine in a tightly closed container away from heat and moisture and out of the reach of children and pets.

How Should I Take This Drug?
Take this drug exactly as directed by your doctor. If you do not understand the instructions, ask your doctor or nurse to explain them to you.

 Read the following information. If you do not understand it or if any of it causes you special concern, check with your doctor.

Before taking this drug, tell your doctor if you are taking any other prescription or over-the-counter drugs, including vitamins and herbals.

Should I avoid any other medicines, foods, alcohol, and/or activities?
Your prescription and nonprescription medicines may interact with other drugs, causing harm. Certain foods or alcohol can also interact with drug products. Never begin taking a new medicine—prescription or nonprescription—without asking your doctor or nurse if it will interact with alcohol, food, or other medicines. Some drugs can cause drowsiness and affect activities such as driving.

Precautions:
Kanamycin sulfate can cause injury to the nerve for hearing (eighth cranial nerve, auditory). Tell your doctor or nurse right away if you feel dizzy, or have difficulty walking, ringing in your ears (tinnitus), a roaring sound in your ears, or any decrease in hearing. The drug should be stopped and changed to another effective drug without these side effects.

Kanamycin sulfate can injure your kidneys. Your doctor will monitor blood tests to find this early, if it occurs. Make sure you tell your doctor if you have ever had any kidney problems.

All antibiotics can cause allergic reactions. Stop the drug and tell your doctor or nurse right away if you develop a rash, hives, red blotches on your skin, difficulty breathing, or chest pain.

Use of antibiotics can change the normal organisms in your body. Women are at risk of getting fungal infections. Tell your nurse or doctor if you get vaginal itching or discharge.

Use in pregnancy only if infection is life-threatening and no safer drug exists.

Tell your doctor if you have any drug allergies, especially to antibiotic drugs.

Tell all the doctors, dentists, and pharmacists you visit that you are taking this drug.

- Most of the following side effects probably will not occur.
- Your doctor or nurse will want to discuss specific care instructions with you.
- They can help you understand these side effects and help you deal with them.

Side Effects:

More Common Side Effects
Nausea
Headache
Feeling drowsy or sleepy

Less Common Side Effects
Dizziness
Ringing in the ears (tinnitus)
Roaring sound in the ears
Difficulty walking
Decreased appetite

Rare Side Effects
Diarrhea related to infection of the intestinal lining (pseudomembranous colitis)
Decreased hearing
Rash
Hives
Vomiting
Tingling of the skin
Decreased white blood cell count with increased risk of infection
Decreased platelet count with increased risk of bleeding
Decreased red blood cell count with increased risk of anemia and tiredness (fatigue)

Side Effects / Symptoms of the Drug
Stop the drug and call your doctor or nurse right away if you develop a rash, hives, fever, or chills. This can be a serious reaction and needs to be treated right away.

Stop the drug and call your doctor or nurse right away if you get diarrhea that does not stop, abdominal cramping, and blood and/or pus in the stool. This needs to be treated right away.

Stop the drug and call your doctor or nurse right away if you get ringing in your ears (tinnitus), a roaring sound in your ears, or hearing loss.

Other side effects not listed above can also occur in some patients.
Tell your doctor or nurse if you develop any problems.

FDA Approval: Yes

kaolin/pectin

Trade Names:
Kaodene, Kaopectate, K-P, K-Pek

Type of Drug:
Kaolin/pectin is an antidiarrheal drug.

How Drug Works:
Kaolin/pectin decreases fluid in the stool, which reduces diarrhea.

How Drug Is Given:
Kaolin/pectin is a liquid or concentrated suspension taken by mouth. The dose and frequency depend on how severe your diarrhea is. Keep the medicine in a tightly closed container away from heat and moisture and out of the reach of children and pets.

How Should I Take This Drug?
Take this drug exactly as directed by your doctor. If you do not understand the instructions, ask your doctor or nurse to explain them to you.

 Read the following information. If you do not understand it or if any of it causes you special concern, check with your doctor.

Before taking this drug, tell your doctor if you are taking any other prescription or over-the-counter drugs, including vitamins and herbals.

Should I avoid any other medicines, foods, alcohol, and/or activities?
Your prescription and nonprescription medicines may interact with other drugs, causing harm. Certain foods or alcohol can also interact with drug products. Never begin taking a new medicine—prescription or nonprescription—without asking your doctor or nurse if it will interact with alcohol, food, or other medicines. Some drugs can cause drowsiness and affect activities such as driving.

Precautions:
To decrease the diarrhea, modify your diet. Try to eat small, frequent meals that are warm or at room temperature. Avoid foods that cause gas (such as broccoli or beans), fatty foods (such as bacon or cheeses), citrus fruits and juices, and high-lactose foods (such as milk or ice cream). Eat foods high in sodium and potassium (such as soups, sports drinks, and bananas). Eat foods high in soluble fiber (such as rice or bananas). Avoid foods high in insoluble fiber (such as cereal or nuts). Try to drink at least eight 8 oz glasses of water a day. To add calories, dilute with fruit juice.

Tell your doctor if you are also taking lincomycin or digoxin. Talk to your doctor about possible drug interactions.

Tell all the doctors, dentists, and pharmacists you visit that you are taking this drug.
- Most of the following side effects probably will not occur.
- Your doctor or nurse will want to discuss specific care instructions with you.
- They can help you understand these side effects and help you deal with them.

Side Effects:

More Common Side Effects
Brief constipation

Other side effects not listed above can also occur in some patients.
Tell your doctor or nurse if you develop any problems.

FDA Approval: Yes

ketoconazole

Trade Name:
Nizoral

Type of Drug:
Ketoconazole is an antifungal drug.

How Drug Works:
Ketoconazole stops fungi from reproducing and kills the organisms at higher doses.

How Drug Is Given:
Ketoconazole is given by mouth as a pill once a day, or it can be used as a cream or shampoo. Ketoconazole given as a pill needs acid in the stomach to work. If you are taking medicines that stop the acid (antacids, cimetidine, ranitidine, fotidine, or sulcralfate), then take the ketoconazole at least 2 hours before taking these other medicines. If your stomach does not make acid (achlorhydria), then take the pill with a cola beverage. The dose and number of doses depend on the infection being treated. Keep the medicine in a tightly closed container away from heat and moisture and out of the reach of children and pets.

How Should I Take This Drug?
Take this drug exactly as directed by your doctor. If you do not understand the instructions, ask your doctor or nurse to explain them to you.

 Read the following information. If you do not understand it or if any of it causes you special concern, check with your doctor.

Before taking this drug, tell your doctor if you are taking any other prescription or over-the-counter drugs, including vitamins and herbals.

Should I avoid any other medicines, foods, alcohol, and/or activities?
Your prescription and nonprescription medicines may interact with other drugs, causing harm. Certain foods or alcohol can also interact with drug products. Never begin taking a new medicine—prescription or non-prescription—without asking your doctor or nurse if it will interact with alcohol, food, or other medicines. Some drugs can cause drowsiness and affect activities such as driving.

Precautions:
Tell your doctor if you are taking rifampin, isoniazid, warfarin (Coumadin), cyclosporine, phenytoin (Dilantin), theophylline, terfenadine, or corticosteroids. Talk to your doctor about possible drug interactions.

All drugs used to fight microorganisms can cause allergic reactions. Stop the drug and tell your nurse or doctor right away if you develop a rash, hives, red blotches on your skin, difficulty breathing, or chest pain.

Tell all the doctors, dentists, and pharmacists you visit that you are taking this drug.

• Most of the following side effects probably will not occur.
• Your doctor or nurse will want to discuss specific care instructions with you.
• They can help you understand these side effects and help you deal with them.

Side Effects:

More Common Side Effects
Nausea

Less Common Side Effects
Diarrhea
Vomiting

Rare Side Effects
Abdominal pain
Constipation
Increased liver function blood tests
Breast enlargement in men
Rash
Hives
Dizziness
Nervousness
Difficulty sleeping
Fever
Sleepiness
Decreased sexual ability

Side Effects / Symptoms of the Drug
Call your doctor or nurse if you develop a rash, fever, or chills. You need to be evaluated.

Other side effects not listed above can also occur in some patients.
Tell your doctor or nurse if you develop any problems.

FDA Approval: Yes

ketorolac tromethamine

Trade Name:
Toradol

Type of Drug:
Ketorolac tromethamine is a nonopioid analgesic that belongs to the general class of drugs called nonsteroidal anti-inflammatory drugs (NSAIDs).

How Drug Works:
Ketorolac tromethamine blocks the synthesis of prostaglandins. This prevents pain receptors from passing the pain message to the brain so that pain perception is decreased. This drug reduces inflammation. It also reduces fever by helping the body to dilate blood vessels so that heat is lost from the body. It is the only NSAID that can be given by injection.

How Drug Is Given:
Ketorolac tromethamine is given as an injection in a muscle or vein, or by mouth as a pill. It is given as a single dose, or 4 times a day at least 4 to 6 hours apart for up to 5 days. The pill should be taken with a full glass of water, together with food or with an antacid. You should sit up for 15 to 30 minutes after taking the pill. The dose is standard, but it is larger when only a single dose is given. Keep the medicine in a tightly closed container away from heat and moisture and out of the reach of children and pets.

How Should I Take This Drug?
Take this drug exactly as directed by your doctor. If you do not understand these instructions, ask your doctor or nurse to explain them to you.

 Read the following information. If you do not understand it or if any of it causes you special concern, check with your doctor.

Before taking this drug, tell your doctor if you are taking any other prescription or over-the-counter drugs, including vitamins and herbals.

Should I avoid any other medicines, foods, alcohol, and/or activities?
Your prescription and nonprescription medicines may interact with other drugs, causing harm. Certain foods or alcohol can also interact with drug products. Never begin taking a new medicine—prescription or nonprescription—without asking your doctor or nurse if it will interact with alcohol, food, or other medicines. Some drugs can cause drowsiness and affect activities such as driving.

Precautions:
Ketorolac tromethamine is used for acute, short-term relief of pain. It is not to be used for chronic pain.

DO NOT take aspirin or other nonsteroidal anti-inflammatory drugs with ketorolac tromethamine. This may increase the risk of stomach irritation and bleeding.

DO NOT take ketorolac tromethamine if you have a peptic or duodenal ulcer, if you are allergic to aspirin, or if you have kidney or liver disease. Talk to your doctor about this.

Tell your doctor if you are taking medicine such as Coumadin to decrease blood clotting or steroids, such as prednisone. It is important to talk with your doctor about risk for bleeding.

Tell all the doctors, dentists, and pharmacists you visit that you are taking this drug.
- Most of the following side effects probably will not occur.
- Your doctor or nurse will want to discuss specific care instructions with you.
- They can help you understand these side effects and help you deal with them.

Side Effects:

More Common Side Effects
Heartburn
Dizziness
Drowsiness
Lightheadedness

Less Common Side Effects
Nausea
Loss of appetite
Constipation
Bloating
Peptic ulcers
Headache
Tiredness (fatigue)
Confusion
Mood swings

Vomiting
Diarrhea
Sores in mouth or on lips
Abdominal pain
Bleeding from gastrointestinal tract
Nervousness
Anxiety
Depression

Rare Side Effects
Decreased hearing
Changes in vision
Double vision
Cataracts
Jaundice
Hepatitis
Kidney damage
Rash
Itching
Decreased white blood cell count with increased risk of infection
Decreased platelet count with increased risk of bleeding
Decreased red blood cell count with increased risk of anemia and tiredness (fatigue)
Liver damage

Side Effects / Symptoms of the Drug
Call your doctor or nurse right away if you have bleeding from the gastrointestinal tract such as vomiting blood or coffee-ground material, blood in stool, or black, tarry stools. Stop taking ketorolac tromethamine until after you talk with your doctor.

Call your doctor or nurse right away if you have dizziness, ringing in your ears, nausea, vomiting, headache, or sweating. These symptoms usually occur when too much of the medicine is taken. Stop taking ketorolac tromethamine until you talk to your doctor or nurse.

Other side effects not listed above can also occur in some patients.
Tell your doctor or nurse if you develop any problems.

FDA Approval: Yes

lactulose

Trade Names:
Cholac, Constilac, Constulose, Duphalac

Type of Drug:
Lactulose belongs to the general class of laxatives used to treat constipation.

How Drug Works:
Lactulose pulls water into the large intestines causing distention. This stimulates the normal forward movement of the intestines (peristalsis), resulting in a bowel movement within 24 to 48 hours. It is also used to lower blood ammonia levels in liver failure.

How Drug Is Given:
Lactulose is a liquid taken by mouth. It is very sweet and can be taken with water or juice to decrease the sweetness. Keep the medicine in a tightly closed container away from heat and moisture and out of the reach of children and pets.

How Should I Take This Drug?
Take this drug exactly as directed by your doctor. If you do not understand the instructions, ask your doctor or nurse to explain them to you.

 Read the following information. If you do not understand it or if any of it causes you special concern, check with your doctor.

Before taking this drug, tell your doctor if you are taking any other prescription or over-the-counter drugs, including vitamins and herbals.

Should I avoid any other medicines, foods, alcohol, and/or activities?
Your prescription and nonprescription medicines may interact with other drugs, causing harm. Certain foods or alcohol can also interact with drug products. Never begin taking a new medicine—prescription or nonprescription—without asking your doctor or nurse if it will interact with alcohol, food, or other medicines. Some drugs can cause drowsiness and affect activities such as driving.

Precautions:
To prevent constipation, try to drink 2 to 3 quarts of fluid daily, increase the amount of bran, fruits, and vegetables in your diet (try to eat 5 servings of fruits and vegetables daily), eat vegetable fiber or cereal, and do gentle exercise as tolerated.

Talk to your doctor before taking lactulose if you have nausea, vomiting, abdominal pain, blood in the stool, or haven't had a bowel movement in several days. There may be something else wrong besides constipation.

Some laxatives can cause diarrhea, which can cause loss of fluids, nutrients, and electrolytes. It is important to replace the fluid that you lose through diarrhea. Try to drink 2 to 3 quarts of fluid a day. Fluids with electrolytes, such as chicken soup or sports drinks, are helpful in replacing potassium and salt that are lost in diarrhea. Take the laxative as prescribed by your doctor.

If you use laxatives all the time, the body forgets the normal process of moving your bowels. You then depend upon the laxative for a bowel movement.

If you are taking opioid pain relievers, you will need to take a laxative regularly.

Tell all the doctors, dentists, and pharmacists you visit that you are taking this drug.
- Most of the following side effects probably will not occur.
- Your doctor or nurse will want to discuss specific care instructions with you.
- They can help you understand these side effects and help you deal with them.

Side Effects:

More Common Side Effects
Abdominal bloating

Gas

Abdominal pain

Loss of normal reflexes to move bowels when laxatives are used on a long-term basis

Less Common Side Effects
Dehydration due to fluid loss in diarrhea

Diarrhea

Loss of electrolytes

Nausea

Rare Side Effects
Vomiting

Cramps

Other side effects not listed above can also occur in some patients.
Tell your doctor or nurse if you develop any problems.

FDA Approval: Yes

levofloxacin

Trade Name:
Levaquin

Type of Drug:
Levofloxacin is an antibiotic that belongs to a group of drugs called fluoroquinolones.

How Drug Works:
Levofloxacin prevents bacteria from making copies of DNA, so new bacteria cannot be made. Levofloxacin is used to treat sensitive gram-negative and some gram-positive bacteria. It is used to treat sinusitis, bronchitis, pneumonia, skin infections, and complicated urinary tract infections.

How Drug Is Given:
Levofloxacin is a pill taken by mouth once a day with an 8 oz glass of water. Take the pill, with or without food, for 7 to 10 days as directed by your doctor. If also taking antacids, sulcrafate, iron, or vitamins with zinc, take the levofloxacin 2 hours before or after. Drink an 8 oz glass of water every hour. It can also be given by an injection in the vein over 1 hour. The dose depends on your weight, the infection being treated, and how well your kidneys are working.

How Should I Take This Drug?
Take this drug exactly as directed by your doctor. If you do not understand the instructions, ask your doctor or nurse to explain them to you.

 Read the following information. If you do not understand it or if any of it causes you special concern, check with your doctor.

Before taking this drug, tell your doctor if you are taking any other prescription or over-the-counter drugs, including vitamins and herbals.

Should I avoid any other medicines, foods, alcohol, and/or activities?
Your prescription and nonprescription medicines may interact with other drugs, causing harm. Certain foods or alcohol can also interact with drug products. Never begin taking a new medicine—prescription or nonprescription—without asking your doctor or nurse if it will interact with alcohol, food, or other medicines. Some drugs can cause drowsiness and affect activities such as driving.

Precautions:
If you are also taking antacids that contain magnesium or aluminum, iron, or sucralfate, take them 2 hours before or after your levofloxacin dose. If you take a vitamin containing zinc, take it at least 2 hours before or after your levofloxacin dose.

Tell your doctor if you have any allergies, especially to antibiotic drugs.

All antibiotics can cause allergic reactions. Stop the drug and tell your doctor or nurse right away if you develop a rash, hives, red blotches on your skin, or difficulty breathing.

Tell your doctor or nurse if you are taking oral diabetic medicines or insulin for diabetes mellitus. Levofloxacin may lower your blood sugar.

Use of antibiotics can change the normal organisms in your body. Women are at risk of getting fungal infections. Tell your nurse or doctor if you get vaginal itching or discharge.

Tell your doctor if you are also taking warfarin (Coumadin), cimetidine, cyclosporine, phenytoin (Dilantin), or theophylline. There may be serious drug interactions.

Levofloxacin can increase your sensitivity to direct sunlight. Try to avoid direct sunlight, wear sunscreen, and keep your head, arms, and legs covered when outside.

Tell all the doctors, dentists, and pharmacists you visit that you are taking this drug.

- Most of the following side effects probably will not occur.
- Your doctor or nurse will want to discuss specific care instructions with you.
- They can help you understand these side effects and help you deal with them.

Side Effects:

More Common Side Effects
Vaginal itching
Vaginal candidiasis (fungal infection)

Less Common Side Effects
Vomiting
Abdominal pain
Diarrhea
Loss of appetite

Rare Side Effects
Diarrhea related to infection of the intestinal lining (pseudomembranous colitis)
Dizziness
Tiredness
Lightheadedness
Rash
Hives
Flushing
Increased sensitivity to sunlight

Side Effects / Symptoms of the Drug
Do not drive a car or operate heavy machinery until you know the effect levofloxacin has on you. If you are dizzy, lightheaded, or feel tired, you should not drive or operate heavy machinery.

Stop the drug and call your doctor or nurse right away if you develop a rash, fever, muscle aches, diarrhea with abdominal cramping, or blood or pus in your stool. This can be a serious reaction and needs to be treated right away.

Other side effects not listed above can also occur in some patients.
Tell your doctor or nurse if you develop any problems.

FDA Approval: Yes

levorphanol tartrate

Trade Name:
Levo-Dromoran

Type of Drug:
Levorphanol tartrate is a man-made opioid analgesic.

How Drug Works:
Levorphanol tartrate relieves moderate to severe pain and is similar to morphine. It binds to opioid receptors in the brain and central nervous system (CNS), altering the perception of pain as well as the emotional response to pain.

How Drug Is Given:
Levorphanol tartrate is a pill taken by mouth. It comes as a short-acting form (4 hours) or as a long-acting form (12 to 24 hours). Take it as directed by your doctor with an 8 oz glass of water. The dose depends on how much is needed to control your pain. Keep the medicine in a tightly closed container away from heat and moisture and out of the reach of children and pets. It can also be given by an injection in a vein.

How Should I Take This Drug?
Take this drug exactly as directed by your doctor. If you do not understand the instructions, ask your doctor or nurse to explain them to you.

 Read the following information. If you do not understand it or if any of it causes you special concern, check with your doctor.

Before taking this drug, tell your doctor if you are taking any other prescription or over-the-counter drugs, including vitamins and herbals.

Should I avoid any other medicines, foods, alcohol, and/or activities?
Your prescription and nonprescription medicines may interact with other drugs, causing harm. Certain foods or alcohol can also interact with drug products. Never begin taking a new medicine—prescription or nonprescription—without asking your doctor or nurse if it will interact with alcohol, food, or other medicines. Some drugs can cause drowsiness and affect activities such as driving.

Precautions:
Take the smallest effective dose to prevent development of tolerance and physical dependence. Tolerance (larger doses needed to give the same effect) can develop as well as physical dependence (body goes into withdrawal if drug is suddenly stopped). This is different from addiction, which is psychological dependence (take drug for psychological effect, not for relief of pain). Tell your doctor or nurse if you still are in pain even though you are taking the medicine as directed.

Since levorphanol tartrate affects the central nervous system (CNS), it is important not to take other drugs or substances that are known CNS depressants such as alcohol, sedatives, and hypnotics.

Acetaminophen or aspirin may be combined with levorphanol tartrate to increase the pain relief action.

You should be on a bowel regimen to prevent constipation while you are taking opioid pain relievers. Talk to your nurse or doctor about this.

Tell all the doctors, dentists, and pharmacists you visit that you are taking this drug.

- Most of the following side effects probably will not occur.
- Your doctor or nurse will want to discuss specific care instructions with you.
- They can help you understand these side effects and help you deal with them.

ide Effects:

More Common Side Effects
Constipation
Drowsiness
Sedation
Nausea
Dry mouth

Less Common Side Effects
Changes in mood
Euphoria
Depression
Mental clouding
Decreased rate of breathing
Vomiting
Delayed digestion
Decreased blood pressure when changing position
Decreased heart rate

Rare Side Effects
Bowel rupture due to constipation
Decreased sexual interest
Impotence
Difficulty urinating
Facial flushing
Itching
Perspiration

Side Effects / Symptoms of the Drug
Drink fluids (8 oz every 1 to 2 hours in sips) to prevent constipation. Also, try to eat foods high in fiber such as bran. You may need to take a stool softener, bulk-forming agent, and/or laxative to help keep your bowel movements regular.

Call your doctor or nurse right away if you have not moved your bowels in 2 days.

Abruptly stopping the drug can cause anxiety, dizziness, nausea and vomiting, and tiredness. The drug should be gradually discontinued.

> *Other side effects not listed above can also occur in some patients.*
> **Tell your doctor or nurse if you develop any problems.**

FDA Approval: Yes

linezolid

Trade Name:
Zyvox

Type of Drug:
Linezolid is an antibiotic that belongs to a group of drugs called oxazolidinones, a new class of antibiotics.

How Drug Works:
Linezolid prevents bacteria from making proteins. This causes the bacteria to die. Linezolid has a different way of attacking bacteria, so they cannot develop a resistance to it. Linezolid is used to treat gram-positive organisms, especially those that are resistant to other antibiotics such as vancomycin.

How Drug Is Given:
Linezolid is a pill or liquid taken by mouth with an 8 oz glass of water twice a day for 10 to 14 days. It can also be given as an injection in a vein over 30 to 60 minutes. The dose and how long you take it depends on the type of infection being treated. Gently swish the liquid a few times before pouring the dose; do not shake. Keep the medicine in a tightly closed container away from heat and moisture and out of the reach of children and pets.

How Should I Take This Drug?
Take this drug exactly as directed by your doctor. If you do not understand the instructions, ask your doctor or nurse to explain them to you.

 Read the following information. If you do not understand it or if any of it causes you special concern, check with your doctor.

Before taking this drug, tell your doctor if you are taking any other prescription or over-the-counter drugs, including vitamins and herbals.

Should I avoid any other medicines, foods, alcohol, and/or activities?
Your prescription and nonprescription medicines may interact with other drugs, causing harm. Certain foods or alcohol can also interact with drug products. Never begin taking a new medicine—prescription or nonprescription—without asking your doctor or nurse if it will interact with alcohol, food, or other medicines. Some drugs can cause drowsiness and affect activities such as driving.

Precautions:
Tell your doctor if you have any drug allergies, especially to antibiotic drugs, erythromycin in particular.

All antiobiotics can cause allergic reactions. Stop the drug and tell your doctor or nurse right away if you develop a rash, hives, fever and chills, red blotches on your skin, or difficulty breathing.

Use of antibiotics can change the normal organisms in your body. Women are at risk for fungal infections. Tell your nurse or doctor if you have vaginal itching or discharge.

Linezolid may interact with other drugs. Make sure you tell your doctor about all the medicines you are taking.

Tell all the doctors, dentists, and pharmacists you visit that you are taking this drug.
- Most of the following side effects probably will not occur.
- Your doctor or nurse will want to discuss specific care instructions with you.
- They can help you understand these side effects and help you deal with them.

Side Effects:

More Common Side Effects
Nausea
Vomiting
Loss of appetite

Less Common Side Effects
Red blotches on the skin
Itching of the skin
Rash
Muscle aches
Vaginal itching

Rare Side Effects
Diarrhea related to infection of the lining of the intestines (pseudomembranous colitis)
Swelling of ankles
Severe allergic reaction with fever, chills, rash, swelling of throat or face, and difficulty breathing
Headache
Decreased hearing
Ringing in ears (tinnitis)

Side Effects / Symptoms of the Drug
Stop the drug and call your doctor or nurse right away if you develop a rash, fever, chills, or swelling of lips or face. This can be serious.

Other side effects not listed above can also occur in some patients.
Tell your doctor or nurse if you develop any problems.

FDA Approval: Yes

loperamide hydrochloride

Trade Name:
Imodium

Type of Drug:
Loperamide hydrochloride is an antidiarrhea drug.

How Drug Works:
Loperamide hydrochloride slows the movement of the intestines. This allows water to be absorbed from the stool, so the stool becomes more firm.

How Drug Is Given:
Loperamide hydrochloride is a capsule taken by mouth. The first dose is 2 capsules taken after a loose stool, followed by 1 capsule after every loose stool after that. Do not take more than 4 capsules unless your doctor directs you to take more than this. Drink a lot of water, sports drinks, and/or soups to replace the fluid lost with diarrhea. The dose is the same for all adults. Keep the medicine in a tightly closed container away from heat and moisture and out of the reach of children and pets.

How Should I Take This Drug?
Take this drug exactly as directed by your doctor. If you do not understand the instructions, ask your doctor or nurse to explain them to you.

 Read the following information. If you do not understand it or if any of it causes you special concern, check with your doctor.

Before taking this drug, tell your doctor if you are taking any other prescription or over-the-counter drugs, including vitamins and herbals.

Should I avoid any other medicines, foods, alcohol, and/or activities?
Your prescription and nonprescription medicines may interact with other drugs, causing harm. Certain foods or alcohol can also interact with drug products. Never begin taking a new medicine—prescription or non-prescription—without asking your doctor or nurse if it will interact with alcohol, food, or other medicines. Some drugs can cause drowsiness and affect activities such as driving.

Precautions:
Tell your doctor if you have ulcerative colitis. The drug should not be used for diarrhea from infection of the intestines caused by antibiotics (pseudomembranous colitis).

To decrease the diarrhea, modify your diet. Try to eat small, frequent meals that are warm or at room temperature. Avoid foods that cause gas (such as broccoli or beans), fatty foods (such as bacon or cheeses), citrus fruits and juices, and high-lactose foods (such as milk or ice cream). Eat foods high in sodium and potassium (such as soups or sports drinks). Eat foods high in soluble fiber (such as rice or bananas). Avoid foods high in insoluble fiber (such as cereal or nuts). Try to drink at least eight 8 oz glasses of water a day. To add calories, dilute with fruit juice.

Take as directed by your nurse or doctor. This drug is often given to prevent or stop the diarrhea associated with irinotecan chemotherapy. If the diarrhea does not go away after 48 hours, call your doctor or nurse.

Tell all the doctors, dentists, and pharmacists you visit that you are taking this drug.

- Most of the following side effects probably will not occur.
- Your doctor or nurse will want to discuss specific care instructions with you.
- They can help you understand these side effects and help you deal with them.

Side Effects:

More Common Side Effects
Nausea

Less Common Side Effects
Vomiting
Abdominal pain
Drowsiness
Dizziness
Tiredness (fatigue)

Rare Side Effects
Rash

Other side effects not listed above can also occur in some patients.
Tell your doctor or nurse if you develop any problems.

FDA Approval: Yes

lorazepam

Trade Name:
Ativan

Type of Drug:
Lorazepam belongs to a general class of antianxiety drugs called benzodiazepines.

How Drug Works:
Lorazepam binds to certain receptors in the brain and spinal cord to bring about reduced anxiety, cause muscle relaxation, and prevent seizures. Lorazepam may also be used to prevent nausea and vomiting following chemotherapy. Lorazepam causes amnesia (difficulty remembering an event).

How Drug Is Given:
Lorazepam can be taken as a pill by mouth or under the tongue, or as an injection under the skin or in a muscle. The dose depends on the reason you are taking it and how well it works. Keep the medicine in a tightly closed container away from heat and moisture and out of the reach of children and pets.

How Should I Take This Drug?
Take this drug exactly as directed by your doctor. If you do not understand the instructions, ask your doctor or nurse to explain them to you.

 Read the following information. If you do not understand it or if any of it causes you special concern, check with your doctor.

Before taking this drug, tell your doctor if you are taking any other prescription or over-the-counter drugs, including vitamins and herbals.

Should I avoid any other medicines, foods, alcohol, and/or activities?
Your prescription and nonprescription medicines may interact with other drugs, causing harm. Certain foods or alcohol can also interact with drug products. Never begin taking a new medicine—prescription or nonprescription—without asking your doctor or nurse if it will interact with alcohol, food, or other medicines. Some drugs can cause drowsiness and affect activities such as driving.

Precautions:
Tell your doctor if you are taking any of the following drugs as they may have serious interactions with lorazepam: oral contraceptives, isoniazid (INH), ketoconazole, cimetidine, digoxin, levodopa, or a tricyclic antidepressant drug.

You should not take this drug if you have acute angle closure glaucoma.

Take lorazepam only as directed by your doctor. It may cause psychological dependence (addiction) and physical dependence (body goes into withdrawal if drug is suddenly stopped). When taken as directed by your doctor or nurse, this will not be a problem.

Abruptly stopping the drug can cause anxiety, dizziness, nausea and vomiting, and tiredness. The drug should be gradually stopped.

When you start taking the drug, you may feel drowsy, dizzy, confused, weak, or have a headache. This should go away after a few days of taking the drug. If not, talk to your doctor; your dose may need to be reduced.

The drug should not be given to women who are pregnant or breastfeeding.

Since lorazepam affects the central nervous system (CNS), it is important not to take other drugs or substances that are known CNS depressants such as alcohol, sedatives, and hypnotics.

Tell all the doctors, dentists, and pharmacists you visit that you are taking this drug.
- Most of the following side effects probably will not occur.
- Your doctor or nurse will want to discuss specific care instructions with you.
- They can help you understand these side effects and help you deal with them.

Side Effects:

More Common Side Effects
Drowsiness (when first starting the drug)
Tiredness (when first starting the drug)
Confusion (when first starting the drug)
Weakness (when first starting the drug)
Headache (when first starting the drug)

Less Common Side Effects
Nausea
Dry mouth
Constipation
Lack of coordination
Decreased mental alertness
Change in heart rate
Change in blood pressure

Rare Side Effects
Vivid dreams
Bizarre behavior
Vomiting
Change in weight
Palpitations
Swelling of feet
Hives
Rash

Side Effects / Symptoms of the Drug
When you start taking the drug, you may feel drowsy, dizzy, confused, weak, or have a headache. Do not drive or operate heavy machinery if you are drowsy or dizzy. This should go away after a few days of taking the drug. If it does not, talk to your doctor; your dose may need to be reduced.

Be careful walking around or changing position if you are drowsy. Stop the drug and call your doctor or nurse if the drowsiness does not go away, or if you have trouble walking or moving because of it.

Tell your doctor or nurse if you get fine tremors, feel like your body is rigid, or have difficulty speaking or swallowing. You can be given another medicine to lessen these problems.

Other side effects not listed above can also occur in some patients.
Tell your doctor or nurse if you develop any problems.

FDA Approval: Yes

magnesium citrate

Trade Names:
Citrate of magnesium, MagCitrate

Type of Drug:
Magnesium citrate is a saline laxative used to treat constipation.

How Drug Works:
Magnesium citrate pulls water from the tissues into the small intestines. This stimulates the normal forward movement of the intestines (peristalsis), resulting in a bowel movement within 3 to 6 hours.

How Drug Is Given:
Magnesium citrate is a liquid taken by mouth, mixed with water or juice. The dose depends on how well it works and the reason you are taking it. Refrigerate the medicine before using. Keep the medicine in a tightly closed container away from heat and moisture and out of the reach of children and pets.

How Should I Take This Drug?
Take this drug exactly as directed by your doctor. If you do not understand the instructions, ask your doctor or nurse to explain them to you.

 Read the following information. If you do not understand it or if any of it causes you special concern, check with your doctor.

Before taking this drug, tell your doctor if you are taking any other prescription or over-the-counter drugs, including vitamins and herbals.

Should I avoid any other medicines, foods, alcohol, and/or activities?
Your prescription and nonprescription medicines may interact with other drugs, causing harm. Certain foods or alcohol can also interact with drug products. Never begin taking a new medicine—prescription or non-prescription—without asking your doctor or nurse if it will interact with alcohol, food, or other medicines. Some drugs can cause drowsiness and affect activities such as driving.

Precautions:
To prevent constipation, try to drink 2 to 3 quarts of fluid a day, increase the amount of fruits and vegetables in your diet (try to eat 5 servings daily), eat bran cereals, and do gentle exercise as tolerated.

Some laxatives can cause diarrhea that can result in loss of fluids, nutrients, and electrolytes. It is important to replace the fluid that you lose through diarrhea. Try to drink 2 to 3 quarts of fluid a day. Fluids with electrolytes, such as broth or sports drinks, are helpful in replacing potassium and salt that are lost in diarrhea.

If you use laxatives all the time, your body may forget the normal process of moving the bowels. You then get dependent on the laxative.

If you are taking opioid pain relievers, you will need to take a laxative regularly.

Talk to your doctor before taking magnesium citrate if you have nausea, vomiting, abdominal pain, blood in the stool, or are impacted. There may be something else wrong besides constipation.

Tell all the doctors, dentists, and pharmacists you visit that you are taking this drug.

- Most of the following side effects probably will not occur.
- Your doctor or nurse will want to discuss specific care instructions with you.
- They can help you understand these side effects and help you deal with them.

Side Effects:

More Common Side Effects
Loss of normal reflexes to move bowels when laxatives are used on a long-term basis
Nausea
Abdominal pain

Less Common Side Effects
Diarrhea
Dehydration resulting from diarrhea
Loss of electrolytes

Other side effects not listed above can also occur in some patients.
Tell your doctor or nurse if you develop any problems.

FDA Approval: Yes

megestrol acetate

Trade Name:
Megace

Type of Drug:
Megestrol acetate is a synthetic progestin (female hormone) used to treat anorexia and cachexia.

How Drug Works:
The exact mechanism by which megestrol acetate works to stimulate appetite and weight gain is unknown at this time. Weight gain seems to be from increased fat storage rather than water gain.

How Drug Is Given:
Megestrol acetate is a liquid taken by mouth. The liquid is a higher dose and is taken once a day to increase appetite. The dose can be lowered if your body responds well to it. Keep the medicine in a tightly closed container away from heat and moisture and out of the reach of children and pets.

How Should I Take This Drug?
Take this drug exactly as directed by your doctor. If you do not understand the instructions, ask your doctor or nurse to explain them to you.

 Read the following information. If you do not understand it or if any of it causes you special concern, check with your doctor.

Before taking this drug, tell your doctor if you are taking any other prescription or over-the-counter drugs, including vitamins and herbals.

Should I avoid any other medicines, foods, alcohol, and/or activities?
Your prescription and nonprescription medicines may interact with other drugs, causing harm. Certain foods or alcohol can also interact with drug products. Never begin taking a new medicine—prescription or nonprescription—without asking your doctor or nurse if it will interact with alcohol, food, or other medicines. Some drug products can cause drowsiness and affect activities such as driving.

Precautions:
When megestrol is given for anorexia, more side effects are likely to occur than when the drug is used to treat cancer because the dose for anorexia is much larger.

Tell all the doctors, dentists, and pharmacists you visit that you are taking this drug.
- -
- Most of the following side effects probably will not occur.
- Your doctor or nurse will want to discuss specific care instructions with you.
- They can help you understand these side effects and help you deal with them.

Side Effects:

More Common Side Effects
Weight gain

Less Common Side Effects
Breakthrough vaginal bleeding

Rare Side Effects
Deep vein thrombosis (blood clots in legs) or blood clots in lungs
Carpal tunnel syndrome
Nausea
Vomiting
Tumor flare (temporary increase in symptoms associated with the cancer, such as bone pain)

Side Effects / Symptoms of the Drug
Call your doctor or nurse right away if you develop pain in your calf, red streaks on your lower legs, difficulty breathing, or chest pain. Let your doctor or nurse know if you are retaining fluid (swelling in your ankles, lower legs, or hands).

Other side effects not listed above can also occur in some patients.
Tell your doctor or nurse if you develop any problems.

FDA Approval: Yes

meperidine hydrochloride

Trade Names:
Demerol, Mepergan Fortis

Type of Drug:
Meperidine hydrochloride is a synthetic opioid analgesic, similar to morphine.

How Drug Works:
Meperidine hydrochloride relieves moderate to severe acute pain. It binds to opioid receptors in the brain and central nervous system (CNS), altering the perception of pain as well as the emotional response to pain.

How Drug Is Given:
Meperidine hydrochloride can be given by an injection in a vein, in the muscle, or under the skin. It can also be given as a pill by mouth. The dose depends on the reason the medicine is being given and how well your pain goes away with the dose.

How Should I Take This Drug?
Take this drug exactly as directed by your doctor. If you do not understand the instructions, ask your doctor or nurse to explain them to you.

 Read the following information. If you do not understand it or if any of it causes you special concern, check with your doctor.

Before taking this drug, tell your doctor if you are taking any other prescription or over-the-counter drugs, including vitamins and herbals.

Should I avoid any other medicines, foods, alcohol, and/or activities?
Your prescription and nonprescription medicines may interact with other drugs, causing harm. Certain foods or alcohol can also interact with drug products. Never begin taking a new medicine—prescription or nonprescription—without asking your doctor or nurse if it will interact with alcohol, food, or other medicines. Some drugs can cause drowsiness and affect activities such as driving.

Precautions:
Take the smallest effective dose to prevent development of tolerance (larger doses needed to give the same effect) as well as physical dependence (body goes into withdrawal if drug is suddenly stopped). This is different from addiction, which is psychological dependence (take drug for psychological effect, not for relief of pain). Tell your doctor or nurse if you still are in pain even though you are taking the medicine as directed.

Since meperidine hydrochloride affects the central nervous system (CNS), it is important not to take other drugs or substances that are known CNS depressants such as alcohol, sedatives, and hypnotics.

Acetaminophen or aspirin may be combined with meperidine hydrochloride to increase pain relief.

You should be on a bowel regimen to prevent constipation while you are taking opioid pain relievers. Talk to your nurse or doctor about this.

Meperidine hydrochloride is used to relieve acute pain, such as postoperative pain. It should not be used to manage chronic pain related to cancer. The pain relief is short acting, and frequent use can cause dangerous side effects.

Tell all the doctors, dentists, and pharmacists you visit that you are taking this drug.
- Most of the following side effects probably will not occur.
- Your doctor or nurse will want to discuss specific care instructions with you.
- They can help you understand these side effects and help you deal with them.

Side Effects:

More Common Side Effects
Constipation
Drowsiness
Sedation
Nausea
Vomiting
Dizziness
Dry mouth

Less Common Side Effects
Changes in mood
Euphoria
Mental clouding
Decreased breathing rate
Decreased blood pressure when changing position
Delayed digestion
Decreased heart rate

Rare Side Effects
Difficulty urinating
Seizures
Decreased sexual interest
Impotence

Side Effects / Symptoms of the Drug
Drink fluids (8 oz every hour in sips) to prevent constipation. Also, try to eat foods high in fiber such as bran, fruits, and vegetables. You may need to take a stool softener, bulk-forming agent, and/or laxative to help keep your bowel movements regular.

Call your doctor or nurse right away if you have not moved your bowels in 2 days.

Abruptly stopping the drug can cause anxiety, dizziness, nausea and vomiting, and tiredness. The drug should be gradually stopped.

Other side effects not listed above can also occur in some patients.
Tell your doctor or nurse if you develop any problems.

FDA Approval: Yes

methadone

Trade Names:
Dolophine, Methadose

Type of Drug:
Methadone is a synthetic opioid analgesic, similar to morphine.

How Drug Works:
Methadone relieves moderate to severe pain. It binds to opioid receptors in the brain and central nervous system (CNS), altering the perception of pain as well as the emotional response to pain.

How Drug Is Given:
Methadone is given as a pill or liquid by mouth, or as an injection in a vein, muscle, or under the skin. The dose depends on how well your pain is managed by the dose. Keep the medicine in a tightly closed container away from heat and moisture and out of the reach of children and pets.

How Should I Take This Drug?
Take this drug exactly as directed by your doctor. If you do not understand the instructions, ask your doctor or nurse to explain them to you.

 Read the following information. If you do not understand it or if any of it causes you special concern, check with your doctor.

Before taking this drug, tell your doctor if you are taking any other prescription or over-the-counter drugs, including vitamins and herbals.

Should I avoid any other medicines, foods, alcohol, and/or activities?
Your prescription and nonprescription medicines may interact with other drugs, causing harm. Certain foods or alcohol can also interact with drug products. Never begin taking a new medicine—prescription or nonprescription—without asking your doctor or nurse if it will interact with alcohol, food, or other medicines. Some drugs can cause drowsiness and affect activities such as driving.

Precautions:
Take the smallest effective dose to prevent development of tolerance (larger doses needed to give the same effect) as well as physical dependence (body goes into withdrawal if drug is suddenly stopped). This is different from addiction, which is psychological dependence (take drug for psychological effect, not for relief of pain). Tell your doctor or nurse if you still have pain even though you are taking the medicine as directed.

Since methadone affects the central nervous system (CNS), it is important not to take other drugs or substances that are known CNS depressants such as alcohol, sedatives, and hypnotics.

Acetaminophen or aspirin may be combined with methadone to increase the pain relief action.

You should be on a bowel regimen to prevent constipation while you are taking opioid pain relievers. Talk to your nurse or doctor about this.

Tell all the doctors, dentists, and pharmacists you visit that you are taking this drug.
- Most of the following side effects probably will not occur.
- Your doctor or nurse will want to discuss specific care instructions with you.
- They can help you understand these side effects and help you deal with them.

Side Effects:

More Common Side Effects
Constipation
Drowsiness
Sedation
Nausea
Dizziness
Dry mouth

Less Common Side Effects
Vomiting
Changes in mood
Euphoria
Depression
Mental clouding
Decreased breathing rate
Decreased blood pressure when changing position
Delayed digestion
Decreased heart rate

Rare Side Effects
Difficulty urinating
Seizures
Decreased sexual interest
Impotence

Side Effects / Symptoms of the Drug
Drink fluids (8 oz every hour in sips) to prevent constipation. Also, try to eat foods high in fiber such as bran, fruits, and vegetables. You may need to take a stool softener, bulk-forming agent, and/or laxative to help keep your bowel movements regular.

Call your doctor or nurse right away if you have not moved your bowels in 2 days.

Abruptly stopping the drug can cause anxiety, dizziness, nausea and vomiting, and tiredness. The drug should be gradually stopped.

Other side effects not listed above can also occur in some patients.
Tell your doctor or nurse if you develop any problems.

FDA Approval: Yes

methylcellulose

Trade Name:
Citrucel

Type of Drug:
Methylcellulose is a bulk-producing laxative used to treat constipation.

How Drug Works:
Methylcellulose absorbs water, which expands in the intestines. This stimulates the normal forward movement of the intestines (peristalsis), resulting in a bowel movement within 12 to 24 hours. Methylcellulose may also be used to slow down diarrhea.

How Drug Is Given:
Methylcellulose is a powder mixed in at least 8 oz of juice or water. Drink it right after mixing or it will become too thick. Keep container tightly closed away from heat and moisture and out of the reach of children and pets.

How Should I Take This Drug?
Take this drug exactly as directed by your doctor. If you do not understand the instructions, ask your doctor or nurse to explain them to you.

 Read the following information. If you do not understand it or if any of it causes you special concern, check with your doctor.

Before taking this drug, tell your doctor if you are taking any other prescription or over-the-counter drugs, including vitamins and herbals.

Should I avoid any other medicines, foods, alcohol, and/or activities?
Your prescription and nonprescription medicines may interact with other drugs, causing harm. Certain foods or alcohol can also interact with drug products. Never begin taking a new medicine—prescription or nonprescription—without asking your doctor or nurse if it will interact with alcohol, food, or other medicines. Some drugs can cause drowsiness and affect activities such as driving.

Precautions:
Methylcellulose is not absorbed by the gastrointestinal tract, so there are few side effects.

To prevent constipation, try to drink 2 to 3 quarts of fluid a day, increase the amount of fruits and vegetables in your diet (5 servings of fruits and vegetables daily), eat bran cereals, and do gentle exercise as tolerated.

Tell all the doctors, dentists, and pharmacists you visit that you are taking this drug.

- Most of the following side effects probably will not occur.
- Your doctor or nurse will want to discuss specific care instructions with you.
- They can help you understand these side effects and help you deal with them.

Side Effects:

More Common Side Effects
Nausea

Less Common Side Effects
Vomiting
Cramps

Other side effects not listed above can also occur in some patients.
Tell your doctor or nurse if you develop any problems.

FDA Approval: Yes

metoclopramide

Trade Name:
Reglan

Type of Drug:
Metoclopramide belongs to the general class of drugs called substituted benzamides, which are used to treat nausea and vomiting.

How Drug Works:
When given at low doses, metoclopramide increases emptying of the stomach, thus decreasing the chance of developing nausea and vomiting due to food remaining in the stomach. When given at high doses, metoclopramide blocks the messages to the part of the brain responsible for nausea and vomiting resulting from chemotherapy.

How Drug Is Given:
Metoclopramide is a pill given by mouth usually 30 minutes before a meal and at bedtime. It can also be given as an injection in a vein. Keep the medicine in a tightly closed container away from heat and moisture and out of the reach of children and pets.

How Should I Take This Drug?
Take this drug exactly as directed by your doctor. If you do not understand the instructions, ask your doctor or nurse to explain them to you.

 Read the following information. If you do not understand it or if any of it causes you special concern, check with your doctor.

Before taking this drug, tell your doctor if you are taking any other prescription or over-the-counter drugs, including vitamins and herbals.

Should I avoid any other medicines, foods, alcohol, and/or activities?
Your prescription and nonprescription medicines may interact with other drugs, causing harm. Certain foods or alcohol can also interact with drug products. Never begin taking a new medicine—prescription or nonprescription—without asking your doctor or nurse if it will interact with alcohol, food, or other medicines. Some drugs can cause drowsiness and affect activities such as driving.

Precautions:
Metoclopramide may cause extrapyramidal side effects. These include restlessness, tongue protrusion, and involuntary movements. These side effects stop immediately when you are given diphenhydramine.

Metoclopramide is given before and after chemotherapy to prevent nausea and vomiting. It is often combined with other drugs such as dexamethasone and diphenhydramine. It may also be given in low doses following cisplatin chemotherapy to prevent delayed nausea and vomiting.

Tell all the doctors, dentists, and pharmacists you visit that you are taking this drug.

- Most of the following side effects probably will not occur.
- Your doctor or nurse will want to discuss specific care instructions with you.
- They can help you understand these side effects and help you deal with them.

Side Effects:

More Common Side Effects
Feeling sedated
Sleepiness
Restlessness
Diarrhea
Dry mouth

Rare Side Effects
Rash
Hives
Decreased blood pressure

Side Effects / Symptoms of the Drug
Be careful getting up, changing position, or when walking.

Other side effects not listed above can also occur in some patients.
Tell your doctor or nurse if you develop any problems.

FDA Approval: Yes

metronidazole hydrochloride

Trade Name:
Flagyl

Type of Drug:
Metronidazole hydrochloride belongs to a general class of drugs called antibiotics.

How Drug Works:
Metronidazole hydrochloride interferes with bacteria and protozoa's ability to make DNA so they are unable to reproduce. It is used to treat gram-negative and gram-positive bacteria and protozoa.

How Drug Is Given:
Metronidazole hydrochloride is a pill taken once in a single dose, or more likely, 3 times a day for 7 to 14 days as directed by your doctor. Take with food or milk to lessen stomach upset. It can also be given as an injection in a vein over 30 minutes. The dose depends on your weight, the type of infection being treated, and how well your liver is working. Do not drink alcohol while taking the medicine. Keep the medicine in a tightly closed container away from heat and moisture and out of the reach of children and pets.

 Read the following information. If you do not understand it or if any of it causes you special concern, check with your doctor.

Before taking this drug, tell your doctor if you are taking any other prescription or over-the-counter drugs, including vitamins and herbals.

Should I avoid any other medicines, foods, alcohol, and/or activities?
Your prescription and nonprescription medicines may interact with other drugs, causing harm. Certain foods or alcohol can also interact with drug products. Never begin taking a new medicine—prescription or non-prescription—without asking your doctor or nurse if it will interact with alcohol, food, or other medicines. Some drugs can cause drowsiness and affect activities such as driving.

Precautions:
Tell your doctor if you are taking the anticoagulant warfarin (Coumadin), phenobarbital, phenytoin (Dilantin), or cimetidine. Talk to your doctor about possible drug interactions.

Tell your doctor if you have any drug allergies, especially to antibiotic drugs.

All antibiotics can cause allergic reactions. Stop the drug and tell your doctor or nurse right away if you develop a rash, hives, red blotches on your skin, difficulty breathing, or chest pain.

Use of antibiotics can change the normal organisms in your body. Women are at risk of getting fungal infections. Tell your nurse or doctor if you get vaginal itching or discharge.

This drug should not be used during the first 3 months of pregnancy or by mothers who are breastfeeding. It should be used cautiously in patients with a history of blood disorders, liver disease, central nervous system (CNS) disorders, and alcoholism.

DO NOT drink alcohol while taking metronidazole hydrochloride, as it causes a serious reaction (nausea, vomiting, headache, flushing, abdominal cramping, and sweating). Do not drink alcohol for 48 hours after the last drug dose.

Tell all the doctors, dentists, and pharmacists you visit that you are taking this drug.

- Most of the following side effects probably will not occur.
- Your doctor or nurse will want to discuss specific care instructions with you.
- They can help you understand these side effects and help you deal with them.

Side Effects:

More Common Side Effects
Nausea
Headache
Loss of appetite
Metallic taste in mouth after taking the pill

Less Common Side Effects
Vomiting
Diarrhea
Heartburn
Constipation
Numbness and tingling in hands and/or feet
Darkened urine
Change in pattern of urination
Vaginal itching or discharge
Vaginal candidiasis (fungal infection)
Irritation of vein where drug is given

Rare Side Effects
Diarrhea related to infection of the intestinal lining (pseudomembranous colitis)
Dizziness
Difficulty walking
Confusion
Mood changes
Rash
Itching
Flushing
Joint pain
Decreased sexual interest
Dryness of vagina

Side Effects / Symptoms of the Drug
Stop the drug and call your doctor or nurse right away if you develop a rash, hives, fever, and chills. This can be a serious reaction and needs to be treated right away.

Stop the drug and call your doctor or nurse right away if you get diarrhea that does not stop, abdominal cramping, and blood and/or pus in the stool. This needs to be treated right away.

Other side effects not listed above can also occur in some patients.
Tell your doctor or nurse if you develop any problems.

FDA Approval: Yes

mezlocillin sodium

Trade Name:
Mezlin

Type of Drug:
Mezlocillin sodium is an antibiotic that belongs to a group of drugs called penicillins.

How Drug Works:
Mezlocillin sodium prevents bacteria from making their protein wall, which causes the cells to die. It is used to treat serious gram-negative infections of the lungs, urinary tract, and skin.

How Drug Is Given:
Mezlocillin sodium is given as an injection in a vein 4 to 6 times a day. The dose depends on the infection being treated, your weight, and how well your kidneys are working. Mezlocillin sodium can also be given as an injection in a muscle.

 Read the following information. If you do not understand it or if any of it causes you special concern, check with your doctor.

Before taking this drug, tell your doctor if you are taking any other prescription or over-the-counter drugs, including vitamins and herbals.

Should I avoid any other medicines, foods, alcohol, and/or activities?
Your prescription and nonprescription medicines may interact with other drugs, causing harm. Certain foods or alcohol can also interact with drug products. Never begin taking a new medicine—prescription or non-prescription—without asking your doctor or nurse if it will interact with alcohol, food, or other medicines. Some drugs can cause drowsiness and affect activities such as driving.

Precautions:
All antibiotics can cause allergic reactions. Stop the drug and tell your doctor or nurse right away if you develop a rash, hives, red blotches on your skin, or difficulty breathing.

Use of antibiotics can change the normal organisms in your body. Women are at risk of getting fungal infections. Tell your nurse or doctor if you get vaginal itching or discharge.

This drug should be used with caution by women who are pregnant or breastfeeding.

Tell your doctor if you have any drug allergies, especially to antibiotic drugs.

Tell all the doctors, dentists, and pharmacists you visit that you are taking this drug.
- -
- Most of the following side effects probably will not occur.
- Your doctor or nurse will want to discuss specific care instructions with you.
- They can help you understand these side effects and help you deal with them.

Side Effects:

More Common Side Effects
Nausea

Less Common Side Effects
Vomiting
Diarrhea
Vaginal itching
Irritation of the vein used for giving the drug
Low blood potassium level
Vaginal candidiasis (fungal infection)

Rare Side Effects
Rash
Hives
Itching
Fever
Chills
Darkening and peeling of skin
Diarrhea related to infection of the intestinal lining (pseudomembranous colitis)
Decreased white blood cell count with increased risk of infection
Decreased red blood cell count with increased risk of tiredness (fatigue) and anemia
Dizziness
Headache
Sleepiness

Side Effects / Symptoms of the Drug
Stop the drug and call your doctor or nurse right away if you develop a rash, fever, chills, or peeling skin. This can be a serious reaction and needs to be treated right away.

Stop the drug and call your doctor or nurse right away if you get diarrhea that does not stop, abdominal cramping, and blood and/or pus in the stool. This needs to be treated right away.

Other side effects not listed above can also occur in some patients.
Tell your doctor or nurse if you develop any problems.

FDA Approval: Yes

miconazole nitrate

Trade Name:
Monistat

Type of Drug:
Miconazole nitrate is an antifungal drug.

How Drug Works:
Miconazole nitrate prevents fungi from reproducing and kills the organisms at higher doses.

How Drug Is Given:
Miconazole nitrate is given in a number of ways. Given as an injection in the vein over 30 to 60 minutes, the dose and length of treatment depend on the infection being treated. Miconazole nitrate is also given as a vaginal suppository or as a cream or powder applied to the skin. Keep the medicine in a tightly closed container away from heat and moisture and out of the reach of children and pets.

How Should I Take This Drug?
Take this drug exactly as directed by your doctor. If you do not understand the instructions, ask your doctor or nurse to explain them to you.

 Read the following information. If you do not understand it or if any of it causes you special concern, check with your doctor.

Before taking this drug, tell your doctor if you are taking any other prescription or over-the-counter drugs, including vitamins and herbals.

Should I avoid any other medicines, foods, alcohol, and/or activities?
Your prescription and nonprescription medicines may interact with other drugs, causing harm. Certain foods or alcohol can also interact with drug products. Never begin taking a new medicine—prescription or non-prescription—without asking your doctor or nurse if it will interact with alcohol, food, or other medicines. Some drugs can cause drowsiness and affect activities such as driving.

Precautions:
Tell your doctor if you are taking rifampin, isoniazid, warfarin (Coumadin), cyclosporine, phenytoin (Dilantin), or oral anticoagulants (Coumadin). Talk to your doctor about possible drug interactions.

All drugs used to fight microorganisms can cause allergic reactions. Stop the drug and tell your nurse or doctor right away if you develop a rash, hives, red blotches on your skin, or difficulty breathing.

When given for an infection throughout your body (systemic), the first dose is usually given in a hospital setting so you can be watched closely for any reaction.

The intravenous form of the drug is used for systemic fungal infections. The suppositories and vaginal cream are used to treat fungal infections of the vagina. Cream and powder may also be used for affected skin areas, as directed by your doctor.

Tell all the doctors, dentists, and pharmacists you visit that you are taking this drug.
- Most of the following side effects probably will not occur.
- Your doctor or nurse will want to discuss specific care instructions with you.
- They can help you understand these side effects and help you deal with them.

Side Effects:

More Common Side Effects
Pain and irritation at place of injection
Mild nausea
Burning in the vagina (when using suppository)

Less Common Side Effects
Vomiting
Loss of appetite
Dizziness
Diarrhea
Bitter taste
Flushing of face
Anxiety
Blurred vision
Headache

Rare Side Effects
Severe allergic reaction
Decreased red blood cell count with increased risk of anemia and tiredness (fatigue)
Rash
Itching
Fever
Chills

Side Effects / Symptoms of the Drug
Call your doctor or nurse right away if you develop rash, fever, or chills. Your doctor needs to evaluate you.

Other side effects not listed above can also occur in some patients.
Tell your doctor or nurse if you develop any problems.

FDA Approval: Yes

mineral oil

Trade Name:
Fleet Mineral Oil

Type of Drug:
Mineral oil is a lubricant laxative used to treat constipation.

How Drug Works:
Mineral oil lubricates the intestinal surface so that water is not absorbed into the tissue. The water swells the intestines, stimulating the normal forward movement of the intestines (peristalsis), which results in a bowel movement within 6 to 8 hours.

How Drug Is Given:
Mineral oil is taken as a liquid by mouth on an empty stomach at bedtime. It can also be taken as a rectal enema. The dose is the same for all adults and depends on how well it works. Keep the medicine in a tightly closed container away from heat and moisture and out of the reach of children and pets.

How Should I Take This Drug?
Take this drug exactly as directed by your doctor. If you do not understand the instructions, ask your doctor or nurse to explain them to you.

 Read the following information. If you do not understand it or if any of it causes you special concern, check with your doctor.

Before taking this drug, tell your doctor if you are taking any other prescription or over-the-counter drugs, including vitamins and herbals.

Should I avoid any other medicines, foods, alcohol, and/or activities?
Your prescription and nonprescription medicines may interact with other drugs, causing harm. Certain foods or alcohol can also interact with drug products. Never begin taking a new medicine—prescription or non-prescription—without asking your doctor or nurse if it will interact with alcohol, food, or other medicines. Some drugs can cause drowsiness and affect activities such as driving.

Precautions:
Do not take mineral oil if you are also taking docusate calcium, docusate potassium, and docusate sodium. These drugs will cause the mineral oil to be absorbed into the body.

To prevent constipation, try to drink 2 to 3 quarts of fluid a day, increase the amount of fruits and vegetables in your diet (5 servings of fruits and vegetables daily), eat bran cereal, and do gentle exercise as tolerated.

Some laxatives can cause diarrhea that can result in loss of fluids, nutrients, and electrolytes. It is important to replace the fluid that you lose through diarrhea. Try to drink 2 to 3 quarts of fluid a day. Fluids with electrolytes, such as chicken broth or sports drinks, are helpful in replacing potassium and salt that are lost in diarrhea. Take this medicine as instructed by your doctor.

If you use laxatives all the time, your body may forget the normal process of moving the bowels. You then get dependent upon the laxative.

If you are taking opioid pain relievers, you will need to take a laxative regularly.

This drug should not be used for more than 1 week.

Patients with an intestinal obstruction, fecal impaction, or ulcerative bowel disease, or if there is nausea, vomiting, or abdominal pain should not use this drug.

Tell all the doctors, dentists, and pharmacists you visit that you are taking this drug.
- Most of the following side effects probably will not occur.
- Your doctor or nurse will want to discuss specific care instructions with you.
- They can help you understand these side effects and help you deal with them.

Side Effects:

More Common Side Effects
Loss of normal reflexes to move bowels when laxatives are used for a long time
Nausea
Cramps

Less Common Side Effects
Vomiting
Diarrhea

Other side effects not listed above can also occur in some patients.
Tell your doctor or nurse if you develop any problems.

FDA Approval: Yes

minocycline hydrochloride

Trade Names:
Minocin, Vectrin, Dynacin

Type of Drug:
Minocycline hydrochloride belongs to the group of drugs called antibiotics.

How Drug Works:
Minocycline hydrochloride prevents bacteria from making proteins, which causes the bacteria to die. It is active against gram-positive and gram-negative bacteria and organisms called mycobacteria and chlamydia.

How Drug Is Given:
Minocycline hydrochloride is taken as a pill, capsule, or liquid by mouth 2 to 4 times a day for 5 to 15 days. Take it with or without food at about the same time each day. Shake the liquid before pouring the dose. It can also be given as an injection in a vein over 1 to 6 hours, 1 to 2 times a day. The dose depends on the infection being treated, your weight, and how well your kidneys are working. The first day's dose is usually twice the next day's dose to get the amount of drug in the blood at an effective level to kill the organisms. If you are also taking iron, take it 2 hours before minocycline hydrochloride or 3 hours after the dose. Keep the medicine in a tightly closed container away from heat and moisture and out of the reach of children and pets.

How Should I Take This Drug?
Take this drug exactly as directed by your doctor. If you do not understand the instructions, ask your doctor or nurse to explain them to you.

 Read the following information. If you do not understand it or if any of it causes you special concern, check with your doctor.

Before taking this drug, tell your doctor if you are taking any other prescription or over-the-counter drugs, including vitamins and herbals.

Should I avoid any other medicines, foods, alcohol, and/or activities?
Your prescription and nonprescription medicines may interact with other drugs, causing harm. Certain foods or alcohol can also interact with drug products. Never begin taking a new medicine—prescription or nonprescription—without asking your doctor or nurse if it will interact with alcohol, food, or other medicines. Some drugs can cause drowsiness and affect activities such as driving.

Precautions:
Tell your doctor if you have any drug allergies, especially to antibiotic drugs.

All antibiotics can cause allergic reactions.

Use of antibiotics can change the normal organisms in your body. Women are at risk for fungal infections. Tell your nurse or doctor if you have vaginal itching or discharge.

Minocycline hydrochloride can interact with other medicines. Make sure that you tell your doctor about all the medicines you are taking, especially if you are taking warfarin (Coumadin), medicines to stop diarrhea, iron, lithium, or oral contraceptives.

Minocycline hydrochloride can decrease the effectivess of oral contraceptives and cause break-through bleeding. If you are taking oral contraceptives, make sure that you also use a barrier method of birth control.

Minocycline hydrochloride can cause dizziness, lightheadedness, or unsteadiness. Make sure that you are careful and hold onto something to prevent falling when you first take minocycline hydrochloride. If this side effect does not go away, tell your doctor or nurse.

Minocycline hydrochloride may darken the skin and lining of the mouth (mucous membranes).

If you have myasthenia gravis, minocycline hydrochloride may increase muscle weakness. Talk to your doctor about this.

Minocycline hydrochloride causes an exaggerated sunburn (photosensitivity). Wear a hat and clothing to cover all skin areas that are exposed to the sun. Avoid direct sunlight if possible, or wear protective clothing if you have to be out in the sun.

Tell all the doctors, dentists, and pharmacists you visit that you are taking this drug.

- Most of the following side effects probably will not occur.
- Your doctor or nurse will want to discuss specific care instructions with you.
- They can help you understand these side effects and help you deal with them.

Side Effects:

More Common Side Effects
Nausea
Diarrhea
Loss of appetite
Increased skin sensitivity to the sun
Pain and redness at the intravenous injection site
Irritation of the vein used for intravenous injection
Lightheadedness
Dizziness
Headache

Less Common Side Effects
Vomiting
Abdominal discomfort
Heartburn
Swelling of the tongue
Vaginal itching

Rare Side Effects
Hairy tongue
Red or dark rash with peeling of the skin
Severe allergic reaction with fever, chills, rash, red blotches on the skin, swelling of throat or face, and difficulty breathing
Joint aches
Liver problems
Diarrhea related to infection of the intestinal lining (pseudomembranous colitis)
Decreased white blood cell count with increased risk of infection
Decreased red blood cell count with increased risk of tiredness and anemia
Decreased platelet count with risk of bleeding

Side Effects / Symptoms of the Drug
Stop the drug and tell your doctor or nurse right away if you develop fever, chills, rash, or red blotches on the skin.

Other side effects not listed above can also occur in some patients.
Tell your doctor or nurse if you develop any problems.

FDA Approval: Yes

mirtazapine

Trade Name:
Remeron

Type of Drug:
Mirtazapine belongs to a general class of drugs called antidepressants.

How Drug Works:
Mirtazapine increases the amount of serotonin and norepinephrine in the brain so that the feeling of depression is prevented or relieved.

How Drug Is Given:
Mirtazapine is a pill given by mouth once a day at bedtime, or in 2 divided doses morning and evening, with or without food. The dose depends on how well the medicine works, and your doctor may increase the dose gradually to get a better effect. Keep the medicine in a tightly closed container away from heat and moisture and out of the reach of children and pets.

How Should I Take This Drug?
Take this drug exactly as directed by your doctor. If you do not understand the instructions, ask your doctor or nurse to explain them to you.

 Read the following information. If you do not understand it or if any of it causes you special concern, check with your doctor.

Before taking this drug, tell your doctor if you are taking any other prescription or over-the-counter drugs, including vitamins and herbals.

Should I avoid any other medicines, foods, alcohol, and/or activities?
Your prescription and nonprescription medicines may interact with other drugs, causing harm. Certain foods or alcohol can also interact with drug products. Never begin taking a new medicine—prescription or nonprescription—without asking your doctor or nurse if it will interact with alcohol, food, or other medicines. Some drugs can cause drowsiness and affect activities such as driving.

Precautions:
Tell your doctor if you have epilepsy, liver or kidney problems, heart disease, low blood pressure, acute narrow angle glaucoma, enlarged prostate or problems in passing your urine, or diabetes mellitus. This drug should be used cautiously if you have any of these problems.

Stop the drug and tell your doctor right away if you develop jaundice (yellow eyes or skin).

It may take 2 weeks or longer for the antidepressant effect to work.

Mirtazapine causes sedation and drowsiness, especially during the first 2 weeks of starting the drug. It can help you sleep at night, and this effect starts right away. Many people find taking the drug at bedtime best.

When first taking mirtazapine, do not drive a car or operate heavy machinery until the effect is known.

Abruptly stopping the drug can cause nausea, headache, and malaise. The drug should be gradually stopped.

Mirtazapine affects the central nervous system (CNS), so it is important not to take other drugs or substances that are known to suppress the CNS such as alcohol, sedatives, and hypnotics.

Tell all the doctors, dentists, and pharmacists you visit that you are taking this drug.

- Most of the following side effects probably will not occur.
- Your doctor or nurse will want to discuss specific care instructions with you.
- They can help you understand these side effects and help you deal with them.

Side Effects:

More Common Side Effects
Increased appetite
Weight gain
Drowsiness
Decreased mental alertness

Less Common Side Effects
Swelling of feet and hands

Rare Side Effects
Low blood pressure when moving from lying to sitting or standing positions
Seizures
Low white blood cell count with risk for infection
Abnormal liver function tests (which is temporary)
Skin rash

Side Effects / Symptoms of the Drug
Stop the drug and call your doctor or nurse right away if you develop a rash or feel that you want to hurt yourself.

Stop the drug and call your doctor or nurse right away if you get tremors in your hands or feet, have a seizure, or become jaundiced (yellowing of eyes or skin).

Other side effects not listed above can also occur in some patients.
Tell your doctor or nurse if you develop any problems.

FDA Approval: Yes

morphine

Trade Names:
Astramorph, Duramorph, Infumorph, Kadian Morphine Sulfate Sustained Release, MS Contin, MSIR, Oramorph, Roxanol

Type of Drug:
Morphine is an opioid analgesic used to relieve moderate to severe pain.

How Drug Works:
Morphine binds to opioid receptors in the brain and central nervous system (CNS), altering the perception of pain as well as the emotional response to pain.

How Drug Is Given:
Morphine comes in a number of preparations. It is usually taken as a pill by mouth. It comes in a short-acting form (3 to 4 hours) or a long-acting form (12 to 24 hours). Take the pill or liquid with a full glass of water, with or without food. Make sure to shake the liquid before pouring the dose. Try to drink an 8 oz glass of water or fluid every hour to help prevent constipation. It can also be given by an injection in a vein or the spinal cord, in a pump connected to a vein, as a liquid, or as a rectal suppository. When taking a suppository, open the package and dip the tip in water. If you are right-handed, lie down on your left side, bring your knees up near your chest, and insert the suppository in your rectum about an inch. Stay in this position for about 15 minutes, then get up and wash your hands well. The dose depends on how much is needed to control your pain. Keep the medicine in a tightly closed container away from heat and moisture and out of the reach of children and pets.

How Should I Take This Drug?
Take this drug exactly as directed by your doctor. If you do not understand the instructions, ask your doctor or nurse to explain them to you.

 Read the following information. If you do not understand it or if any of it causes you special concern, check with your doctor.

Before taking this drug, tell your doctor if you are taking any other prescription or over-the-counter drugs, including vitamins and herbals.

Should I avoid any other medicines, foods, alcohol, and/or activities?
Your prescription and nonprescription medicines may interact with other drugs, causing harm. Certain foods or alcohol can also interact with drug products. Never begin taking a new medicine—prescription or nonprescription—without asking your doctor or nurse if it will interact with alcohol, food, or other medicines. Some drugs can cause drowsiness and affect activities such as driving.

Precautions:
Take the smallest effective dose to prevent development of tolerance (larger doses needed to give the same effect) as well as physical dependence (body goes into withdrawal if drug is suddenly stopped). This is different from addiction, which is psychological dependence (take drug for psychological effect, not for relief of pain). Tell your doctor or nurse if you are still in pain even though you are taking the medicine as directed.

Acetaminophen or aspirin may be combined with morphine to increase the pain relief action.

You should be on a bowel regimen to prevent constipation while you are taking opioid pain relievers. Talk to your nurse or doctor about this.

Since morphine affects the central nervous system (CNS), it is important not to take other drugs or substances that are known CNS depressants such as alcohol, sedatives, and hypnotics.

Tell all the doctors, dentists, and pharmacists you visit that you are taking this drug.

- Most of the following side effects probably will not occur.
- Your doctor or nurse will want to discuss specific care instructions with you.
- They can help you understand these side effects and help you deal with them.

Side Effects:

More Common Side Effects
Constipation
Drowsiness
Sedation
Nausea
Dizziness
Dry mouth

Less Common Side Effects
Vomiting
Changes in mood
Euphoria
Depression
Mental clouding
Decreased breathing rate
Decreased blood pressure when changing position
Delayed digestion
Decreased heart rate

Rare Side Effects
Difficulty urinating
Decreased sexual interest
Impotence

Side Effects / Symptoms of the Drug

Drink fluids (8 oz every hour in sips) to prevent constipation. Also, try to eat foods high in fiber such as bran, fruits, and vegetables. You may need to take a stool softener, bulk-forming agent, and/or laxative to help keep your bowel movements regular.

Call your doctor or nurse right away if you have not moved your bowels in 2 days.

Abruptly stopping the drug can cause anxiety, dizziness, nausea and vomiting, and tiredness. The drug should be gradually discontinued.

Other side effects not listed above can also occur in some patients.
Tell your doctor or nurse if you develop any problems.

FDA Approval: Yes

nafcillin sodium

Trade Name:
Unipen

Type of Drug:
Nafcillin sodium is a semisynthetic penicillin that belongs to a general class of drugs called antibiotics.

How Drug Works:
Nafcillin sodium prevents bacteria from making their cell walls, which causes the cells to die. It is used to treat gram-positive infections and bacteria that are resistant to penicillin.

How Drug Is Given:
Nafcillin sodium is a pill taken by mouth with an 8 oz glass of water 4 times a day for 10 to 14 days. Take with 8 oz of water on an empty stomach, 1 hour before or 2 hours after a meal. It can also be given as an injection in a vein over 30 to 60 minutes 6 times a day. The dose and how long you take it depends on your weight and the type of infection being treated. Keep the medicine in a tightly closed container away from heat and moisture and out of the reach of children and pets.

How Should I Take This Drug?
Take this drug exactly as directed by your doctor. If you do not understand the instructions, ask your doctor or nurse to explain them to you.

 Read the following information. If you do not understand it or if any of it causes you special concern, check with your doctor.

Before taking this drug, tell your doctor if you are taking any other prescription or over-the-counter drugs, including vitamins and herbals.

Should I avoid any other medicines, foods, alcohol, and/or activities?
Your prescription and nonprescription medicines may interact with other drugs, causing harm. Certain foods or alcohol can also interact with drug products. Never begin taking a new medicine—prescription or non-prescription—without asking your doctor or nurse if it will interact with alcohol, food, or other medicines. Some drugs can cause drowsiness and affect activities such as driving.

Precautions:
All antibiotics can cause allergic reactions. Stop the drug and tell your doctor or nurse right away if you develop a rash, hives, red blotches on your skin, or difficulty breathing.

Use of antibiotics can change the normal organisms in your body. Women are at risk of getting fungal infections. Tell your nurse or doctor if you get vaginal itching or discharge.

Nafcillin sodium should be used with caution by women who are pregnant or breastfeeding.

Tell your doctor if you have any drug allergies, especially to antibiotic drugs. You should not take this drug if you are allergic to penicillin.

Tell all the doctors, dentists, and pharmacists you visit that you are taking this drug.

- Most of the following side effects probably will not occur.
- Your doctor or nurse will want to discuss specific care instructions with you.
- They can help you understand these side effects and help you deal with them.

Side Effects:

More Common Side Effects
Nausea
Vaginal itching
Vaginal candidiasis (fungal infection)

Less Common Side Effects
Vomiting
Diarrhea
Irritation of vein used for giving the drug

Rare Side Effects
Rash
Hives
Itching
Fever
Chills
Muscle aches
Swelling of feet
Darkening and peeling of skin
Diarrhea related to infection of the intestinal lining (pseudomembranous colitis)
Decreased white blood cell count with increased risk of infection
Decreased red blood cell count with increased risk of tiredness and anemia

Side Effects / Symptoms of the Drug
Stop the drug and call your doctor or nurse right away if you develop a rash, fever, chills, or peeling skin. This can be a serious reaction and needs to be treated right away.

Stop the drug and call your doctor or nurse right away if you get diarrhea that does not stop, abdominal cramping, or blood and/or pus in the stool. This needs to be treated right away.

Other side effects not listed above can also occur in some patients.
Tell your doctor or nurse if you develop any problems.

FDA Approval: Yes

nefazodone hydrochloride

Trade Name:
Serzone

Type of Drug:
Nefazodone hydrochloride belongs to a general class of antidepressant/antianxiety drugs.

How Drug Works:
Nefazodone hydrochloride works by increasing the amount of serotonin and norepinephrine in the brain, so that the feeling of depression is prevented or relieved.

How Drug Is Given:
Nefazodone hydrochloride is a pill usually taken 2 times a day on an empty stomach. If you are changing from another antidepressant (monamine oxidase inhibitor), you should wait at least 2 weeks before starting nefazodone hydrochloride. If you change from nefazodone hydrochloride to a monamine oxidase inhibitor–type antidepressant, you must wait 7 days after stopping nefazodone hydrochloride before starting the new drug. The dose depends on the dose that is effective, and your doctor may need to slowly increase the dose of the medicine. The dose also depends on your age and how well your liver is working. Keep the medicine in a tightly closed container away from heat and moisture and out of the reach of children and pets.

How Should I Take This Drug?
Take this drug exactly as directed by your doctor. If you do not understand the instructions, ask your doctor or nurse to explain them to you.

 Read the following information. If you do not understand it or if any of it causes you special concern, check with your doctor.

Before taking this drug, tell your doctor if you are taking any other prescription or over-the-counter drugs, including vitamins and herbals.

Should I avoid any other medicines, foods, alcohol, and/or activities?
Your prescription and nonprescription medicines may interact with other drugs, causing harm. Certain foods or alcohol can also interact with drug products. Never begin taking a new medicine—prescription or nonprescription—without asking your doctor or nurse if it will interact with alcohol, food, or other medicines. Some drugs can cause drowsiness and affect activities such as driving.

Precautions:
Tell your doctor if you are taking terfenadine, astemizole, cisapride, or any other antidepressants that are monoamine oxidase inhibitors. You cannot take any of these drugs with nefazodone hydrochloride, as very serious side effects can occur.

Tell your doctor if you are taking any of the following drugs as they may have serious interactions with nefazodone hydrochloride: alprazolam, digoxin, propranolol, or triazolam.

Once you start taking nefazodone hydrochloride, it may take a few weeks before you feel the full effect of the drug.

Drowsiness and dizziness usually go away in 1 to 2 weeks. Tell your doctor or nurse if these symptoms do not go away.

Tell all the doctors, dentists, and pharmacists you visit that you are taking this drug.
- Most of the following side effects probably will not occur.
- Your doctor or nurse will want to discuss specific care instructions with you.
- They can help you understand these side effects and help you deal with them.

Side Effects:

More Common Side Effects
Dizziness
Drowsiness
Difficulty sleeping
Dry mouth
Nausea
Constipation
Headache
Feeling "blah"

Less Common Side Effects
Lightheadedness
Heartburn

Rare Side Effects
Agitation
Blurred vision
Confusion
Decreased ability to concentrate
Difficulty remembering
Sensation of pins and needles in hands and/or feet
Lack of coordination
Tremors
Twitching
Abnormal dreams
Decreased blood pressure when changing position
Increased heart rate
Increased blood pressure
Vomiting
Diarrhea
Frequent urination
Bone pain
Mouth sores
Peptic ulcer

Side Effects / Symptoms of the Drug
Be careful walking around or changing position if you are drowsy. Do not drive or operate heavy machinery if you are drowsy or dizzy. Stop the drug and call your doctor or nurse if the drowsiness does not go away, or if you have trouble walking or moving because of it.

Other side effects not listed above can also occur in some patients.
Tell your doctor or nurse if you develop any problems.

FDA Approval: Yes

nortriptyline hydrochloride

Trade Names:
Aventyl, Pamelor

Type of Drug:
Nortriptyline hydrochloride belongs to a general class of tricyclic antidepressant drugs.

How Drug Works:
Nortriptyline hydrochloride stops the uptake of serotonin in the nerve endings, thus increasing the amount of serotonin and norepinephrine available in the brain. This decreases the feeling of depression. Nortriptyline hydrochloride also may increase pain relief when given with opioid analgesics.

How Drug Is Given:
Nortriptyline hydrochloride is a pill given by mouth once a day at bedtime, so you will sleep better. Once you start taking the pills, it may take up to 2 weeks to feel the full effect. Other benefits like sleeping better and decreased pain will happen right away. The dose depends on your age, how well the medicine helps you, and how well your liver is working. Your doctor may need to gradually increase the dose. In addition, the doctor will monitor the drug level in the blood. Keep the medicine in a tightly closed container away from heat and moisture and out of the reach of children and pets.

 Read the following information. If you do not understand it or if any of it causes you special concern, check with your doctor.

Before taking this drug, tell your doctor if you are taking any other prescription or over-the-counter drugs, including vitamins and herbals.

Should I avoid any other medicines, foods, alcohol, and/or activities?
Your prescription and nonprescription medicines may interact with other drugs, causing harm. Certain foods or alcohol can also interact with drug products. Never begin taking a new medicine—prescription or non-prescription—without asking your doctor or nurse if it will interact with alcohol, food, or other medicines. Some drugs can cause drowsiness and affect activities such as driving.

Precautions:
Tell your doctor if you are taking any of the following drugs as they may have serious interactions with nortriptyline hydrochloride: other antidepressant drugs (monoamine oxidase inhibitors), sedatives, cimetidine, barbiturates, or warfarin (Coumadin).

Since nortriptyline hydrochloride affects the central nervous system (CNS), it is important not to take other drugs or substances that are known CNS depressants such as alcohol, sedatives, and hypnotics.

Tell your doctor if you have had a heart attack (myocardial infarction), have a seizure disorder, or have benign prostatic hypertrophy. You should not take this drug.

Tell your doctor if you have urinary retention, narrow-angle glaucoma, hyperthyroidism, liver problems, or have thoughts of suicide. This drug should be used very cautiously if you have any of these conditions.

Abruptly stopping the drug can cause anxiety, dizziness, nausea and vomiting, and tiredness. The drug should be gradually stopped.

Side effects in the elderly may be more severe. These include dry mouth, constipation, confusion, disorientation, and hallucinations.

When you start taking the drug, you may feel drowsy, dizzy, confused, or weak. This should go away after 1 to 2 weeks of taking the drug. If it does not, talk to your doctor. Your dose may need to be reduced.

Tell all the doctors, dentists, and pharmacists you visit that you are taking this drug.
- Most of the following side effects probably will not occur.
- Your doctor or nurse will want to discuss specific care instructions with you.
- They can help you understand these side effects and help you deal with them.

Side Effects:

More Common Side Effects
Drowsiness
Tiredness (fatigue)
Dizziness
Dry mouth
Vomiting
Diarrhea
Abdominal cramping

Less Common Side Effects
Confusion
Disorientation
Nausea
Changes in appetite
Urinary retention

Rare Side Effects
Hallucinations
Fine tremors
Rigidity
Difficulty speaking
Difficulty swallowing
Numbness and tingling in hands and/or feet
Blurred vision
Decrease in blood pressure when changing position
Change in the electrical activity of the heart by EKG (electrocardiogram)
Increased blood pressure
Increased heart rate
Rash
Hives
Increased sensitivity to sunlight

Side Effects / Symptoms of the Drug
Be careful walking around or changing position if you are drowsy. Do not drive a car or operate heavy machinery if you are drowsy or dizzy. Stop the drug and call your doctor or nurse if the drowsiness does not go away, or if you have trouble walking or moving because of it.

Tell your doctor or nurse if you get fine tremors, feel like your body is rigid, or have difficulty speaking or swallowing. You can be given another medicine to lessen these problems.

Other side effects not listed above can also occur in some patients.
Tell your doctor or nurse if you develop any problems.

FDA Approval: Yes

nystatin

Trade Names:
Mycostatin, Nilstat

Type of Drug:
Nystatin belongs to the general class of antifungal drugs.

How Drug Works:
Nystatin injures fungus so that the cell dies. It is used for the treatment of candidiasis involving the lining of the mouth, intestine, and vagina.

How Drug Is Given:
Nystatin is taken by mouth as a liquid or as a suppository that can be sucked to treat a mouth or throat infection. Shake the liquid before using the stopper to measure the dose. First, rinse your mouth to clean it of any food. Take the dose in your mouth and swish for 1 to 2 minutes, then swallow or spit out the liquid, as directed by your doctor. Don't rinse your mouth or eat for 15 to 30 minutes. If you have trouble rinsing your mouth, talk with your doctor or nurse to see if you can suck the suppositories instead of taking the liquid. They are equally effective. The suppository can also be inserted in the vagina to treat an infection in that area. Keep the medicine in a tightly closed container away from heat and moisture and out of the reach of children and pets.

How Should I Take This Drug?
Take this drug exactly as directed by your doctor. If you do not understand the instructions, ask your doctor or nurse to explain them to you.

 Read the following information. If you do not understand it or if any of it causes you special concern, check with your doctor.

Before taking this drug, tell your doctor if you are taking any other prescription or over-the-counter drugs, including vitamins and herbals.

Should I avoid any other medicines, foods, alcohol, and/or activities?
Your prescription and nonprescription medicines may interact with other drugs, causing harm. Certain foods or alcohol can also interact with drug products. Never begin taking a new medicine—prescription or nonprescription—without asking your doctor or nurse if it will interact with alcohol, food, or other medicines. Some drugs can cause drowsiness and affect activities such as driving.

Tell all the doctors, dentists, and pharmacists you visit that you are taking this drug.

- Most of the following side effects probably will not occur.
- Your doctor or nurse will want to discuss specific care instructions with you.
- They can help you understand these side effects and help you deal with them.

Side Effects:

Rare Side Effects
Nausea
Vomiting
Diarrhea

Other side effects not listed above can also occur in some patients.
Tell your doctor or nurse if you develop any problems.

FDA Approval: Yes

octreotide acetate

Trade Name:
Sandostatin

Type of Drug:
Octreotide acetate acts like somatostatin, a naturally occurring hormone that helps regulate many functions in the body. It is used to treat diarrhea caused by AIDS, chemotherapy, and radiation. It is also used to control some symptoms of carcinoid syndrome (such as flushing, wheezing, and diarrhea) and to treat graft-versus-host disease.

How Drug Works:
Octreotide acetate has many effects. It slows the time the stool passes through the intestines. This allows water to be absorbed from the stool, so the stool becomes more firm. It also blocks the release of serotonin, gastrin, and pancreatic enzymes. Octreotide is usually used for diarrhea when other treatments have not worked and other treatable causes have been excluded.

How Drug Is Given:
Octreotide acetate is given as an injection under the skin. A preparation is also available for giving it in the muscle. You or a family member may be taught to give the injection. After the right dose is found, most patients can take the shot once a month. Keep the syringes, needles, and supplies in a safe place, out of the reach of chlidren and pets. The medicine should be kept in its original container in the refrigerator; you should take it out 1 hour before the shot is due. The dose depends on the amount that works, and the number of doses depends on why you are taking the medicine. Keep the used syringes and needles in a special container. Ask your nurse or doctor about this, and when you should bring the filled container back to the office. Octreotide acetate can also be given as an injection in a vein 1 to 4 times a day, or as a continuous infusion for 24 hours.

How Should I Take This Drug?
Take this drug exactly as directed by your doctor. If you do not understand the instructions, ask your doctor or nurse to explain them to you.

 Read the following information. If you do not understand it or if any of it causes you special concern, check with your doctor.

Before taking this drug, tell your doctor if you are taking any other prescription or over-the-counter drugs, including vitamins and herbals.

Should I avoid any other medicines, foods, alcohol, and/or activities?
Your prescription and nonprescription medicines may interact with other drugs, causing harm. Certain foods or alcohol can also interact with drug products. Never begin taking a new medicine—prescription or non-prescription—without asking your doctor or nurse if it will interact with alcohol, food, or other medicines. Some drugs can cause drowsiness and affect activities such as driving.

Precautions:
To help decrease diarrhea, change your diet. Try to eat small, frequent meals that are warm or at room temperature. Avoid foods that cause gas (such as broccoli or beans), fatty foods (such as bacon or cheeses), citrus fruits and juices, and high-lactose foods (such as milk or ice cream). Eat foods high in sodium and potassium (such as soups, sports drinks, and bananas). Eat foods high in soluble fiber (such as rice or bananas). Avoid foods high in insoluble fiber (such as cereal or nuts). Try to drink at least eight oz glasses of water a day. To add calories, dilute with fruit juice.

Tell your doctor if you are taking cyclosporine, insulin, oral hypoglycemic agents (for diabetes), beta blockers, or calcium channel blockers (heart medicines). Talk with your doctor about possible drug interactions.

Tell all the doctors, dentists, and pharmacists you visit that you are taking this drug.
- -
- Most of the following side effects probably will not occur.
- Your doctor or nurse will want to discuss specific care instructions with you.
- They can help you understand these side effects and help you deal with them.

Side Effects:

More Common Side Effects
Nausea
Bruising at place of injection

Less Common Side Effects
Abdominal pain
Decreased absorption of fat from intestines
Decreased appetite
Headache

Rare Side Effects
Anxiety
Joint or muscle aches
Rash
Dizziness
Lightheadedness
Swelling of feet
Headache
Facial flushing
Changes in blood sugar level

Side Effects / Symptoms of the Drug
Tell your doctor or nurse if the diarrhea does not go away after 1 to 2 doses, as the dose of the drug may have to be increased.

Other side effects not listed above can also occur in some patients.
Tell your doctor or nurse if you develop any problems.

FDA Approval: Yes

ondansetron hydrochloride

Trade Name:
Zofran

Type of Drug:
Ondansetron hydrochloride belongs to a general class of drugs called serotonin antagonists. It is an antinausea medicine.

How Drug Works:
Ondansetron hydrochloride blocks the serotonin pathway to the vomiting center in the brain so the brain no longer receives a vomiting message.

How Drug Is Given:
Ondansetron hydrochloride is taken by mouth as a pill, on the tongue as a tablet that dissolves, as a liquid, or as an injection in a vein over 30 minutes. Take the pill, tablet, or liquid 1 hour before the chemotherapy is given. Shake the liquid before pouring the dose. The dose depends on the type of chemotherapy you are receiving and whether you have had problems with nausea and vomiting in the past. Keep the medicine in a tightly closed container away from heat and moisture and out of the reach of children and pets.

How Should I Take This Drug?
Take this drug exactly as directed by your doctor. If you do not understand the instructions, ask your doctor or nurse to explain them to you.

 Read the following information. If you do not understand it or if any of it causes you special concern, check with your doctor.

Before taking this drug, tell your doctor if you are taking any other prescription or over-the-counter drugs, including vitamins and herbals.

Should I avoid any other medicines, foods, alcohol, and/or activities?
Your prescription and nonprescription medicines may interact with other drugs, causing harm. Certain foods or alcohol can also interact with drug products. Never begin taking a new medicine—prescription or nonprescription—without asking your doctor or nurse if it will interact with alcohol, food, or other medicines. Some drugs can cause drowsiness and affect activities such as driving.

Tell all the doctors, dentists, and pharmacists you visit that you are taking this drug.
- Most of the following side effects probably will not occur.
- Your doctor or nurse will want to discuss specific care instructions with you.
- They can help you understand these side effects and help you deal with them.

Side Effects:

Less Common Side Effects
Diarrhea
Constipation
Headache

Rare Side Effects
Abnormal liver function test results that pass very quickly

Other side effects not listed above can also occur in some patients.
Tell your doctor or nurse if you develop any problems.

FDA Approval: Yes

oxacillin sodium

Trade Names:
Bactocill, Prostaphlin

Type of Drug:
Oxacillin sodium is a semisynthetic penicillin that belongs to a general class of drugs called antibiotics.

How Drug Works:
Oxacillin sodium prevents bacteria from making their cell walls, so the cells die. It is used to treat gram-positive infections and bacteria that are resistent to penicillin.

How Drug Is Given:
Oxacillin sodium is taken by mouth 4 times a day for 10 to 14 days. Take with 8 oz of water on an empty stomach, 1 hour before or 2 hours after a meal. It can also be given as an injection in a vein over 30 minutes 6 times a day. The dose and how long you take it depends on your weight and the type of infection being treated. Keep the medicine in a tightly closed container away from heat and moisture and out of the reach of children and pets.

How Should I Take This Drug?
Take this drug exactly as directed by your doctor. If you do not understand the instructions, ask your doctor or nurse to explain them to you.

 Read the following information. If you do not understand it or if any of it causes you special concern, check with your doctor.

Before taking this drug, tell your doctor if you are taking any other prescription or over-the-counter drugs, including vitamins and herbals.

Should I avoid any other medicines, foods, alcohol, and/or activities?
Your prescription and nonprescription medicines may interact with other drugs, causing harm. Certain foods or alcohol can also interact with drug products. Never begin taking a new medicine—prescription or nonprescription—without asking your doctor or nurse if it will interact with alcohol, food, or other medicines. Some drugs can cause drowsiness and affect activities such as driving.

Precautions:
Tell your doctor if you have any drug allergies, especially to antibiotic drugs. You should not take this drug if you are allergic to penicillin.

All antibiotics can cause allergic reactions. Stop the drug and tell your doctor or nurse right away if you develop a rash, hives, red blotches on your skin, difficulty breathing, or chest pain.

Use of antibiotics can change the normal organisms in your body. Women are at risk for fungal infections. Tell your nurse or doctor if you get vaginal itching or discharge.

This drug should be used with caution by women who are pregnant or breastfeeding.

Tell all the doctors, dentists, and pharmacists you visit that you are taking this drug.

- Most of the following side effects probably will not occur.
- Your doctor or nurse will want to discuss specific care instructions with you.
- They can help you understand these side effects and help you deal with them.

Side Effects:

More Common Side Effects
Nausea
Vaginal itching
Vaginal candidiasis (fungal infection)

Less Common Side Effects
Vomiting
Diarrhea
Sores in mouth
Irritation of the vein used to give the drug

Rare Side Effects
Rash
Hives
Fever
Chills
Itching
Muscle aches
Swelling of feet
Darkening and peeling of skin
Diarrhea related to infection of the intestinal lining (pseudomembranous colitis)
Decreased white blood cell count with increased risk of infection
Seizures
Decreased red blood cell count with increased risk of tiredness and anemia
Blood in urine
Abnormal liver function blood tests
Inflammation of liver (hepatitis)

Side Effects / Symptoms of the Drug
Stop the drug and call your doctor or nurse right away if you develop a rash, fever, chills, or peeling skin. This can be a serious reaction and needs to be treated right away.

Stop the drug and call your doctor or nurse right away if you get diarrhea that does not stop, abdominal cramping, or blood and/or pus in the stool. This needs to be treated right away.

Other side effects not listed above can also occur in some patients.
Tell your doctor or nurse if you develop any problems.

FDA Approval: Yes

oxazepam

Trade Name:
Serax

Type of Drug:
Oxazepam belongs to a general class of antianxiety drugs called benzodiazepines.

How Drug Works:
Oxazepam binds to certain receptors in the brain and spinal cord to bring about reduced anxiety, muscle relaxation, and prevention of seizures.

How Drug Is Given:
Oxazepam is a pill taken by mouth with or without food. The dose is the same for all adults. In addition, the dose may be adjusted to meet your needs. Keep the medicine in a tightly closed container away from heat and moisture and out of the reach of children and pets.

How Should I Take This Drug?
Take this drug exactly as directed by your doctor. If you do not understand the instructions, ask your doctor or nurse to explain them to you.

 Read the following information. If you do not understand it or if any of it causes you special concern, check with your doctor.

Before taking this drug, tell your doctor if you are taking any other prescription or over-the-counter drugs, including vitamins and herbals.

Should I avoid any other medicines, foods, alcohol, and/or activities?
Your prescription and nonprescription medicines may interact with other drugs, causing harm. Certain foods or alcohol can also interact with drug products. Never begin taking a new medicine—prescription or nonprescription—without asking your doctor or nurse if it will interact with alcohol, food, or other medicines. Some drugs can cause drowsiness and affect activities such as driving.

Precautions:
Tell your doctor if you are taking any of the following drugs as they may have serious interactions with oxazepam: oral contraceptives, isoniazid, ketoconazole, cimetidine, digoxin, levodopa, or a tricyclic antidepressant drug.

Abruptly stopping the drug can cause anxiety, dizziness, nausea and vomiting, and tiredness. The drug should be gradually stopped.

Take oxazepam only as directed by your doctor. Diazepam may cause psychological dependence (addiction) and physical dependence (body goes into withdrawal if drug is suddenly stopped). When taken as directed by your doctor or nurse, this will not be a problem.

Women who are pregnant or breastfeeding should not take this drug.

Since oxazepam affects the central nervous system (CNS), it is important not to take other drugs or substances that are known CNS depressants such as alcohol, sedatives, and hypnotics.

Tell all the doctors, dentists, and pharmacists you visit that you are taking this drug.
- Most of the following side effects probably will not occur.
- Your doctor or nurse will want to discuss specific care instructions with you.
- They can help you understand these side effects and help you deal with them.

Side Effects:

More Common Side Effects
Drowsiness
Tiredness (fatigue)
Weakness
Dry mouth
Constipation

Less Common Side Effects
Nausea
Vomiting
Change in weight
Lack of coordination
Decreased mental alertness

Rare Side Effects
Decrease in blood pressure
Rash
Itching
Hives
Abnormal liver function blood tests

Side Effects / Symptoms of the Drug
Be careful walking around or changing position if you are drowsy. Do not drive or operate heavy machinery if you are drowsy or dizzy. Call your doctor or nurse if the drowsiness does not go away, or if you have trouble walking or moving because of it.

Other side effects not listed above can also occur in some patients.
Tell your doctor or nurse if you develop any problems.

FDA Approval: Yes

oxycodone

Trade Names:
Endodan, Oxycontin, Percocet, Percodan, Roxiprin

Type of Drug:
Oxycodone is a synthetic opioid analgesic, similar to morphine.

How Drug Works:
Oxycodone relieves moderate to moderately severe pain. It binds to opioid receptors in the brain and central nervous system (CNS), altering the perception of pain as well as the emotional response to it. It also suppresses the cough reflex.

How Drug Is Given:
Oxycodone comes in a number of preparations to take by mouth. Oxycodone by itself is an immediate-release pill that lasts 3 to 4 hours. Sustained-release pills (like Oxycontin) are taken every 12 hours. Try to drink an 8 oz glass of water or fluid every hour to help prevent constipation. You should take a laxative so that you move your bowels at least every other day. The dose depends on how much is needed to control your pain. Keep the medicine in a tightly closed container away from heat and moisture and out of the reach of children and pets.

How Should I Take This Drug?
Take this drug exactly as directed by your doctor. If you do not understand the instructions, ask your doctor or nurse to explain them to you.

 Read the following information. If you do not understand it or if any of it causes you special concern, check with your doctor.

Before taking this drug, tell your doctor if you are taking any other prescription or over-the-counter drugs, including vitamins and herbals.

Should I avoid any other medicines, foods, alcohol, and/or activities?
Your prescription and nonprescription medicines may interact with other drugs, causing harm. Certain foods or alcohol can also interact with drug products. Never begin taking a new medicine—prescription or nonprescription—without asking your doctor or nurse if it will interact with alcohol, food, or other medicines. Some drugs can cause drowsiness and affect activities such as driving.

Precautions:
Take the smallest effective dose to prevent development of tolerance and physical dependence. Tolerance (larger doses needed to give the same effect) can develop as well as physical dependence (body goes into withdrawal if drug is suddenly stopped). This is different from addiction, which is psychological dependence (take drug for psychological effect, not for relief of pain). Tell your doctor or nurse if you still have pain even though you are taking the medicine as directed.

Since oxycodone affects the central nervous system (CNS), it is important not to take other drugs or substances that are known CNS depressants such as alcohol, sedatives, and hypnotics.

Acetaminophen or aspirin may be combined with oxycodone to increase the pain relief action.

You should be on a bowel regimen to prevent constipation while you are taking opioid pain relievers. Talk to your nurse or doctor about this.

Tell all the doctors, dentists, and pharmacists you visit that you are taking this drug.
- Most of the following side effects probably will not occur.
- Your doctor or nurse will want to discuss specific care instructions with you.
- They can help you understand these side effects and help you deal with them.

Side Effects:

More Common Side Effects
Constipation
Drowsiness
Sedation
Nausea
Dizziness
Dry mouth

Less Common Side Effects
Vomiting
Changes in mood
Euphoria
Depression
Confusion
Decreased breathing rate
Decreased blood pressure when changing position
Delayed digestion
Decreased heart rate

Rare Side Effects
Difficulty urinating
Decreased sexual interest
Impotence

Side Effects / Symptoms of the Drug
Drink fluids (8 oz every hour in sips) to prevent constipation. Also, try to eat foods high in fiber such as bran, fruits, and vegetables. You may need to take a stool softener, bulk-forming agent, and/or laxative to help keep your bowel movements regular.

Call your doctor or nurse right away if you have not moved your bowels in 2 days.

Abruptly stopping the drug can cause anxiety, dizziness, nausea and vomiting, and tiredness. The drug should be gradually discontinued.

Other side effects not listed above can also occur in some patients.
Tell your doctor or nurse if you develop any problems.

FDA Approval: Yes

pamidronate disodium

Trade Name:
Aredia

Type of Drug:
Pamidronate disodium belongs to a specific class of calcium-lowering agents called biphosphonates used to treat hypercalcemia (high calcium level in the blood).

How Drug Works:
Pamidronate disodium stops bone breakdown, so calcium is not released from the bones into the blood. It is used to treat bone metastases from breast cancer.

How Drug Is Given:
Pamidronate disodium is given by injection in a vein over 2 to 4 hours. The dose is the same for all adults. You may also get fluids by vein to help your kidneys make urine.

 Read the following information. If you do not understand it or if any of it causes you special concern, check with your doctor.

Before taking this drug, tell your doctor if you are taking any other prescription or over-the-counter drugs, including vitamins and herbals.

Should I avoid any other medicines, foods, alcohol, and/or activities?
Your prescription and nonprescription medicines may interact with other drugs, causing harm. Certain foods or alcohol can also interact with drug products. Never begin taking a new medicine—prescription or non-prescription—without asking your doctor or nurse if it will interact with alcohol, food, or other medicines. Some drugs can cause drowsiness and affect activities such as driving.

Tell all the doctors, dentists, and pharmacists you visit that you are taking this drug.

- Most of the following side effects probably will not occur.
- Your doctor or nurse will want to discuss specific care instructions with you.
- They can help you understand these side effects and help you deal with them.

Side Effects:

More Common Side Effects
Fever lasting for a short time 24 to 48 hours after infusion
Pain at place of injection
Irritation of vein used for giving the drug

Less Common Side Effects
Nausea
Constipation
Decreased appetite

Rare Side Effects
Vomiting
Abdominal discomfort

Other side effects not listed above can also occur in some patients.
Tell your doctor or nurse if you develop any problems.

FDA Approval: Yes

paroxetine hydrochloride

Trade Name:
Paxil

Type of Drug:
Paroxetine hydrochloride belongs to a general class of antidepressant drugs.

How Drug Works:
Paroxetine hydrochloride appears to increase the activity of serotonin in the brain and central nervous system (CNS) by stopping the uptake of serotonin by the nerves. This decreases the feeling of depression.

How Drug Is Given:
Paroxetine hydrochloride is a pill taken once a day in the morning, with or without food. The dose depends on your response to the lowest dose, your age, and how well your kidneys and liver are working. If you are changing from another antidepressant (monamine oxidase inhibitor), you should wait at least 2 weeks before starting paroxetine hydrochloride. If you change from paroxetine hydrochloride to a monamine oxidase inhibitor–type antidepressant, you must wait 14 days after stopping paroxetine hydrochloride before starting the new drug. Keep the medicine in a tightly closed container away from heat and moisture and out of the reach of children and pets.

How Should I Take This Drug?
Take this drug exactly as directed by your doctor. If you do not understand the instructions, ask your doctor or nurse to explain them to you.

  Read the following information. If you do not understand it or if any of it causes you special concern, check with your doctor.

Before taking this drug, tell your doctor if you are taking any other prescription or over-the-counter drugs, including vitamins and herbals.

Should I avoid any other medicines, foods, alcohol, and/or activities?
Your prescription and nonprescription medicines may interact with other drugs, causing harm. Certain foods or alcohol can also interact with drug products. Never begin taking a new medicine—prescription or nonprescription—without asking your doctor or nurse if it will interact with alcohol, food, or other medicines. Some drugs can cause drowsiness and affect activities such as driving.

Precautions:
It may take a few weeks to find the right dose for you. Your doctor will start you off at a smaller dose then increase it weekly if you do not feel better.

Tell your doctor if you are taking tryptophan, other antidepressant drugs (monoamine oxidase inhibitors), or sumatriptan. You cannot take paroxetine hydrochloride if you are taking any of these drugs.

Tell your doctor if you are taking any of the following drugs as they may have serious interactions with paroxetine hydrochloride: warfarin (Coumadin), lithium, theophylline, or digoxin.

Women who are pregnant or breastfeeding should not take this drug.

Paroxetine hydrochloride should be taken in the morning as a single daily dose. If you are changing from another antidepressant (monoamine oxidase inhibitor), you should wait at least 2 weeks before starting paroxetine hydrochloride. If you change from paroxetine hydrochloride to a monoamine oxidase inhibitor–type antidepressant, you must wait 14 days after stopping paroxetine hydrochloride before starting the new drug.

Tell all the doctors, dentists, and pharmacists you visit that you are taking this drug.

- Most of the following side effects probably will not occur.
- Your doctor or nurse will want to discuss specific care instructions with you.
- They can help you understand these side effects and help you deal with them.

Side Effects:

More Common Side Effects
Sweating

Less Common Side Effects
Sleepiness
Dizziness
Difficulty sleeping
Tremors
Nervousness
Feeling "blah"
Nausea
Decreased appetite
Decreased sexual ability

Rare Side Effects
Headache
Confusion
Feeling anxious
Numbness and tingling in fingers and toes

Side Effects / Symptoms of the Drug
Do not drive or operate heavy machinery if you are drowsy or dizzy. Call your doctor or nurse if the drowsiness does not go away, or if you have trouble walking or moving because of it.

Other side effects not listed above can also occur in some patients.
Tell your doctor or nurse if you develop any problems.

FDA Approval: Yes

penicillin G

Trade Names:
PenG Potassium, PenG Sodium

Type of Drug:
Penicillin G is an antibiotic that is a natural penicillin.

How Drug Works:
Penicillin G prevents bacteria from manufacturing their cell wall, so the bacteria die. It is used to treat many gram-positive and some gram-negative bacteria.

How Drug Is Given:
Penicillin G is taken as a pill or liquid by mouth, or by injection in a vein over 30 to 60 minutes. Take the pill or liquid on an empty stomach at about the same time each day, 1 hour before or 2 hours after eating. Avoid acidic fruit juices like orange or grapefruit for 1 hour before or after taking the medicine. Shake the liquid well before pouring the dose. The dose and number of doses depend on your weight and the infection being treated. Keep the medicine in a tightly closed container away from heat and moisture and out of the reach of children and pets.

How Should I Take This Drug?
Take this drug exactly as directed by your doctor. If you do not understand the instructions, ask your doctor or nurse to explain them to you.

 Read the following information. If you do not understand it or if any of it causes you special concern, check with your doctor.

Before taking this drug, tell your doctor if you are taking any other prescription or over-the-counter drugs, including vitamins and herbals.

Should I avoid any other medicines, foods, alcohol, and/or activities?
Your prescription and nonprescription medicines may interact with other drugs, causing harm. Certain foods or alcohol can also interact with drug products. Never begin taking a new medicine—prescription or non-prescription—without asking your doctor or nurse if it will interact with alcohol, food, or other medicines. Some drugs can cause drowsiness and affect activities such as driving.

Precautions:
All antibiotics can cause allergic reactions. Stop the drug and tell your doctor or nurse right away if you develop a rash, hives, red blotches on your skin, difficulty breathing, or chest pain.

Use of antibiotics can change the normal organisms in your body. Women are at risk of getting fungal infections. Tell your nurse or doctor if you get vaginal itching or discharge.

Women who are pregnant or breastfeeding should use this drug with caution.

Tell your doctor if you have any drug allergies, especially to antibiotic drugs. You should not take this drug if you are allergic to penicillin.

Tell all the doctors, dentists, and pharmacists you visit that you are taking this drug.
- Most of the following side effects probably will not occur.
- Your doctor or nurse will want to discuss specific care instructions with you.
- They can help you understand these side effects and help you deal with them.

Side Effects:

More Common Side Effects
Nausea
Vaginal itching
Vaginal candidiasis (fungal infection)

Less Common Side Effects
Vomiting
Diarrhea
Irritation of the vein used for giving the drug
Irritation and pain at the place of injection

Rare Side Effects
Rash
Hives
Itching
Fever
Chills
Redness of skin
Darkening and peeling of skin
Swelling of feet and/or hands
Diarrhea related to infection of the intestinal lining (pseudomembranous colitis)
Decreased white blood cell count with increased risk of infection
Decreased platelet count with increased risk of bleeding
Decreased red blood cell count with increased risk of tiredness (fatigue) and anemia
Seizures

Side Effects / Symptoms of the Drug
Stop the drug right away and call your doctor or nurse if you develop a rash, fever, chills, or peeling skin. This can be a serious reaction and needs to be treated right away.

Stop the drug and call your doctor or nurse right away if you get diarrhea that does not stop, abdominal cramping, or blood and/or pus in the stool. This needs to be treated right away.

Other side effects not listed above can also occur in some patients.
Tell your doctor or nurse if you develop any problems.

FDA Approval: Yes

perphenazine

Trade Name:
Trilafon

Type of Drug:
Perphenazine belongs to the general class of drugs called phenothiazines. It is an antipsychotic drug used for treatment of psychotic illness, schizophrenia, alcoholism, and hiccoughs; it is used to prevent nausea and vomiting caused by chemotherapy.

How Drug Works:
Perphenazine blocks certain messages to the brain. With nausea and vomiting, it blocks the "vomiting" message from being sent to the chemoreceptor trigger zone (CTZ). The patient does not receive a nausea message.

How Drug Is Given:
Perphenazine is taken as a pill or liquid by mouth 1 hour before, or by injection in a vein over 5 to 20 minutes before chemotherapy. It is also taken every 4 to 6 hours as needed to treat or prevent nausea and vomiting as directed by your doctor. The dose is the same for all adults. Keep the medicine in a tightly closed container away from heat and moisture and out of the reach of children and pets.

How Should I Take This Drug?
Take this drug exactly as directed by your doctor. If you do not understand the instructions, ask your doctor or nurse to explain them to you.

 Read the following information. If you do not understand it or if any of it causes you special concern, check with your doctor.

Before taking this drug, tell your doctor if you are taking any other prescription or over-the-counter drugs, including vitamins and herbals.

Should I avoid any other medicines, foods, alcohol, and/or activities?
Your prescription and nonprescription medicines may interact with other drugs, causing harm. Certain foods or alcohol can also interact with drug products. Never begin taking a new medicine—prescription or nonprescription—without asking your doctor or nurse if it will interact with alcohol, food, or other medicines. Some drugs can cause drowsiness and affect activities such as driving.

Precautions:
Perphenazine may make you feel very sleepy. Do not drive or operate heavy machinery when you are drowsy.

Perphenazine may cause extrapyramidal side effects. These include restlessness, tongue protrusion, and involuntary movements. These side effects are immediately stopped when you are given diphenhydramine.

Tell all the doctors, dentists, and pharmacists you visit that you are taking this drug.
- Most of the following side effects probably will not occur.
- Your doctor or nurse will want to discuss specific care instructions with you.
- They can help you understand these side effects and help you deal with them.

Side Effects:

More Common Side Effects
Sedation
Sleepiness
Dry mouth
Constipation

Less Common Side Effects
Blurred vision
Restlessness
Involuntary muscle movements
Tremors
Increased appetite
Weight gain

Rare Side Effects
Jaundice
Rash
Hives
Increased sensitivity to sunlight

Side Effects / Symptoms of the Drug
Be careful getting up, changing position, or walking.

Other side effects not listed above can also occur in some patients.
Tell your doctor or nurse if you develop any problems.

FDA Approval: Yes

piperacillin sodium

Trade Name:
Piperacil

Type of Drug:
Piperacillin sodium is a semisynthetic penicillin that belongs to a general class of drugs called antibiotics.

How Drug Works:
Piperacillin sodium prevents bacteria from making their cell wall, causing the bacteria to die. It is used to treat many gram-positive and some gram-negative bacteria that cause infections of the lungs, urinary tract, and skin.

How Drug Is Given:
Piperacillin sodium is given by injection in a vein over 30 to 60 minutes, or in the muscle. The dose and how long you take it depends on your weight and the type of infection being treated.

 Read the following information. If you do not understand it or if any of it causes you special concern, check with your doctor.

Before taking this drug, tell your doctor if you are taking any other prescription or over-the-counter drugs, including vitamins and herbals.

Should I avoid any other medicines, foods, alcohol, and/or activities?
Your prescription and nonprescription medicines may interact with other drugs, causing harm. Certain foods or alcohol can also interact with drug products. Never begin taking a new medicine—prescription or non-prescription—without asking your doctor or nurse if it will interact with alcohol, food, or other medicines. Some drugs can cause drowsiness and affect activities such as driving.

Precautions:
All antibiotics can cause allergic reactions. Stop the drug and tell your doctor or nurse right away if you develop a rash, hives, red blotches on your skin, or difficulty breathing.

Use of antibiotics can change the normal organisms in your body. Women are at risk of getting fungal infections. Tell your nurse or doctor if you get vaginal itching or discharge.

Women who are pregnant or breastfeeding should use this drug with caution.

Tell your doctor if you have any drug allergies, especially to antibiotic drugs. You should not take this drug if you are allergic to penicillin.

Side Effects:

More Common Side Effects
Nausea
Vaginal itching
Vaginal candidiasis (fungal infection)

Less Common Side Effects
Vomiting
Diarrhea
Irritation of vein used for giving the drug
Abnormal blood potassium level

Rare Side Effects
Rash
Hives
Itching
Fever
Chills
Darkening of the skin and peeling
Muscle aches
Swelling of hands and/or feet
Diarrhea related to infection of the intestinal lining (pseudomembranous colitis)
Decreased white blood cell count with increased risk of infection
Decreased red blood cell count with increased risk of anemia and tiredness (fatigue)
Dizziness
Headache
Sleepiness

Side Effects / Symptoms of the Drug
Stop the drug and call your doctor or nurse right away if you develop rash, fever, chills, or peeling skin. This can be a serious reaction and needs to be treated right away.

Stop the drug and call your doctor or nurse right away if you get diarrhea that does not stop, abdominal cramping, or blood and/or pus in the stool. This needs to be treated right away.

Other side effects not listed above can also occur in some patients.
Tell your doctor or nurse if you develop any problems.

FDA Approval: Yes

piperacillin sodium combined with tazobactam sodium

Trade Names:
Tazocin, Zosyn

Type of Drug:
Piperacillin sodium combined with tazobactam sodium is an antibiotic that belongs to the class of drugs called penicillins. It is used to treat serious gram-negative bacterial infections. The tazobactam sodium helps this antibiotic kill bacteria that are resistant to other antibiotics.

How Drug Works:
Piperacillin sodium combined with tazobactam sodium stops bacteria from making their cell wall, causing the bacteria to die. Penicillins are able to do this because they contain a special beta-lactam ring. Some bacteria contain an enzyme that breaks down the beta-lactam ring so that the antibiotic no longer kills the bacteria. Tazobactam stops this enzyme so that the bacteria can still be destroyed by the piperacillin (antibiotic).

How Drug Is Given:
Piperacillin sodium combined with tazobactam sodium is given as an injection in the vein over 30 to 60 minutes or in the muscle. The dose and how long you take it depends on your weight and the type of infection being treated.

 Read the following information. If you do not understand it or if any of it causes you special concern, check with your doctor.

Before taking this drug, tell your doctor if you are taking any other prescription or over-the-counter drugs, including vitamins and herbals.

Should I avoid any other medicines, foods, alcohol, and/or activities?
Your prescription and nonprescription medicines may interact with other drugs, causing harm. Certain foods or alcohol can also interact with drug products. Never begin taking a new medicine—prescription or non-prescription—without asking your doctor or nurse if it will interact with alcohol, food, or other medicines. Some drugs can cause drowsiness and affect activities such as driving.

Precautions:
Tell your doctor if you have any drug allergies, especially to penicillins or other antibiotics.

All antibiotics can cause allergic reactions. Stop the drug and tell your doctor or nurse right away if you develop a rash, hives, red blotches on your skin, fever and chills, difficulty breathing, or swelling of face and lips.

Use of antibiotics can change the normal organisms in your body. Women are at risk for fungal infections. Tell your nurse or doctor if you have vaginal itching or discharge.

Tell all the doctors, dentists, and pharmacists you visit that you are taking this drug.
- Most of the following side effects probably will not occur.
- Your doctor or nurse will want to discuss specific care instructions with you.
- They can help you understand these side effects and help you deal with them.

Side Effects:

More Common Side Effects
Nausea
Diarrhea
Pain at the injection site
Redness at the injection site

Less Common Side Effects
Vomiting
Vaginal itching

Rare Side Effects
Diarrhea related to infection of the intestinal lining (pseudomembranous colitis)
Red blotching of skin
Itching
Muscle aches
Redness of skin
Allergic reaction with rash, fever and chills, and swelling of throat or face
Decreased white blood cell count with increased risk of infection
Decreased red blood cell count with increased risk of tiredness and anemia
Decreased clotting of the blood with risk of bleeding
Dizziness
Headache
Sleepiness
Seizures

Side Effects / Symptoms of the Drug
Stop the drug and call your doctor or nurse right away if you develop severe diarrhea, fever and/or chills, or rash.

Other side effects not listed above can also occur in some patients.
Tell your doctor or nurse if you develop any problems.

FDA Approval: Yes

prochlorperazine

Trade Name:
Compazine

Type of Drug:
Prochlorperazine belongs to a general class of drugs called phenothiazines. It is an antinausea medicine.

How Drug Works:
Prochlorperazine is useful in preventing nausea and vomiting resulting from chemotherapy. It blocks messages to the part of the brain responsible for nausea and vomiting.

How Drug Is Given:
Prochlorperazine is given by mouth as a pill, long-acting capsule, liquid, rectal suppository, or an injection in a vein over 5 to 15 minutes or in a muscle. If you are taking antacids, take the prochlorperazine at least 2 hours before or after the antacid. If you are taking the suppository, open the package and dip the tip of the suppository in water. If you are right-handed, lie down on your left side, bring your knees up near your chest, and insert the suppository in your rectum about an inch. Stay in this position for about 15 minutes, then get up and wash your hands well. The dose depends on the reason you are taking it and how well it has worked at the lowest dose. Keep the medicine in a tightly closed container away from heat and moisture and out of the reach of children and pets.

How Should I Take This Drug?
Take this drug exactly as directed by your doctor. If you do not understand the instructions, ask your doctor or nurse to explain them to you.

 Read the following information. If you do not understand it or if any of it causes you special concern, check with your doctor.

Before taking this drug, tell your doctor if you are taking any other prescription or over-the-counter drugs, including vitamins and herbals.

Should I avoid any other medicines, foods, alcohol, and/or activities?
Your prescription and nonprescription medicines may interact with other drugs, causing harm. Certain foods or alcohol can also interact with drug products. Never begin taking a new medicine—prescription or nonprescription—without asking your doctor or nurse if it will interact with alcohol, food, or other medicines. Some drugs can cause drowsiness and affect activities such as driving.

Precautions:
Prochlorperazine may make you feel very sleepy. Do not drive or operate heavy machinery when you are drowsy.

Prochlorperazine may cause extrapyramidal side effects. These include restlessness, tongue protrusion, and involuntary movements. These side effects are immediately stopped when you are given diphenhydramine.

Tell all the doctors, dentists, and pharmacists you visit that you are taking this drug.
- Most of the following side effects probably will not occur.
- Your doctor or nurse will want to discuss specific care instructions with you.
- They can help you understand these side effects and help you deal with them.

Side Effects:

More Common Side Effects
Dry mouth
Constipation
Sedation
Sleepiness

Less Common Side Effects
Blurred vision
Restlessness
Involuntary muscle movements
Tremors
Increased appetite
Weight gain
Decreased blood pressure when changing position
Increased heart rate
Changes in electrical activity of heart (EKG changes)

Rare Side Effects
Jaundice
Rash
Hives
Increased sensitivity to sunlight

Side Effects / Symptoms of the Drug
Be careful when getting up, changing position, or walking.

Other side effects not listed above can also occur in some patients.
Tell your doctor or nurse if you develop any problems.

FDA Approval: Yes

promethazine hydrochloride

Trade Names:
Anergan, Phenameth, Phenergan

Type of Drug:
Promethazine hydrochloride belongs to a general class of antinausea drugs called antihistamines.

How Drug Works:
Promethazine hydrochloride has sedative, antihistamine, and mild antinausea properties. It has a depressant effect on the central nervous system (CNS), but the specific mechanism is not known.

How Drug Is Given:
Promethazine hydrochloride is given as a pill or liquid by mouth, as a rectal suppository, or as an injection in a vein over 5 minutes or in a muscle. Shake the liquid well before pouring the dose. If you are taking the suppository, open the pckage and dip the tip of the suppository in water. If you are right-handed, lie down on your left side, bring your knees up near your chest, and insert the suppository in your rectum about an inch. Stay in this position for about 15 minutes, then get up and wash your hands well. The dose depends on the reason you are taking it. Keep the medicine in a tightly closed container away from heat and moisture and out of the reach of children and pets.

How Should I Take This Drug?
Take this drug exactly as directed by your doctor. If you do not understand the instructions, ask your doctor or nurse to explain them to you.

 Read the following information. If you do not understand it or if any of it causes you special concern, check with your doctor.

Before taking this drug, tell your doctor if you are taking any other prescription or over-the-counter drugs, including vitamins and herbals.

Should I avoid any other medicines, foods, alcohol, and/or activities?
Your prescription and nonprescription medicines may interact with other drugs, causing harm. Certain foods or alcohol can also interact with drug products. Never begin taking a new medicine—prescription or non-prescription—without asking your doctor or nurse if it will interact with alcohol, food, or other medicines. Some drugs can cause drowsiness and affect activities such as driving.

Precautions:
Promethazine hydrochloride may make you feel very sleepy. Do not drive or operate heavy machinery when you are drowsy.

Promethazine hydrochloride may cause increased risk of confusion, sedation, and drowsiness in the elderly. This drug should be used cautiously in the elderly. It is important to protect against falls or injury.

Tell all the doctors, dentists, and pharmacists you visit that you are taking this drug.
- Most of the following side effects probably will not occur.
- Your doctor or nurse will want to discuss specific care instructions with you.
- They can help you understand these side effects and help you deal with them.

Side Effects:

More Common Side Effects
Drowsiness
Dry mouth
Constipation

Less Common Side Effects
Confusion
Sedation
Restlessness
Tremors
Blurred vision
Decreased blood pressure

Rare Side Effects
Nausea
Vomiting
Difficulty urinating

Side Effects / Symptoms of the Drug
Be careful when getting up, changing position, or walking.

Other side effects not listed above can also occur in some patients.
Tell your doctor or nurse if you develop any problems.

FDA Approval: Yes

psyllium hydrophilic muciloid

Trade Names:
Fiberall, Hydrocil, Metamucil, Perdiem Fiber, Reguloid

Type of Drug:
Psyllium hydrophilic muciloid is a bulk-producing laxative made of plant fiber and is used to treat constipation.

How Drug Works:
Psyllium hydrophilic muciloid absorbs water, which expands in the intestines. This stimulates the normal forward movement of the intestines (peristalsis), resulting in a bowel movement within 12 to 24 hours. It is also soothing to the intestines if they are inflamed (demulcent effect).

How Drug Is Given:
Psyllium hydrophilic muciloid is given by mouth. Mix the powder in 8 oz of juice or water and drink it right away. Otherwise it will get too thick to drink. The dose is the same for all adults, but the number of doses depends on how well it works for you. Keep the medicine in a tightly closed container away from heat and moisture and out of the reach of children and pets.

How Should I Take This Drug?
Take this drug exactly as directed by your doctor. If you do not understand the instructions, ask your doctor or nurse to explain them to you.

 Read the following information. If you do not understand it or if any of it causes you special concern, check with your doctor.

Before taking this drug, tell your doctor if you are taking any other prescription or over-the-counter drugs, including vitamins and herbals.

Should I avoid any other medicines, foods, alcohol, and/or activities?
Your prescription and nonprescription medicines may interact with other drugs, causing harm. Certain foods or alcohol can also interact with drug products. Never begin taking a new medicine—prescription or nonprescription—without asking your doctor or nurse if it will interact with alcohol, food, or other medicines. Some drugs can cause drowsiness and affect activities such as driving.

Precautions:
Psyllium hydrophilic muciloid is not absorbed by the gastrointestinal tract, so there are few side effects. However, the powder may contain sugar. If you have diabetes mellitus, select powder without sugar.

To prevent constipation, try to drink 2 to 3 quarts of fluid a day, increase the amount of fruits and vegetables in your diet (5 servings of fruits and vegetables daily), eat bran cereal, and do gentle exercise as tolerated.

Tell your doctor if you are taking salicylates, nitrofurantoin, or digoxin. Talk with your doctor about possible drug interactions.

Talk to your doctor before taking psyllium hydrophilic muciloid if you have nausea, vomiting, abdominal pain, or bleeding, or if you are impacted. There may be something else wrong besides constipation.

Tell all the doctors, dentists, and pharmacists you visit that you are taking this drug.

- Most of the following side effects probably will not occur.
- Your doctor or nurse will want to discuss specific care instructions with you.
- They can help you understand these side effects and help you deal with them.

Side Effects:

More Common Side Effects
Nausea

Less Common Side Effects
Vomiting

Obstruction of esophagus, stomach, intestines if this medicine is not properly diluted or drunk immediately after mixing, or if you are dehydrated

---
Other side effects not listed above can also occur in some patients.
Tell your doctor or nurse if you develop any problems.

FDA Approval: Yes

quinupristin and dalfopristin

Trade Name:
Synercid

Type of Drug:
Quinupristin and dalfopristin in combination are in the streptogram class of antibiotics, one of the newer classes of antibiotics.

How Drug Works:
Quinupristin and dalfopristin are two drugs that when combined have a greater effect on bacteria. The drug prevents the cell from making proteins, which causes the bacteria to die. Quinupristin and dalfopristin in combination are effective against gram-positive bacteria and some bacteria that are resitant to other antibiotics, such as vancomycin.

How Drug Is Given:
Quinupristin and dalfopristin are given together as an injection in a vein over 60 minutes 2 to 3 times a day. The dose depends on your weight and type and severity of the infection.

 Read the following information. If you do not understand it or if any of it causes you special concern, check with your doctor.

Before taking this drug, tell your doctor if you are taking any other prescription or over-the-counter drugs, including vitamins and herbals.

Should I avoid any other medicines, foods, alcohol, and/or activities?
Your prescription and nonprescription medicines may interact with other drugs, causing harm. Certain foods or alcohol can also interact with drug products. Never begin taking a new medicine—prescription or nonprescription—without asking your doctor or nurse if it will interact with alcohol, food, or other medicines. Some drugs can cause drowsiness and affect activities such as driving.

Precautions:
Tell your doctor if you have any drug allergies, especially to antibiotic drugs.

All antibiotics can cause allergic reactions. Stop the drug and tell your doctor or nurse right away if you develop a rash, hives, fever and chills, red blotches on your skin, swelling of face or lips, or difficulty breathing.

Use of antibiotics can change the normal organisms in your body. Women are at risk for fungal infections. Tell your nurse or doctor if you have vaginal itching or discharge.

Quinupristin and dalfopristin in combination can interact with other drugs. Be sure to tell your doctor about all the medicines you are taking.

Tell all the doctors, dentists, and pharmacists you visit that you are taking this drug.

- Most of the following side effects probably will not occur.
- Your doctor or nurse will want to discuss specific care instructions with you.
- They can help you understand these side effects and help you deal with them.

Side Effects:

More Common Side Effects
Redness, pain, and swelling at injection site
Nausea
Diarrhea
Vaginal itching

Less Common Side Effects
Abdominal pain
Vomiting
Heartburn
Constipation
Irritation of the lining of the mouth
Allergic reaction with rash, fever, chills, red blotching of skin, swelling of face, or difficulty
  breathing
White patches in the mouth
Muscle aches
Aching in the joints

Side Effects / Symptoms of the Drug
Stop the drug and call your doctor or nurse right away if you develop a rash, fever, chills, swelling
of lips or face, or difficulty breathing. This can be serious.

Other side effects not listed above can also occur in some patients.
Tell your doctor or nurse if you develop any problems.

FDA Approval: Yes

rofecoxib

Trade Name:
Vioxx

Type of Drug:
Rofecoxib is a nonopioid analgesic that belongs to the general class of drugs known as nonsteroidal anti-inflammatory drugs (NSAIDs).

How Drug Works:
Rofecoxib blocks prostaglandins (natural substances in the body that cause pain) from being produced. This prevents pain receptors from passing the pain message to the brain so that the perception of pain is reduced. It also reduces inflammation and fever. The drug is used for the treatment of osteoarthritis, management of acute pain, and treatment of painful menstrual periods in women.

How Drug Is Given:
Rofecoxib is a pill taken once a day by mouth with or without food. The dose depends on why you are taking it and how well it works for you. Keep the medicine in a tightly closed container away from heat and moisture and out of the reach of children and pets.

How Should I Take This Drug?
Take this drug exactly as directed by your doctor. If you do not understand the instructions, ask your doctor or nurse to explain them to you.

 Read the following information. If you do not understand it or if any of it causes you special concern, check with your doctor.

Before taking this drug, tell your doctor if you are taking any other prescription or over-the-counter drugs, including vitamins and herbals.

Should I avoid any other medicines, foods, alcohol, and/or activities?
Your prescription and nonprescription medicines may interact with other drugs, causing harm. Certain foods or alcohol can also interact with drug products. Never begin taking a new medicine—prescription or non-prescription—without asking your doctor or nurse if it will interact with alcohol, food, or other medicines. Some drugs can cause drowsiness and affect activities such as driving.

Precautions:
Tell your doctor if you have problems with your liver or kidneys. Your dose may need to be decreased; the drug should not be taken if you have severe liver or kidney problems.

Drug or blood-clotting levels may need to be checked more frequently if you are also taking Coumadin, a blood-thinning medicine, or lithium.

You should not take rofecoxib if you are also taking methotrexate.

Rofecoxib may decrease the effect of your diuretic if you are taking lasix or a thiazide diuretic; it may also decrease the blood pressure-lowering effect of angiotensin converting enzyme (ACE) inhibitors, such as lisinopril. Doses of these drugs may need to be increased while taking rofecoxib. Talk to your doctor about this.

Bleeding of the gastrointestinal tract occurs rarely, especially in people who smoke, drink alcohol, take aspirin or steroid pills, take medicine such as Coumadin to stop the blood from clotting, or have taken non-steroidal pills for a long time.

Women should not take this drug if they are pregnant or breastfeeding.

Tell all the doctors, dentists, and pharmacists you visit that you are taking this drug.

• Most of the following side effects probably will not occur.
• Your doctor or nurse will want to discuss specific care instructions with you.
• They can help you understand these side effects and help you deal with them.

Side Effects:

Less Common Side Effects
Fluid weight gain
Heartburn
Hypertension

Rare Side Effects

Constipation
Passing gas
Vomiting
Bleeding in the esophagus,
  stomach, or intestines
Irritation of the sinuses
Decreased kidney function

Increase in blood liver function values
Dry mouth
Rupture of stomach or duodenal ulcers
Difficulty sleeping
Dizziness
Lung infection
Severe allergic reaction with hives,
itching, rash, or difficulty breathing

Side Effects / Symptoms of the Drug

Stop the drug and call your doctor or nurse right away if you have gnawing or burning stomach pain, black or tarry stools, or vomiting.

Report unexplained weight gain or swelling of the feet (edema).

Stop the drug and report signs and symptoms of liver failure right away. This includes nausea; increased tiredness; drowsiness and feeling sleepy; itching; flu-like symptoms of fever, headache and malaise; jaundice or yellowing of the skin and eyes; or pain in the right upper part of the abdomen.

Stop the drug and call your doctor or nurse right away if you have hives or itching of the skin; call an ambulance to go to the emergency room if you have difficulty breathing.

Other side effects not listed above can also occur in some patients.
Tell your doctor or nurse if you develop any problems.

FDA Approval: Yes

salsalate

Trade Names:
Disalcid, Salflex, Salsalate

Type of Drug:
Salsalate is a nonopioid analgesic that belongs to the general class of drugs called nonsteroidal anti-inflammatory drugs (NSAIDs).

How Drug Works:
Salsalate blocks the synthesis of prostaglandins. This prevents pain receptors from passing the pain message to the brain so that pain perception is decreased. This drug reduces inflammation and also reduces fever by helping the body to dilate blood vessels so that heat is lost from the body. Salsalate is derived from salicylic acid but has fewer side effects than aspirin.

How Drug Is Given:
Salsalate is a pill given by mouth with food, 8 oz of water, or milk. Do not take with antacids. The dose depends on why you are taking it and how well it works for you. Keep the medicine in a tightly closed container away from heat and moisture and out of the reach of children and pets.

How Should I Take This Drug?
Take this drug exactly as directed by your doctor. If you do not understand the instructions, ask your doctor or nurse to explain them to you.

 Read the following information. If you do not understand it or if any of it causes you special concern, check with your doctor.

Before taking this drug, tell your doctor if you are taking any other prescription or over-the-counter drugs, including vitamins and herbals.

Should I avoid any other medicines, foods, alcohol, and/or activities?
Your prescription and nonprescription medicines may interact with other drugs, causing harm. Certain foods or alcohol can also interact with drug products. Never begin taking a new medicine—prescription or nonprescription—without asking your doctor or nurse if it will interact with alcohol, food, or other medicines. Some drugs can cause drowsiness and affect activities such as driving.

Precautions:
DO NOT take aspirin or other nonsteroidal anti-inflammatory drugs with salsalate. This may increase the risk of gastrointestinal side effects.

DO NOT take salsalate if you are allergic to aspirin or have severe kidney or liver disease. Talk to your doctor about this.

Tell your doctor if you are taking medicine such as Coumadin to stop blood from clotting or steroids such as prednisone. It is important to talk with your doctor about risk for bleeding.

Do not drink alcohol while taking salsalate, as this may increase risk of bleeding.

Tell all the doctors, dentists, and pharmacists you visit that you are taking this drug.
- Most of the following side effects probably will not occur.
- Your doctor or nurse will want to discuss specific care instructions with you.
- They can help you understand these side effects and help you deal with them.

Side Effects:

More Common Side Effects
Dizziness

Less Common Side Effects
Nausea
Heartburn
Liver toxicity
Loss of appetite
Increased risk of peptic ulcer
Ringing in the ears (tinnitus)
Vomiting
Diarrhea
Confusion
Feeling sleepy or drowsy
Headache
Sweating

Rare Side Effects
Decreased hearing
Allergic reaction
Increased bleeding time
Decreased white blood cell count with increased risk of infection
Decreased platelet count with increased risk of bleeding
Rash

Side Effects / Symptoms of the Drug
Call your doctor or nurse right away if you have bleeding from the gastrointestinal tract such as vomiting blood or coffee-ground material, blood in your stool, or black, tarry stools. Stop taking salsalate until after you talk with your doctor.

Call your doctor or nurse right away if you have dizziness, ringing in your ears, nausea, vomiting, headache, or sweating. These symptoms usually occur when too much of the medicine is taken. Stop taking salsalate until you talk to your doctor or nurse.

> **Other side effects not listed above can also occur in some patients.**
> **Tell your doctor or nurse if you develop any problems.**

FDA Approval: Yes

scopolamine

Trade Names:
Hyoscine hydrobromide, Scopolamine, Transderm-Scop, Transderm-V

Type of Drug:
Scopolamine belongs to a general class of drugs called anticholinergics (antimuscarinics) used to treat nausea and vomiting.

How Drug Works:
Scopolamine appears to prevent nausea and vomiting related to motion sickness by blocking messages that stimulate the part of the brain responsible for nausea and vomiting.

How Drug Is Given:
Scopolamine is usually given as a transdermal patch placed behind the ear. It must be applied at least 4 hours before chemotherapy and gives a fixed amount of medicine continuously for 3 days. Wash your hands before and after applying the patch. The dose is the same for all adults.

How Should I Take This Drug?
Take this drug exactly as directed by your doctor. If you do not understand the instructions, ask your doctor or nurse to explain them to you.

 Read the following information. If you do not understand it or if any of it causes you special concern, check with your doctor.

Before taking this drug, tell your doctor if you are taking any other prescription or over-the-counter drugs, including vitamins and herbals.

Should I avoid any other medicines, foods, alcohol, and/or activities?
Your prescription and nonprescription medicines may interact with other drugs, causing harm. Certain foods or alcohol can also interact with drug products. Never begin taking a new medicine—prescription or nonprescription—without asking your doctor or nurse if it will interact with alcohol, food, or other medicines. Some drugs can cause drowsiness and affect activities such as driving.

Tell all the doctors, dentists, and pharmacists you visit that you are taking this drug.

- Most of the following side effects probably will not occur.
- Your doctor or nurse will want to discuss specific care instructions with you.
- They can help you understand these side effects and help you deal with them.

Side Effects:

More Common Side Effects
Dry mouth

Less Common Side Effects
Drowsiness
Blurred vision
Dilated pupils

Rare Side Effects
Disorientation
Restlessness
Confusion

Other side effects not listed above can also occur in some patients.
Tell your doctor or nurse if you develop any problems.

FDA Approval: Yes

senna

Trade Names:
Black-Draught, Senekot, Senexon

Type of Drug:
Senna is an irritant/stimulant laxative used to treat constipation.

How Drug Works:
Senna stimulates/irritates the smooth muscle of the intestines. Water collects in the intestines. This stimulates the normal forward movement of the intestines (peristalsis), which results in a bowel movement within 6 to 10 hours.

How Drug Is Given:
Senna is given as a pill or rectal suppository. If you are using the suppository, open the package and dip the tip of the suppository in water. If you are right-handed, lie down on your left side, bring your knees up near your chest, and insert the suppository in your rectum about an inch. Stay in this position for about 15 minutes, then get up and wash your hands well. The dose depends on the reason you are taking it and how well it works for you. Keep the medicine in a tightly closed container away from heat and moisture and out of the reach of children and pets.

How Should I Take This Drug?
Take this drug exactly as directed by your doctor. If you do not understand the instructions, ask your doctor or nurse to explain them to you.

 Read the following information. If you do not understand it or if any of it causes you special concern, check with your doctor.

Before taking this drug, tell your doctor if you are taking any other prescription or over-the-counter drugs, including vitamins and herbals.

Should I avoid any other medicines, foods, alcohol, and/or activities?
Your prescription and nonprescription medicines may interact with other drugs, causing harm. Certain foods or alcohol can also interact with drug products. Never begin taking a new medicine—prescription or nonprescription—without asking your doctor or nurse if it will interact with alcohol, food, or other medicines. Some drugs can cause drowsiness and affect activities such as driving.

Precautions:
Talk to your doctor before taking senna if you have nausea, vomiting, abdominal pain, or blood in the stool, or if you are impacted. There may be something else wrong besides constipation.

To prevent constipation, try to drink 2 to 3 quarts of fluid a day, increase the amount of fruits and vegetables in your diet (5 servings of fruits and vegetables daily), eat bran cereal, and do gentle exercise as tolerated.

If you use laxatives all the time, your body may forget the normal process of moving the bowels. You then get dependent on the laxative. If you are taking opioid pain relievers, you will need to take a laxative regularly.

Some laxatives can cause diarrhea, which results in loss of fluids, nutrients, and electrolytes. It is important to replace the fluid that you lose through diarrhea. Try to drink 2 to 3 quarts of fluid a day. Fluids with electrolytes, such as chicken broth or sports drinks, are helpful in replacing potassium and salt that are lost in diarrhea. Take this medicine as instructed by your doctor.

Tell all the doctors, dentists, and pharmacists you visit that you are taking this drug.
- Most of the following side effects probably will not occur.
- Your doctor or nurse will want to discuss specific care instructions with you.
- They can help you understand these side effects and help you deal with them.

Side Effects:

More Common Side Effects
Loss of normal reflexes to move bowels when laxatives are used on a long-term basis
Nausea
Rectal burning as suppository is absorbed

Less Common Side Effects
Vomiting
Abdominal pain
Diarrhea
Dehydration related to diarrhea
Loss of electrolytes

Other side effects not listed above can also occur in some patients.
Tell your doctor or nurse if you develop any problems.

FDA Approval: Yes

sertraline hydrochloride

Trade Name:
Zoloft

Type of Drug:
Sertraline hydrochloride belongs to the general class of antidepressant drugs.

How Drug Works:
Sertraline hydrochloride stops the uptake of serotonin by the nerves, thus making more serotonin available in the brain and central nervous system (CNS). This decreases the feeling of depression.

How Drug Is Given:
Sertraline hydrochloride is a pill given by mouth once a day, either in the morning or evening. If you are changing from another antidepressant (monamine oxidase inhibitor), you should wait at least 2 weeks before starting sertraline hydrochloride. If you change from sertraline hydrochloride to a monamine oxidase inhibitor-type antidepressant, you must wait 14 days after stopping sertraline hydrochloride before starting the new drug. Keep the medicine in a tightly closed container away from heat and moisture and out of the reach of children and pets.

How Should I Take This Drug?
Take this drug exactly as directed by your doctor. If you do not understand the instructions, ask your doctor or nurse to explain them to you.

 Read the following information. If you do not understand it or if any of it causes you special concern, check with your doctor.

Before taking this drug, tell your doctor if you are taking any other prescription or over-the-counter drugs, including vitamins and herbals.

Should I avoid any other medicines, foods, alcohol, and/or activities?
Your prescription and nonprescription medicines may interact with other drugs, causing harm. Certain foods or alcohol can also interact with drug products. Never begin taking a new medicine—prescription or nonprescription—without asking your doctor or nurse if it will interact with alcohol, food, or other medicines. Some drugs can cause drowsiness and affect activities such as driving.

Precautions:
It may take a few weeks to find the right dose for you. Your doctor will start you off at a smaller dose, then increase it in 1 to 2 weeks if you do not feel better.

Tell your doctor if you are taking other antidepressant drugs. You cannot take a monoamine oxidase inhibitor antidepressant drug with sertraline hydrochloride because it is very dangerous.

DO NOT drink alcohol when you are taking sertraline hydrochloride.

Tell your doctor if you are taking any of the following drugs as they may have serious interactions with sertraline hydrochloride: antianxiety drugs (benzodiazepines), tolbutamide, warfarin (Coumadin), or lithium.

Tell all the doctors, dentists, and pharmacists you visit that you are taking this drug.
- Most of the following side effects probably will not occur.
- Your doctor or nurse will want to discuss specific care instructions with you.
- They can help you understand these side effects and help you deal with them.

Side Effects:

More Common Side Effects
Headache
Difficulty sleeping
Nausea
Diarrhea

Less Common Side Effects
Drowsiness
Agitation
Anxiety
Dry mouth
Heartburn
Vomiting

Dizziness
Nervousness
Tremors
Constipation
Changes in appetite
Urinary frequency

Rare Side Effects
Decreased ability to concentrate
Acne
Twitching
Confusion
Lack of coordination
Hair loss
Palpitations
Swelling of feet
Change in blood pressure
Dizziness when getting up from lying or standing position
Changes in taste
Abdominal pain
Difficulty swallowing
Rash
Dry skin
Itching
Change in menstrual periods
Decreased sexual interest
Sweating

Side Effects / Symptoms of the Drug
Be careful walking around or changing position if you are drowsy. Do not drive or operate heavy machinery if you are drowsy or dizzy. Call your doctor or nurse if the drowsiness does not go away, or if you have trouble walking or moving because of it.

Other side effects not listed above can also occur in some patients.
Tell your doctor or nurse if you develop any problems.

FDA Approval: Yes

sorbitol

Trade Name:
Sorbitol

Type of Drug:
Sorbitol is a hyperosmotic laxative used to treat constipation.

How Drug Works:
Sorbitol pulls water into the large intestines causing distention. This stimulates the normal forward movement of the intestines (peristalsis), which results in a bowel movement within 24 to 48 hours.

How Drug Is Given:
Sorbitol is given as a liquid by mouth or as a rectal suppository. It tastes very sweet. Take with water or juice to decrease the sweetness. If you are using the suppository, open the package and dip the tip of the suppository in water. If you are right-handed, lie down on you left side, bring your knees up near your chest, and insert the suppository in your rectum about an inch. Stay in this position for about 15 minutes, then get up and wash your hands well. The dose depends on the reason you are taking it and how well it has worked. Keep the medicine in a tightly closed container away from heat and moisture and out of the reach of children and pets.

How Should I Take This Drug?
Take this drug exactly as directed by your doctor. If you do not understand the instructions, ask your doctor or nurse to explain them to you.

 Read the following information. If you do not understand it or if any of it causes you special concern, check with your doctor.

Before taking this drug, tell your doctor if you are taking any other prescription or over-the-counter drugs, including vitamins and herbals.

Should I avoid any other medicines, foods, alcohol, and/or activities?
Your prescription and nonprescription medicines may interact with other drugs, causing harm. Certain foods or alcohol can also interact with drug products. Never begin taking a new medicine—prescription or nonprescription—without asking your doctor or nurse if it will interact with alcohol, food, or other medicines. Some drugs can cause drowsiness and affect activities such as driving.

Precautions:
Talk to your doctor before taking sorbitol if you have nausea, vomiting, abdominal pain, or blood in the stool, or if you are impacted. There may be something else wrong besides constipation.

Some laxatives can cause diarrhea. It is important to replace the fluid that you lose through diarrhea. Try to drink 2 to 3 quarts of fluid a day. Fluids with electrolytes, such as chicken broth or sports drinks, are helpful in replacing potassium and salt that are lost in diarrhea.

To prevent constipation, try to drink 2 to 3 quarts of fluid a day, increase the amount of fruits and vegetables in your diet (5 servings of fruits and vegetables daily), eat bran cereal, and do gentle exercise as tolerated.

If you use laxatives all the time, your body may forget the normal process of moving the bowels. You then get dependent on the laxative. If you are taking opioid pain relievers, you will need to take a laxative regularly.

This drug should not be used in patients with an intestinal obstruction or unexplained abdominal pain.

Tell all the doctors, dentists, and pharmacists you visit that you are taking this drug.
- -
- Most of the following side effects probably will not occur.
- Your doctor or nurse will want to discuss specific care instructions with you.
- They can help you understand these side effects and help you deal with them.

Side Effects:

More Common Side Effects
Loss of normal reflexes to move bowels when laxatives are used for a long time
Nausea

Less Common Side Effects
Vomiting
Cramping pain
Diarrhea
Dehydration resulting from diarrhea
Loss of electrolytes

Rare Side Effects
Rectal irritation

Other side effects not listed above can also occur in some patients.
Tell your doctor or nurse if you develop any problems.

FDA Approval: Yes

streptomycin sulfate

Trade Name:
Streptomycin

Type of Drug:
Streptomycin sulfate is an antibiotic that belongs to a group of drugs called aminoglycosides.

How Drug Works:
Streptomycin sulfate prevents bacteria from manufacturing their cell walls, so the bacteria die. It is used to treat tuberculosis and other bacteria.

How Drug Is Given:
Streptomycin sulfate is given by an injection in the muscle. The dose depends on the infection being treated, your age, how well your kidneys are working, and the drug level in the blood.

 Read the following information. If you do not understand it or if any of it causes you special concern, check with your doctor.

Before taking this drug, tell your doctor if you are taking any other prescription or over-the-counter drugs, including vitamins and herbals.

Should I avoid any other medicines, foods, alcohol, and/or activities?
Your prescription and nonprescription medicines may interact with other drugs, causing harm. Certain foods or alcohol can also interact with drug products. Never begin taking a new medicine—prescription or non-prescription—without asking your doctor or nurse if it will interact with alcohol, food, or other medicines. Some drugs can cause drowsiness and affect activities such as driving.

Precautions:
All antibiotics can cause allergic reactions. Stop the drug and tell your doctor or nurse right away if you develop a rash, hives, red blotches on your skin, or difficulty breathing.

Use of antibiotics can change the normal organisms in your body. Women are at risk of getting fungal infections. Tell your nurse or doctor if you get vaginal itching or discharge.

Streptomycin sulfate can injure the nerve for hearing (eighth cranial nerve, auditory). Tell your doctor or nurse right away if you feel dizzy, or have difficulty walking, ringing in your ears (tinnitus), a roaring sound in your ears, or any decrease in hearing. The drug should be stopped and changed to another effective drug without this problem.

Streptomycin sulfate can injure your kidneys. Your doctor will monitor blood tests to find this early, if it occurs. Make sure you tell your doctor if you have ever had any kidney problems.

Use in pregnancy only if life-threatening infection is present and no safer drug exists.

Tell your doctor if you have any drug allergies, especially to antibiotic drugs.

Tell all the doctors, dentists, and pharmacists you visit that you are taking this drug.

- Most of the following side effects probably will not occur.
- Your doctor or nurse will want to discuss specific care instructions with you.
- They can help you understand these side effects and help you deal with them.

Side Effects:

More Common Side Effects
Headache

Less Common Side Effects
Tremors

Tiredness (fatigue)

Nausea

Vomiting

Loss of appetite

Irritation at place of injection

Dizziness

Ringing in ears (tinnitus)

Decreased hearing

Vaginal itching

Vaginal candidiasis (fungal infection)

Rare Side Effects
Numbness and tingling in hands and feet

Muscle twitching

Rash

Itching

Hives

Diarrhea related to infection of the intestinal lining (pseudomembranous colitis)

Decreased white blood cell count with increased risk of infection

Decreased platelet count with increased risk of bleeding

Decreased red blood cell count with increased risk of tiredness and anemia

Abnormal kidney function in blood tests

Side Effects / Symptoms of the Drug
Stop the drug and call your doctor or nurse right away if you develop rash, fever, chills, or peeling skin. This can be a serious reaction and needs to be treated right away.

Stop the drug and call your doctor or nurse right away if you get diarrhea that does not stop, abdominal cramping, or blood and/or pus in the stool. This needs to be treated right away.

Other side effects not listed above can also occur in some patients.
Tell your doctor or nurse if you develop any problems.

FDA Approval: Yes

tetracycline hydrochloride

Trade Names:
Achromycin, Panmycin, Robitet, Sumycin, Tetralan

Type of Drug:
Tetracycline hydrochloride is an antibiotic belonging to a group of drugs called tetracyclines.

How Drug Works:
Tetracycline hydrochloride stops bacteria from reproducing, and at higher doses, kills the bacteria. It is used to treat many gram-positive and gram-negative bacteria and some protozoa.

How Drug Is Given:
Tetracycline hydrochloride is a pill taken by mouth 2 to 4 times a day, or given as an injection in a vein or muscle. Take the pill with an 8 oz glass of water on an empty stomach, either 1 hour before or 2 hours after eating food or drinking milk. If taking antacids, take them 1 to 2 hours before the tetracycline hydrochloride. If taking iron, take it 2 hours before or 3 hours afterward. Take the evening dose at least 1 hour before bedtime. The dose depends on the infection being treated. Keep the medicine in a tightly closed container away from heat and moisture and out of the reach of children and pets.

How Should I Take This Drug?
Take this drug exactly as directed by your doctor. If you do not understand the instructions, ask your doctor or nurse to explain them to you.

 Read the following information. If you do not understand it or if any of it causes you special concern, check with your doctor.

Before taking this drug, tell your doctor if you are taking any other prescription or over-the-counter drugs, including vitamins and herbals.

Should I avoid any other medicines, foods, alcohol, and/or activities?
Your prescription and nonprescription medicines may interact with other drugs, causing harm. Certain foods or alcohol can also interact with drug products. Never begin taking a new medicine—prescription or nonprescription—without asking your doctor or nurse if it will interact with alcohol, food, or other medicines. Some drugs can cause drowsiness and affect activities such as driving.

Precautions:
While taking tetracycline hydrochloride, DO NOT take kaopectate, bismuth, or methoxyflurane.

Oral contraceptives may be less effective when taking tetracycline. Women should also use a barrier contraceptive during the course of tetracycline hydrochloride.

Tell your doctor if you are taking lithium or if you have myasthenia gravis. There may be a drug interaction with lithium, and tetracycline hydrochloride may increase the muscle weakness due to myasthenia gravis.

Tell your doctor if you have any drug allergies, especially to antibiotic drugs.

All antibiotics can cause allergic reactions. Stop the drug and tell your doctor or nurse right away if you develop a rash, hives, red blotches on your skin, or difficulty breathing.

Use of antibiotics can change the normal organisms in your body. Women are at risk of getting fungal infections. Tell your nurse or doctor if you get vaginal itching or discharge.

Women who are pregnant or breastfeeding should not use this drug.

Tell all the doctors, dentists, and pharmacists you visit that you are taking this drug.
- Most of the following side effects probably will not occur.
- Your doctor or nurse will want to discuss specific care instructions with you.
- They can help you understand these side effects and help you deal with them.

Side Effects:

More Common Side Effects
Nausea
Diarrhea
Vaginal itching
Vaginal candidiasis (fungal infection)

Less Common Side Effects
Vomiting
Loss of appetite
Abdominal discomfort
Heartburn
Sore tongue
Redness and pain at place of injection

Rare Side Effects
Black, hairy tongue
Rash
Darkening of nail beds
Increased sensitivity to direct sunlight
Darkening and peeling of skin
Injury to liver when drug is given at high doses
Decreased white blood cell count with increased risk of infection
Decreased platelet count with increased risk of bleeding
Decreased red blood cell count with increased risk of tiredness and anemia
Dizziness
Lightheadedness
Headache

Side Effects / Symptoms of the Drug
Stop the drug and call your doctor or nurse right away if you develop rash, fever, chills, or peeling skin. This can be a serious reaction and needs to be treated right away.

Other side effects not listed above can also occur in some patients.
Tell your doctor or nurse if you develop any problems.

FDA Approval: Yes

thiethylperazine

Trade Name:
Torecan

Type of Drug:
Thiethylperazine belongs to a general class of drugs called phenothiazines used to treat nausea and vomiting.

How Drug Works:
Thiethylperazine is useful in preventing nausea and vomiting resulting from chemotherapy. It blocks messages to the part of the brain responsible for nausea and vomiting.

How Drug Is Given:
Thiethylperazine is given as a pill by mouth, by rectal suppository, or by an injection in a vein over 5 to 15 minutes. Take the pill with food or an 8 oz glass of milk to lessen stomach upset. If you are taking the suppository, open the package and dip the tip of the suppository in water. If you are right-handed, lie down on your left side, bring your knees up near your chest, and insert the suppository in your rectum about an inch. Stay in this position for about 15 minutes, then get up and wash your hands well. The dose depends on the reason you are taking it and how well it works for you. Keep the medicine in a tightly closed container away from heat and moisture and out of the reach of children and pets.

How Should I Take This Drug?
Take this drug exactly as directed by your doctor. If you do not understand the instructions, ask your doctor or nurse to explain them to you.

 Read the following information. If you do not understand it or if any of it causes you special concern, check with your doctor.

Before taking this drug, tell your doctor if you are taking any other prescription or over-the-counter drugs, including vitamins and herbals.

Should I avoid any other medicines, foods, alcohol, and/or activities?
Your prescription and nonprescription medicines may interact with other drugs, causing harm. Certain foods or alcohol can also interact with drug products. Never begin taking a new medicine—prescription or nonprescription—without asking your doctor or nurse if it will interact with alcohol, food, or other medicines. Some drugs can cause drowsiness and affect activities such as driving.

Precautions:
Thiethylperazine may cause extrapyramidal side effects. These include restlessness, tongue protrusion, and involuntary movements. These side effects are immediately stopped when you are given diphenhydramine.

Tell all the doctors, dentists, and pharmacists you visit that you are taking this drug.
- Most of the following side effects probably will not occur.
- Your doctor or nurse will want to discuss specific care instructions with you.
- They can help you understand these side effects and help you deal with them.

Side Effects:

More Common Side Effects
Drowsiness (when given by injection)

Less Common Side Effects
Low blood pressure (when given by injection)

Rare Side Effects
Increased heart rate
Changes in electrical activity of heart (EKG changes)

Other side effects not listed above can also occur in some patients.
Tell your doctor or nurse if you develop any problems.

FDA Approval: Yes

ticarcillin disodium

Trade Name:
Ticar

Type of Drug:
Ticarcillin disodium is a semisynthetic penicillin that belongs to a general class of drugs called antibiotics.

How Drug Works:
Ticarcillin disodium prevents bacteria from manufacturing their cell walls, which causes the bacteria to die. It is used to treat many gram-positive and some gram-negative bacteria that cause infections of the lungs, urinary tract, and skin.

How Drug Is Given:
Ticarcillin disodium is given as an injection in a vein over 30 to 60 minutes, 4 to 6 times a day, or in a muscle. The dose and the number of doses depend on your weight, how well your kidneys are working, and the type of infection being treated.

 Read the following information. If you do not understand it or if any of it causes you special concern, check with your doctor.

Before taking this drug, tell your doctor if you are taking any other prescription or over-the-counter drugs, including vitamins and herbals.

Should I avoid any other medicines, foods, alcohol, and/or activities?
Your prescription and nonprescription medicines may interact with other drugs, causing harm. Certain foods or alcohol can also interact with drug products. Never begin taking a new medicine—prescription or nonprescription—without asking your doctor or nurse if it will interact with alcohol, food, or other medicines. Some drugs can cause drowsiness and affect activities such as driving.

Precautions:
All antibiotics can cause allergic reactions. Stop the drug and tell your doctor or nurse right away if you develop a rash, hives, red blotches on your skin, difficulty breathing, or chest pain.

Use of antibiotics can change the normal organisms in your body. Women are at risk of getting fungal infections. Tell your nurse or doctor if you get vaginal itching or discharge.

Tell your doctor if you have any drug allergies, especially to antibiotic drugs. You should not take this drug if you are allergic to penicillin.

Tell all the doctors, dentists, and pharmacists you visit that you are taking this drug.
- Most of the following side effects probably will not occur.
- Your doctor or nurse will want to discuss specific care instructions with you.
- They can help you understand these side effects and help you deal with them.

Side Effects:

More Common Side Effects
Nausea
Vaginal itching
Vaginal candidiasis (fungal infection)

Less Common Side Effects
Vomiting
Diarrhea
Irritation of vein used to give the drug
Decreased blood potassium level

Rare Side Effects
Rash
Hives
Fever
Chills
Muscle aches
Swelling
Darkening and peeling of skin
Diarrhea related to infection of the intestinal lining (pseudomembranous colitis)
Dizziness
Headache
Sleepiness
Itching

Side Effects / Symptoms of the Drug
Stop the drug and call your doctor or nurse right away if you develop rash, fever, chills, or peeling skin. This can be a serious reaction and needs to be treated right away.

Stop the drug and call your doctor or nurse right away if you get diarrhea that does not stop, abdominal cramping, or blood and/or pus in the stool. This needs to be treated right away.

Other side effects not listed above can also occur in some patients.
Tell your doctor or nurse if you develop any problems.

FDA Approval: Yes

tobramycin sulfate

Trade Name:
Nebcin

Type of Drug:
Tobramycin sulfate is an antibiotic that belongs to a group of drugs called aminoglycosides.

How Drug Works:
Tobramycin sulfate prevents bacteria from manufacturing cell walls, which causes the bacteria to die. It is used to treat gram-negative and some gram-positive bacterial infections.

How Drug is Given:
Tobramyacin sulfate is given by injection in a vein 3 times a day. The dose depends on your weight, how well your kidneys are working, and the type of infection being treated.

 Read the following information. If you do not understand it or if any of it causes you special concern, check with your doctor.

Before taking this drug, tell your doctor if you are taking any other prescription or over-the-counter drugs, including vitamins and herbals.

Should I avoid any other medicines, foods, alcohol, and/or activities?
Your prescription and nonprescription medicines may interact with other drugs, causing harm. Certain foods or alcohol can also interact with drug products. Never begin taking a new medicine—prescription or nonprescription—without asking your doctor or nurse if it will interact with alcohol, food, or other medicines. Some drugs can cause drowsiness and affect activities such as driving.

Precautions:
All antibiotics can cause allergic reactions. Stop the drug and tell your doctor or nurse right away if you develop a rash, hives, red blotches on your skin, or difficulty breathing.

Use of antibiotics can change the normal organisms in your body. Women are at risk of getting fungal infections. Tell your nurse or doctor if you get vaginal itching or discharge.

Tobramycin sulfate can injure the nerve for hearing (eighth cranial nerve, auditory). Tell your doctor or nurse right away if you feel dizzy, or have difficulty walking, ringing in your ears, a roaring sound in your ears, or any decrease in hearing. The drug should be stopped and changed to another effective drug without this problem.

Tobramycin sulfate can injure your kidneys. Your doctor will monitor blood tests to find this early, if it occurs. Make sure you tell your doctor if you have ever had any kidney problems.

Use during pregnancy only if infection is life-threatening and no safer drug exists.

Tell your doctor if you have any drug allergies, especially to antibiotic drugs.

Tell all the doctors, dentists, and pharmacists you visit that you are taking this drug.
- Most of the following side effects probably will not occur.
- Your doctor or nurse will want to discuss specific care instructions with you.
- They can help you understand these side effects and help you deal with them.

Side Effects:

More Common Side Effects
Headache

Less Common Side Effects
Dizziness
Dizziness when standing up
Difficulty walking
Ringing in ears (tinnitus)
Roaring sound in ears
Tremors
Tiredness (fatigue)

Rare Side Effects
Hearing loss
Numbness and tingling in hands and feet
Muscle twitching
Rash
Itching
Hives
Fever
Nausea
Vomiting
Loss of appetite
Decreased white blood cell count with increased risk of infection
Decreased platelet count with increased risk of bleeding
Decreased red blood cell count with increased risk of tiredness and anemia
Liver injury
Abnormal kidney function blood tests

Side Effects / Symptoms of the Drug
Stop the drug and call your doctor or nurse right away if you develop rash, fever, chills, or peeling skin. This can be a serious reaction and needs to be treated right away.

Other side effects not listed above can also occur in some patients.
Tell your doctor or nurse if you develop any problems.

FDA Approval: Yes

trazodone hydrochloride

Trade Names:
Desyrel, Trialodine

Type of Drug:
Trazodone hydrochloride belongs to a general class of antidepressant drugs.

How Drug Works:
Trazodone hydrochloride stops the uptake of serotonin by the nerves, making more serotonin available in the brain. This decreases the feeling of depression.

How Drug Is Given:
Trazodone hydrochloride is a pill taken by mouth with food, 1 to 3 times a day. If you are taking a single dose, take it at bedtime to sleep better. The dose depends on your age and on how well the medicine helps you. It may take up to 4 weeks to feel the benefit. Your doctor may gradually increase the dose. Keep the medicine in a tightly closed container away from heat and moisture and out of the reach of children and pets.

How Should I Take This Drug?
Take this drug exactly as directed by your doctor. If you do not understand the instructions, ask your doctor or nurse to explain them to you.

 Read the following information. If you do not understand it or if any of it causes you special concern, check with your doctor.

Before taking this drug, tell your doctor if you are taking any other prescription or over-the-counter drugs, including vitamins and herbals.

Should I avoid any other medicines, foods, alcohol, and/or activities?
Your prescription and nonprescription medicines may interact with other drugs, causing harm. Certain foods or alcohol can also interact with drug products. Never begin taking a new medicine—prescription or nonprescription—without asking your doctor or nurse if it will interact with alcohol, food, or other medicines. Some drugs can cause drowsiness and affect activities such as driving.

Precautions:
Tell your doctor if you are taking any of the following drugs as they may have serious interactions with trazodone hydrochloride: medicines for blood pressure, barbiturates, clonidine, digoxin, other central nervous system (CNS) depressant drugs, other antidepressant medicines (monoamine oxidase inhibitors), and phenytoin (Dilantin).

Since trazodone hydrochloride affects the central nervous system (CNS), it is important not to take other drugs or substances that are known CNS depressants such as alcohol, sedatives, and hypnotics.

Trazodone hydrochloride may make you feel drowsy and/or dizzy when you change your position from lying or sitting to standing. Tell your doctor or nurse if this continues or is severe.

DO NOT take this drug if you are recovering from a heart attack (myocardial infarction) or receiving electroshock therapy.

Trazodone hydrochloride may cause severe sedation and dizziness in the elderly (when changing position).

Take trazodone hydrochloride at bedtime to help you sleep.

Most people will respond within the first 2 weeks of treatment. Others will respond within 2 to 4 weeks.

Tell all the doctors, dentists, and pharmacists you visit that you are taking this drug.

- Most of the following side effects probably will not occur.
- Your doctor or nurse will want to discuss specific care instructions with you.
- They can help you understand these side effects and help you deal with them.

Side Effects:

More Common Side Effects
Drowsiness
Lightheadedness

Dizziness
Decrease in blood pressure when changing
from a lying or sitting position to standing

Less Common Side Effects
Tiredness (fatigue)
Confusion
Excitement
Disorientation
Difficulty remembering

Nightmares
Anger
Decreased ability to concentrate
Nervousness

Rare Side Effects
Hallucinations
Difficulty sleeping
Difficulty speaking
Lack of coordination
Tremors
Numbness or tingling in hands and/or feet
Prolonged or inappropriate penile erections (priapism)
Diarrhea
Nausea
Vomiting
Blurred vision
Heart palpitations
Increased heart rate
Change in blood pressure
Shortness of breath
Chest pain

Side Effects / Symptoms of the Drug

For men, if you develop prolonged or inappropriate penile erections, STOP taking trazodone hydrochloride and call your doctor or nurse right away. If this problem has lasted 24 hours or more, you need to see a urologist (a specialist in this problem).

DO NOT drive or operate heavy machinery until you know the effect of the medicine on you. Trazodone hydrochloride may cause you to feel drowsy, dizzy, have decreased reaction time, and decreased ability to concentrate. It is very dangerous to drive or operate heavy machinery if you feel this way.

Tell your doctor or nurse if you have problems with any of the side effects. He or she will help you find ways to manage them, or perhaps find another effective drug without these problems.

Other side effects not listed above can also occur in some patients.
Tell your doctor or nurse if you develop any problems.

FDA Approval: Yes

trovafloxacin

Trade Name:
Trovan

Type of Drug:
Trovafloxacin is an antibiotic that belongs to a class of drugs called fluoroquinolones.

How Drug Works:
Trovafloxacin interferes with bacterial DNA so that the cells cannot reproduce. This drug is used for many gram-positive and gram-negative bacterial infections. It is used for severe infections only.

How Drug Is Given:
Trovafloxacin is given as an injection in a vein or as a pill by mouth once a day. Take the pill with 8 oz of water 2 hours after a meal or food. This medicine does not work well with the following medicines: antacids with aluminum, magnesium, or calcium; cimetidine; sucralfate; vitamin pills with zinc and iron. Take these other medicines at least 2 hours before or 2 hours after the trovofloxacin. Talk with your nurse about scheduling your medicines. The dose depends on your weight, the infection being treated, and how well your liver is working. This drug should be started in the hospital. Keep the medicine in a tightly closed container away from heat and moisture and out of the reach of children and pets.

How Should I Take This Drug?
Take this drug exactly a directed by your doctor. If you do not understand the instructions, ask your doctor or nurse to explain them to you.

 Read the following information. If you do not understand it or if any of it causes you special concern, check with your doctor.

Before taking this drug, tell your doctor if you are taking any other prescription or over-the-counter drugs, including vitamins and herbals.

Should I avoid any other medicines, foods, alcohol, and/or activities?
Your prescription and nonprescription medicines may interact with other drugs, causing harm. Certain foods or alcohol can also interact with drug products. Never begin taking a new medicine—prescription or nonprescription—without asking your doctor or nurse if it will interact with alcohol, food, or other medicines. Some drugs can cause drowsiness and affect activities such as driving.

Precautions:
Try to decrease the amount of caffeine you drink while taking trovafloxacin as caffeine increases the drug clearance from the body. Side effects such as headache, restlessness, dizziness, hallucinations, and seizures happen more often if you drink a lot of caffeine.

Tell your doctor if you have any drug allergies, especially to antibiotic drugs.

All antibiotics can cause allergic reactions. Stop the drug and tell your doctor or nurse right away if you develop a rash, hives, red blotches on your skin, or difficulty breathing.

Use of antibiotics can change the normal organisms in your body. Women are at risk of getting fungal infections. Tell your nurse or doctor if you get vaginal itching or discharge.

Women who are pregnant or breastfeeding should not use this drug.

Make your doctor aware of any other medications that you are taking.

Tell all the doctors, dentists, and pharmacists you visit that you are taking this drug.
- Most of the following side effects probably will not occur.
- Your doctor or nurse will want to discuss specific care instructions with you.
- They can help you understand these side effects and help you deal with them.

Side Effects:

More Common Side Effects
Nausea
Diarrhea
Headache
Restlessness

Less Common Side Effects
Vomiting
Abdominal discomfort
Loss of appetite
Vaginal itching
Vaginal candidiasis (fungal infection)

Rare Side Effects
Dizziness
Hallucinations
Seizures
Rash
Hives
Flushing
Fever
Chills
Increased sensitivity to direct sunlight

Side Effects / Symptoms of the Drug
Stop the drug and call your doctor or nurse right away if you develop rash, fever, chills, or peeling skin. This can be a serious reaction and needs to be treated right away.

Other side effects not listed above can also occur in some patients.
Tell your doctor or nurse if you develop any problems.

FDA Approval: Yes

valcyclovir hydrochloride

Trade Name:
Valtrex

Type of Drug:
Valcyclovir hydrochloride belongs to the general class of drugs called antivirals.

How Drug Works:
Valcyclovir hydrochloride prevents viruses from reproducing. It is used to treat herpes viruses, herpes zoster (shingles), Epstein-Barr virus, and cytomegalovirus.

How Drug Is Given:
Valcyclovir hydrochloride is a pill taken by mouth, with or without food. The dose depends on the infection being treated and how well your kidneys are working. Keep the medicine in a tightly closed container away from heat and moisture and out of the reach of children and pets.

How Should I Take This Drug?
Take this drug exactly as directed by your doctor. If you do not understand the instructions, ask your doctor or nurse to explain them to you.

 Read the following information. If you do not understand it or if any of it causes you special concern, check with your doctor.

Before taking this drug, tell your doctor if you are taking any other prescription or over-the-counter drugs, including vitamins and herbals.

Should I avoid any other medicines, foods, alcohol, and/or activities?
Your prescription and nonprescription medicines may interact with other drugs, causing harm. Certain foods or alcohol can also interact with drug products. Never begin taking a new medicine—prescription or non-prescription—without asking your doctor or nurse if it will interact with alcohol, food, or other medicines. Some drugs can cause drowsiness and affect activities such as driving.

Precautions:
Tell your doctor if you are also taking cimetidine or probenecid. Talk to your doctor about possible drug interactions.

This drug should not be used if your immune system is suppressed.

Tell all the doctors, dentists, and pharmacists you visit that you are taking this drug.

- Most of the following side effects probably will not occur.
- Your doctor or nurse will want to discuss specific care instructions with you.
- They can help you understand these side effects and help you deal with them.

Side Effects:

More Common Side Effects
Headache

Less Common Side Effects
Nausea

Vomiting

Rare Side Effects
Kidney problems

Side Effects / Symptoms of the Drug
Your doctor or nurse will check your kidney function before starting the drug.

Other side effects not listed above can also occur in some patients.
Tell your doctor or nurse if you develop any problems.

FDA Approval: Yes

vancomycin hydrochloride

Trade Name:
Vancocin

Type of Drug:
Vancomycin hydrochloride belongs to a general class of drugs called antibiotics.

How Drug Works:
Vancomycin hydrochloride prevents bacteria from manufacturing their cell walls, which causes the bacteria to die. It is used to treat many gram-positive bacterial infections.

How Drug Is Given:
Vancomycin hydrochloride is given as an injection in a vein over 1 hour twice a day, or as a pill or liquid by mouth in 4 divided doses. Vancomycin hydrochloride does not work well with cholestryramine or colestipol; if you are taking either of these medicines, separate the vancomycin hydrochloride by 3 to 4 hours. The dose depends on your weight, the infection being treated, how well your kidneys are working, and the medicine level in your blood. Keep the medicine in a tightly closed container away from heat and moisture and out of the reach of children and pets.

How Should I Take This Drug?
Take this drug exactly as directed by your doctor. If you do not understand these instructions, ask your doctor or nurse to explain them to you.

 Read the following information. If you do not understand it or if any of it causes you special concern, check with your doctor.

Before taking this drug, tell your doctor if you are taking any other prescription or over-the-counter drugs, including vitamins and herbals.

Should I avoid any other medicines, foods, alcohol, and/or activities?
Your prescription and nonprescription medicines may interact with other drugs, causing harm. Certain foods or alcohol can also interact with drug products. Never begin taking a new medicine—prescription or nonprescription—without asking your doctor or nurse if it will interact with alcohol, food, or other medicines. Some drugs can cause drowsiness and affect activities such as driving.

Precautions:
All antibiotics can cause allergic reactions. Stop the drug and tell your doctor or nurse right away if you develop a rash, hives, red blotches on your skin, or difficulty breathing.

Use of antibiotics can change the normal organisms in your body. Women are at risk of getting fungal infections. Tell your nurse or doctor if you get vaginal itching or discharge.

Vancomycin hydrochloride can injure the nerve for hearing (eighth cranial nerve, auditory). Tell your doctor or nurse right away if you feel dizzy, have difficulty walking, ringing in your ears, a roaring sound in your ears, or any decrease in hearing. The drug should be stopped and changed to another effective drug without this problem.

Vancomycin hydrochloride can injure your kidneys. Your doctor will monitor blood tests to find this early if it occurs. Make sure you tell your doctor if you have ever had any kidney problems.

If the drug is given too quickly in the vein, you can get a flushing in your neck or a rash over the neck, face, and chest. You may also have wheezing, difficulty breathing, and a decrease in your blood pressure. Tell your doctor or nurse immediately if you feel a flush in your neck or any other problems.

Tell your doctor if you have any drug allergies, especially to antibiotic drugs.

Tell all the doctors, dentists, and pharmacists you visit that you are taking this drug.

- Most of the following side effects probably will not occur.
- Your doctor or nurse will want to discuss specific care instructions with you.
- They can help you understand these side effects and help you deal with them.

Side Effects:

More Common Side Effects
Vaginal itching
Vaginal candidiasis (fungal infection)

Less Common Side Effects
Irritation of vein used for giving the drug
Ringing in ears (tinnitus)
Roaring sound in ears
Increase in kidney function tests

Rare Side Effects
Hearing loss
Kidney injury
Decreased white blood cell count with increased risk of infection
Decreased platelet count with increased risk of bleeding
Rash
Hives
Fever
Chills
Decrease in blood pressure

Side Effects / Symptoms of the Drug
Call your doctor or nurse if you develop rash, fever, or chills. Your doctor needs to evaluate you.

Other side effects not listed above can also occur in some patients.
Tell your doctor or nurse if you develop any problems.

FDA Approval: Yes

venlafaxine hydrochloride

Trade Name:
Effexor

Type of Drug:
Venlafaxine hydrochloride belongs to the general class of antidepressant drugs.

How Drug Works:
Venlafaxine hydrochloride works by increasing the amount of serotonin and norepinephrine in the brain, so that the feeling of depression is prevented or relieved.

How Drug Is Given:
Venlafaxine hydrochloride is taken as a pill by mouth. There are 2 types: immediate release and extended release. The immediate release is taken 2 to 3 times a day with food. The extended release is taken once a day with food. The dose depends on your response to the lowest dose and how well your kidneys and liver are working. Keep the medicine in a tightly closed container away from heat and moisture and out of the reach of children and pets.

How Should I Take This Drug?
Take this drug exactly as directed by your doctor. If you do not understand these instructions, ask your doctor or nurse to explain them to you.

 Read the following information. If you do not understand it or if any of it causes you special concern, check with your doctor.

Before taking this drug, tell your doctor if you are taking any other prescription or over-the-counter drugs, including vitamins and herbals.

Should I avoid any other medicines, foods, alcohol, and/or activities?
Your prescription and nonprescription medicines may interact with other drugs, causing harm. Certain foods or alcohol can also interact with drug products. Never begin taking a new medicine—prescription or non-prescription—without asking your doctor or nurse if it will interact with alcohol, food, or other medicines. Some drugs can cause drowsiness and affect activities such as driving.

Precautions:
If you are currently taking another antidepressant in the monamine oxidase inhibitor (MAOI) class, your doctor will wait about 2 weeks before starting you on venlafaxine hydrochloride. If you change from venlafaxine hydrochloride to an MAOI, your doctor will not start you on the new drug immediately. Your doctor may lower your dose gradually before stopping it completely. You cannot take venlafaxine hydrochloride with an MAOI without the risk of very serious side effects.

Tell your doctor if you are taking cimetidine or haloperidol (Haldol) as they may have serious interactions with venlafaxine hydrochloride.

Women who are pregnant or breastfeeding should not take this drug.

Tell all the doctors, dentists, and pharmacists you visit that you are taking this drug.
- Most of the following side effects probably will not occur.
- Your doctor or nurse will want to discuss specific care instructions with you.
- They can help you understand these side effects and help you deal with them.

Side Effects:

More Common Side Effects
Migraine headache
Dizziness when standing up
Tightness in the jaw
Nausea

Less Common Side Effects
Loss of appetite
Constipation
Problems in sexual function
Feeling "blah"
Neck pain
Hangover like effect
Bone pain
Bruises on skin
Problems urinating

Rare Side Effects
Change in blood pressure
Change in heart rate or heart rhythm
Swelling in feet
Hallucinations
Increased sensitivity to sunlight
Difficulty sleeping
Diarrhea
Difficulty swallowing
Acne
Hives
Dizziness when changing position
Inflammation of veins in the lower leg
Euphoria
Blurred vision
Hair loss
Dry mouth
Heartburn
Upset stomach
Rash
Dry skin

Side Effects / Symptoms of the Drug
Tell your doctor or nurse if you get black and blue spotbruises on the skin, have difficulty in passing your urine, or any other problems that do not go away. Your doctor or nurse will help you find ways to manage these problems, or perhaps find another effective drug without these problems.

Other side effects not listed above can also occur in some patients.
Tell your doctor or nurse if you develop any problems.

FDA Approval: Yes

zolpidem tartrate

Trade Name:
Ambien

Type of Drug:
Zolpidem tartrate is a drug of the hypnotic class that resembles a benzodiazepine drug.

How Drug Works:
Zolpidem tartrate is used to treat insomnia by enhancing the activity of chemicals in the brain. It produces deep sleep and does not have the muscle relaxant or anticonvulsant properties of benzodiazepine drugs.

How Drug Is Given:
Zolpidem tartrate is a pill given by mouth on an empty stomach. The dose depends on the lowest dose that works for you. Keep the medicine in a tightly closed container away from heat and moisture and out of the reach of children and pets.

How Should I Take This Drug?
Take this drug exactly as directed by your doctor. If you do not understand the instructions, ask your doctor or nurse to explain them to you.

 Read the following information. If you do not understand it or if any of it causes you special concern, check with your doctor.

Before taking this drug, tell your doctor if you are taking any other prescription or over-the-counter drugs, including vitamins and herbals.

Should I avoid any other medicines, foods, alcohol, and/or activities?
Your prescription and nonprescription medicines may interact with other drugs, causing harm. Certain foods or alcohol can also interact with drug products. Never begin taking a new medicine—prescription or nonprescription—without asking your doctor or nurse if it will interact with alcohol, food, or other medicines. Some drugs can cause drowsiness and affect activities such as driving.

Precautions:
DO NOT drink alcohol while taking this drug.

Tell your doctor if you are depressed. This drug may make you feel more depressed. If this happens, stop the drug and ask your doctor to find another effective medicine without this problem.

Women who are pregnant or breastfeeding should not take this drug.

Tell all the doctors, dentists, and pharmacists you visit that you are taking this drug.

- Most of the following side effects probably will not occur.
- Your doctor or nurse will want to discuss specific care instructions with you.
- They can help you understand these side effects and help you deal with them.

Side Effects:

More Common Side Effects
Drowsiness
Sleepiness

Less Common Side Effects
Tiredness (fatigue)
Feeling "drugged"
Depression
Anxiety
Irritability

Rare Side Effects
Nausea
Vomiting
Heartburn
Double vision
Lack of coordination
Decreased memory

Side Effects / Symptoms of the Drug
DO NOT drive or operate heavy machinery until you know the effect of the medicine on you. Zolpidem tartrate may cause you to feel drowsy, dizzy, have decreased reaction time, and decreased ability to concentrate. It is very dangerous to drive or operate heavy machinery if you feel this way.

Other side effects not listed above can also occur in some patients.
Tell your doctor or nurse if you develop any problems.

FDA Approval: Yes

Glossary

Ablative therapy: treatment that removes or destroys the function of an organ, for example, removing the ovaries or having some type of chemotherapy that causes the ovaries to stop working.

Absolute neutrophil count (ANC): a calculation by health care providers to determine how likely someone is to develop an infection. Someone with an ANC of 1,000 or less is considered to be neutropenic and at risk of developing an infection. An ANC lower than 500 is considered severe neutropenia.

Adjuvant therapy: treatment used in addition to the main treatment. It usually refers to hormonal therapy, chemotherapy, or radiation added after surgery to increase the chances of curing the disease or keeping it in check.

Agranulocytes: a type of white blood cell that does not contain granules in the cytoplasm of the cell. It includes 3 subtypes: lymphocytes, monocytes, and macrophages.

Alopecia: hair loss. This often occurs as a result of chemotherapy or, less often, from radiation therapy to the head. In most cases, the hair grows back after treatment ends.

Analgesic: a drug that relieves pain.

Androgen: a male sex hormone. Androgens may be used to treat recurrent breast cancer. Their effect is to block the activity of estrogen, thereby slowing the growth of the cancer.

Androgen blocker: use of drugs to disrupt the actions of male hormones.

Anemia: low red blood cell count.

Anorexia: loss of appetite.

Antibacterial: any agent that stops or destroys the growth of bacteria.

Antibiotic: drugs used to kill organisms that cause disease. Antibiotics may be made by living organisms or they may be created in the lab. Since some cancer treatments can reduce the body's ability to fight off infection, antibiotics may be used to treat or prevent these infections.

Antibody: a protein in the blood that defends against foreign agents, such as bacteria. These agents contain certain substances called antigens. Each antibody works against a specific antigen.

Antidepressant: any medicine or other kind of therapy that acts to lessen, prevent, or cure mental depression.

Antiestrogen: a substance (for example, the drug tamoxifen) that blocks the effect of estrogen on tumors. Antiestrogens are used to treat breast cancers that depend on estrogen for growth.

Antifungal: a drug active against fungi.

Antihistamine: a drug or agent that opposes the action of histamine.

Antimetabolites: substances that interfere with the body's chemical processes, such as those creating proteins, DNA, and other chemicals needed for cell growth and reproduction. In treating cancer, antimetabolite drugs disrupt DNA production, which in turn prevents cell division and growth of tumors.

Antineoplastic: anticancer.

Antiviral: a drug effective against viruses that cause disease.

Anxiety: a vague feeling of worry, unease, apprehension, or dread, with a nonspecific source.

Biologic response modifiers: substances that boost the body's immune system to fight against cancer; interferon is one example. Also called biologic therapy.

Blood count: a count of the number of red blood cells and white blood cells in a given sample of blood.

Bone marrow transplantation (BMT): a complex and sometimes risky treatment that may be used when cancer is advanced or has recurred, or as the main treatment in some types of leukemia or lymphoma. A portion of the patient or donor's bone marrow is withdrawn, cleansed, treated, and stored. The patient is given high doses of chemotherapy to kill the cancer cells. The drugs also destroy the remaining bone marrow, thus robbing the body of its natural ability to fight infection. The cleansed marrow is given by transfusion (transplanted) to rescue the patient's immune defenses.

Cachexia: a condition of severe malnutrition, emaciation, and debility.

Cancer: not just one disease but rather a group of diseases. All forms of cancer will cause cells in the body to change and grow out of control. Most types of cancer cells form a lump or mass called a tumor. The tumor can invade and destroy healthy tissue. Cells from the tumor can break away and travel to other parts of the body. There they can continue to grow. This spreading process is called metastasis. When cancer spreads, it is still named after the part of the body where it started. For example, if breast cancer spreads to the lungs, it is still breast cancer, not lung cancer. Some cancers, such as blood cancers, do not form a tumor. Not all tumors are cancer. A tumor that is not cancer is called benign. Benign tumors do not grow and spread the way cancer does. They are usually not a threat to life. Another word for cancerous is malignant.

Catheter: a thin, flexible tube through which fluids enter or leave the body.

Chemoprotective agent: a newer type of drug that protects against specific side effects of certain chemotherapy drugs. For example, dexrazoxane helps prevent heart damage, amifostine helps protect the kidneys, and mesna protects the bladder.

Chemotherapy: treatment with drugs to destroy cancer cells. Chemotherapy is often used with surgery or radiation to treat cancer when the cancer has spread, when it has come back (recurred), or when there is a strong chance that it could recur.

Clinical trials: research studies to test new drugs or other treatments to compare current, standard treatments with others that may be better. Before a new treatment is used on people, it is studied in the lab. If lab studies suggest the treatment will work, the next step is to test its value for patients. These human studies are called clinical trials.

Colony stimulating factors (CSF): types of growth factors that promote growth and division of blood-producing cells in the bone marrow. CSFs are naturally produced in the body. But extra amounts may be given as a treatment to reduce or prevent certain side effects of chemotherapy due to not having enough blood cells.

Control: a goal of cancer treatment if cure is not possible; stopping the cancer from growing and spreading to extend life and provide the best quality of life while you live with cancer.

Corticosteroid: any of a number of steroid substances obtained from the cortex of the adrenal glands. They are sometimes used as an anticancer treatment.

Cure: the goal of chemotherapy and other treatments used to make the tumor or cancer disappear and not return.

Cytokine: a product of cells of the immune system that may stimulate immunity and cause the regression of some cancers.

Cytotoxic: toxic to cells; cell-killing.

Depression: in psychiatry, a mental disorder marked by altered mood, including loss of appetite, feeling of hopelessness, or loss of energy.

DNA: abbreviation for deoxyribonucleic acid. DNA holds genetic information on cell growth, division, and function.

Drug resistance: refers to the ability of cancer cells to become resistant to the effects of the chemotherapy drugs used to treat cancer.

Epidermal Growth Factor Receptor (EGFR): a place on the cell where certain hormones or proteins attach and control how the cell grows, divides into another cell, or makes proteins. In some cancers, these receptors can be "overexpressed" on the surface of a cell, so that the cell gets "turned on" by itself without waiting for the body to tell the cell to divide. It then divides uncontrollably. Agents that block the receptors are being tested to see if this can stop the cells from dividing.

Esophagitis: inflammation or sores in the esophagus (the tube that leads from the throat to the stomach) caused by chemotherapy.

Estrogen: a female sex hormone produced primarily in the ovaries and in small amounts by the adrenal cortex. In breast cancer, estrogen may promote the growth of cancer cells.

Flare: a temporary increase in pain, usually bone pain, in people with metastasis; this occurs when starting specific hormone cancer treatment medicines.

Gene therapy: a new type of treatment in which defective genes are replaced with normal ones. The new genes are delivered into the cells by viruses or proteins.

Granulocytes: white blood cells that contain granules (visible specks) in the cytoplasm of the cell. There are 3 subtypes: neutrophils, eosinophils, and basophils.

Growth factors: a naturally occurring protein that causes cells to grow and divide. Too much growth factor production by some cancer cells helps them grow quickly, and new treatments to block these growth factors are being tested in clinical trials. Other growth factors help normal cells recover from side effects of chemotherapy.

Hematopoietic stem cell transplantation (HSCT): the term used to include bone marrow transplantation (BMT) and peripheral blood stem cell transplantation (PBSCT). These transplants use especially high doses of chemotherapy and/or total body irradiation (TBI) to kill the cancer cells. In the process of using these treatments to wipe out the cancer, normal hematopoietic (blood-forming) stem cells in the bone marrow are also killed. Therefore, stem cells are removed from your blood or bone marrow before treatment and are given back to you once it is completed.

Hemoglobin: the red substance in red blood cells that carries oxygen to other tissues of the body.

Hormone therapy: treatment with hormones, drugs that interfere with hormone production or hormone action, or surgical removal of hormone-producing glands to kill cancer cells or slow their growth. The term also applies to the replacement of other hormones (androgens, thyroid, etc.) that are deficient because of organ failure.

Immunosuppression: the state in which the body's immune system does not respond as it should. This condition may be present at birth, or it may be caused by certain infections (such as human immuno-deficiency virus or HIV) or by certain cancer therapies, such as cancer-cell killing (cytotoxic) drugs, radiation, and bone marrow transplantation.

Immunotherapy: treatments that promote or support the body's immune system response to a disease such as cancer.

Informed consent: a legal document that explains a course of treatment, the risks, benefits, and possible alternatives; the process by which patients agree to treatment.

Interferon: a protein produced by cells. Interferon helps regulate the body's immune system, boosting activity when a threat, such as a virus, is found. Scientists have learned that interferon helps fight against cancer, so it is used to treat some types of cancer.

Intramuscular: within a muscle.

Intravenous: within or into a vein.

Leukopenia: a decrease in the white blood cell count, often a side effect of chemotherapy.

LHRH analogs: stands for **L**euteinizing **H**ormone-**R**eleasing **H**ormone. Man-made hormones that block the production of the male hormone testosterone; sometimes used as a treatment for prostate cancer.

Liposomes: man-made fat globules that are used with chemotherapy drugs to penetrate cancer cells more selectively and decrease possible side effects. Examples of liposomal medicines already in use are Doxil (the encapsulated form of doxorubicin) and DaunoXome (the encapsulated form of daunorubicin).

Lumbar puncture: spinal tap.

Lymphatic system: the tissues and organs (including bone marrow, spleen, thymus, and lymph nodes) that produce and store lymphocytes (cells that fight infection) and the channels that carry the lymph fluid. The entire lymphatic system as an important part of the body's immune system. Invasive cancers sometimes penetrate the lymphatic vessels (channels) and spread (metastasize) to lymph nodes.

- Lymph: clear fluid that flows through lymphatic vessels and contains cells known as lymphocytes. These cells are important in fighting infections and may also have a role in fighting cancer.
- Lymph nodes: small bean-shaped collections of immune system tissue such as lymphocytes, found along lymphatic vessels. They remove cell waste and fluids from lymph and help fight infections. Also called lymph glands.
- Lymphocytes: a type of white blood cell that helps the body fight infection.

Monoclonal antibodies: antibodies made in the laboratory and designed to target specific substances called antigens. Monoclonal antibodies that have been attached to chemotherapy drugs or radioactive substances are being studied to see if they can seek out antigens unique to cancer cells and deliver these treatments directly to the cancer, thus killing the cancer cells without harming healthy tissue. Monoclonal antibodies are also used in other ways, for example, to help find and classify cancer cells.

Mucositis: inflammation of a mucus membrane such as the lining of the mouth.

Myelosuppression: also called bone marrow suppression, damage to the blood cell-producing tissues of the bone marrow. It is one of the most common side effects of chemotherapy.

Nadir: the lowest count that blood cell levels fall to when receiving a cancer treatment that causes bone marrow suppression (myelosuppression) or low blood counts.

Narcotic: a drug that induces stupor and insensibility and relieves pain.

Nausea: an unpleasant feeling or sensation usually preceding vomiting.

Neoadjuvant chemotherapy: chemotherapy given before surgery or radiation to reduce the size of the tumor.

Neutropenia: an abnormally low number of neutrophils, a type of granulocyte (white blood cell). It is the most common factor that makes individuals with cancer at risk for infection.

Nonopioid: medicines used for mild to moderate pain, many of which are over-the counter (without a prescription). Examples include acetaminophen and nonsteroidal anti-inflammatory drugs (NSAIDs), such as aspirin and ibuprofen.

Nonsteroidal anti-inflammatory drugs (NSAIDs): medicines that control mild to moderate pain, inflammation, and fever and can be used either alone or in combination with other medicines.

Ommaya reservoir: a special device that is used for intrathecal (into the brain or spinal fluid) chemotherapy. This device is placed into the skull and then a catheter is inserted into a ventricle (a space inside the brain filled with cerebrospinal fluid).

Oncology: the branch of medicine concerned with the diagnosis and treatment of cancer.

Opioid: also known as narcotics, medicines used for moderate to severe pain and that require a prescription. Examples include morphine, fentanyl, hydromorphone, oxycodone, and codeine.

Oral: of or pertaining to the mouth.

Palliation: treatment that relieves symptoms, such as pain, but is not expected to cure or control the disease. The main purpose is to improve the patient's quality of life.

Parenteral: drugs given intravenously, intramuscularly, or subcutaneously.

Penicillin: one of a group of antibiotics derived from several species of molds. It is a bactericidal, inhibiting the growth of some gram-positive and gram-negative forms of bacteria.

Peripheral blood stem cell transplantation (PBSCT): stem cells are removed from the blood before the patient is treated with large doses of chemotherapy or radiation. After treatment, the cells are given back to the patient in an infusion similar to a blood transfusion.

Pharyngitis: inflammation or sores in the throat caused by chemotherapy.

Platelet: a part of the blood that helps it "stick together" (clot) to promote healing after an injury. Chemotherapy can cause a drop in the platelet count—a condition called thrombocytopenia.

Radiation recall: redness of the skin where radiation therapy has been given in response to certain cancer treatment medicines.

Red blood cells: blood cells that contain hemoglobin, the substance that carries oxygen to other tissues of the body.

Regimen: a strict, regulated plan (such as diet, exercise, or other activity), designed to reach certain goals. In cancer treatment, a plan to treat cancer.

Retching: a rhythmic movement of the diaphragm and stomach muscles controlled by the vomiting center.

Side effects: effects of treatment (other than the effects on the cancer), such as hair loss caused by chemotherapy and fatigue caused by radiation therapy.

Stomatitis: inflammation or ulcers of the mouth area. Stomatitis can be a side effect of some kinds of chemotherapy.

Subcutaneous: beneath the skin.

Systemic therapy: treatment that reaches and affects cells throughout the body; for example, chemotherapy.

Tenckhoff catheter: a catheter specially designed for removing or adding large amounts of fluid from or into the abdominal cavity and is used in intraperitoneal chemotherapy.

Testosterone: the male hormone, made primarily in the testes. It stimulates blood flow, growth in certain tissues, and the secondary sexual characteristics. In men with prostate cancer, it can also encourage growth of the tumor.

Therapeutic index: a wide range of doses that can be used effectively and safely; for example, many over-the-counter medicines.

Therapy: any of the measures taken to treat a disease. Unproven therapy is any therapy that has not been scientifically tested and approved. Use of any unproven therapy instead of standard (proven) therapy is called alternative therapy. Some alternative therapies have dangerous or even life-threatening side effects. For others, the main danger is that a patient may lose the opportunity to benefit from standard therapy. Complementary therapy, on the other hand, refers to therapies used in addition to standard therapy. Some complementary therapies may help relieve certain symptoms of cancer, relieve side effects of standard therapy, or improve a patient's sense of well-being. The ACS recommends that patients considering use of any alternative or complementary therapy discuss this with their health care team.

Thrombocytopenia: a decrease in the number of platelets in the blood; can be a side effect of chemotherapy.

Total body irradiation (TBI): radiation treatment applied to the entire body.

Tyrosine Kinase Inhibitor (TKI): tyrosine kinases help to pass the message telling the cell to divide from the outside of the cell to the center of the cell, where the cell government is (called the nucleus). In some cancers, the message gets sent too many times, and the cell divides uncontrollably. TKIs

Index

Fludara, 102–103
fludarabine phosphate, 102–103
Fluorodeoxyuridine, 100–101
Fluorouracil, 4–5
fluosol DA (20%), 104–105
flutamide, 106–107
fluvestrant, 108–109
fluxoetine hydrochloride, 372–373
Folex, 162–163
Folinic acid, 138–139
Fortaz, 302–303
foscarnet sodium, 374–375
Foscavir, 374–375
ftorafur and uracil (UFT), 224–225
FUDR, 100–101
Fungizone, 256–257
furosemide, 376–377

G

G-CSF, 98–99
gabapentin, 378–379
gallium nitrate, 380–381
ganciclovir, 382–383
Ganite, 380–381
gemcitabine, 110–111
gemtuzumab ozogamicin, 112–113
Gemzar, 110–111
Genapap, 240–241
Genebs, 240–241
Genpril, 394–395
Gentabs, 240–241
Gentamycin, 384–385
gentamycin sulfate, 384–385
Geocillin, 276–277
Geopen, 276–277
Geramycin, 384–385
Gleevec, 124–125
glycerine suppository, 386–387
GM-CSF, 194–195
goserelin acetate, 114–115
granisetron hydrochloride, 388–389

H

Haldol, 390–391
Halenol, 240–241
haloperidol, 390–391
Halotestin, 26–27
Haltran, 394–395
Herceptin, 216–217
Hexadrol, 72–73
Hexalen, 18–19
Hexamenthylmelamine, 18–19
Hycamtin, 210–211
Hydrea, 116–117
Hydrocil, 484–485
hydromorphone, 392–393
hydroxyurea, 116–117
Hyoscine hydrobromide, 492–493
Hypocalcemic agents, 380–381

I

I131 tositumomab, 214–215
Ibuprin, 394–395
ibuprofen, 394–395
Idamycin, 118–119
idarubicin, 118–119
IDEC-Y288, 6–7
idoxifene, 120–121
Ifex, 122–123
IFN-a, 126–127
ifosfamide, 122–123
Illotycin, 358–359
imatinib mesylate, 124–125
imidazole carboxamide, 62–63
imipenem, 396–397
imipramine pamoate, 398–399
Imodium, 420–421
Inapsine, 356–357
Indocin, 400–401
Indocin SR, 400–401
indomethacin, 400–401
Indotech, 400–401
Infumorph, 448–449
Interferon-a 2a, 126–127
Interferon-a 2b, 126–127
interferon alpha, 126–127
interleukin-2, 128–129
interleukin-3, 130–131
interleukin-6, 132–133
Intron A, 126–127
irenotecan, 134–135
Isophosphamide, 122–123
itraconazole, 402–403

K

K-P, 406–407
K-Pek, 406–407
Kadian Morphine Sulfate Sustained
  Release, 448–449
kanamycin sulfate, 404–405
Kantrex, 404–405
Kaodene, 406–407
kaolin/pectin, 406–407
Kaopectate, 406–407
Kefzol, 284–285
ketoconazole, 408–409
ketorolac tromethamine, 410–411
Klonopin, 322–323
Kytril, 388–389

L

L-PAM, 154–155
lactulose, 412–413
Lamotil, 346–347
Lasix, 376–377
Laudanum, 334–335
Laxinate 100, 348–349
letrozole, 136–167
leucovorin, 4
leucovorin calcium, 138–139
Leukeran, 52–53

Leukine, 194–195
leuprolide acetate, 140–141
leuprolide acetate implant, 142–143
Leustatin, 56–57
levamisole hydrochloride, 144–145
Levaquin, 414–415
Levo-Dromoran, 416–417
levofloxacin, 414–415
levorphanol tartrate, 416–417
linezolid, 418–419
Lipo ATRA, 146–147
liposomal amphotericin B, 256–257
liposomal tretinoin, 146–147
Liquiprin, 240–241
lomustine, 148–149
loperamide hydrochloride, 420–421
lorazepam, 422–423
Lupron, 140–141

M

MagCitrate, 424–425
magnesium citrate, 424–425
Mandol, 282–283
Marinol, 354–355
Maxipime, 288
MeCCNU, 164–165
mechloroethamine hydrochloride,
  150–151
Meda Cap, 240–241
Mefoxin, 296–297
Megace, 152–153, 426–427
megestrol acetate, 152–153, 426–427
melphalan hydrochloride, 154–155
menogaril, 156–157
Menogaril, 156–157
Mepergan Fortis, 428–429
meperidine hydrochloride, 428–429
mercaptopurine, 158–159
mesna, 122, 160–161
Mesnex, 160–161
Metamucil, 484–485
methadone, 430–431
Methadose, 430–431
methotrexate, 162–163
methyl-CCNU, 164–165
methylcellulose, 432–433
metoclopramide, 434–435
metronidazole hydrochloride, 436–437
Mexate, 162–163
Mezlin, 438–439
mezlocillin sodium, 438–439
miconazole nitrate, 440–441
Midol 200, 394–395
mineral oil, 348, 442–443
Minocin, 444–445
minocycline hydrochloride, 444–445
Miracalcin, 272–273
mirtazapine, 446–447
Mithracin, 182–183
Mithramycin, 182–183
mitomycin, 166–167